Translational Acupuncture Research

Translational Acupuncture Research

Editor: Ophelia Burnett

FOSTER ACADEMICS

www.fosteracademics.com

www.fosteracademics.com

FOSTER ACADEMICS

Cataloging-in-Publication Data

Translational acupuncture research / edited by Ophelia Burnett.
p. cm.
Includes bibliographical references and index.
ISBN 978-1-64646-634-4
1. Acupuncture. 2. Alternative medicine. 3. Counterirritation. 4. Energy medicine. I. Burnett, Ophelia.
RM184 .T73 2023
615.892--dc23

Foster Academics,
118-35 Queens Blvd., Suite 400,
Forest Hills, NY 11375, USA

ISBN 978-1-64646-634-4 (Hardback)

Contents

Preface

Acupuncture is a type of alternative medicine, which is a significant constituent of conventional Chinese medicine. It involves the insertion of thin needles in one or more parts of body which are left there for fifteen to twenty minutes. It is linked with the application of pressure, heat and laser light. Generally utilized techniques of needling in acupuncture are insertion and de-qi sensation. Stainless steel needles are used in acupuncture, which makes them flexible, rust free and prevents them from breaking. Acupuncture is majorly used to provide pain relief, however, it can be utilized for various other conditions such as sciatica, irritable bowel syndrome and fibromyalgia. The topics covered in this extensive book deal with the core subjects of acupuncture. From theories to research to practical applications, studies related to all contemporary topics of relevance to this field have been included herein. This book includes contributions of experts, which will provide innovative insights into this field to the readers.

This book unites the global concepts and researches in an organized manner for a comprehensive understanding of the subject. It is a ripe text for all researchers, students, scientists or anyone else who is interested in acquiring a better knowledge of this dynamic field.

I extend my sincere thanks to the contributors for such eloquent research chapters. Finally, I thank my family for being a source of support and help.

Editor

1

Bee Venom Acupuncture Attenuates Oxaliplatin-Induced Neuropathic Pain by Modulating Action Potential Threshold in A-Fiber Dorsal Root Ganglia Neurons

Ji Hwan Lee [1,2], Juan Gang [3], Eunhee Yang [4], Woojin Kim [1,2,3,*] and Young-Ho Jin [4,*]

1 Department of Physiology, College of Korean Medicine, Kyung Hee University, Seoul 02453, Korea; mibdna@khu.ac.kr
2 Department of Science in Korean Medicine, Graduate School, Kyung Hee University, Seoul 02453, Korea
3 Department of East-West Medicine, Graduate School, Kyung Hee University, Seoul 02453, Korea; khan2296@naver.com
4 Department of Physiology, College of Medicine, Kyung Hee University, Seoul 02453, Korea; dmsgmls317@gmail.com
* Correspondence: wjkim@khu.ac.kr (W.K.); jinyh@khu.ac.kr (Y.-H.J.)

Abstract: Oxaliplatin is a third-generation platinum-based chemotherapeutic drug widely used in colorectal cancer treatment. Although potent against this tumor, it can induce cold and mechanical allodynia even after a single injection. The currently used drugs to attenuate this allodynia can also cause unwanted effects, which limit their use. Bee venom acupuncture (BVA) is widely used in Korean medicine to treat pain. Although the effect of BVA on oxaliplatin-induced neuropathic pain has been addressed in many studies, its action on dorsal root ganglia (DRG) neurons has never been investigated. A single oxaliplatin injection (6 mg/kg, intraperitoneally) induced cold and mechanical allodynia, and BVA (0.1 and 1 mg/kg, subcutaneous, ST36) dose-dependently decreased allodynia in rats. On acutely dissociated lumbar 4–6 DRG neurons, 10 min application of oxaliplatin (100 μM) shifted the voltage-dependence of sodium conductance toward negative membrane potentials in A- but not C-fibers. The resting membrane potential remained unchanged, but the action potential threshold decreased significantly compared to that of the control ($p < 0.05$). However, 0.1 μg/mL of BVA administration increased the lowered action potential threshold. In conclusion, these results suggest that BVA may attenuate oxaliplatin-induced neuropathic pain by altering the action potential threshold in A-fiber DRG neurons.

Keywords: action potential; allodynia; bee venom acupuncture; oxaliplatin; voltage-gated sodium channel

Key Contribution: BVA attenuates oxaliplatin-induced neuropathic pain by modulating the action potential threshold in myelinated A-fiber DRG neurons.

1. Introduction

Oxaliplatin is a chemotherapeutic drug widely used in the treatment of advanced metastatic colorectal cancer [1], which is the second highest cause of death due to cancer after lung carcinoma [2]. Despite its effect on tumor size reduction, its use can be limited due to peripheral neuropathy rapidly occurring after infusion in up to 80–90% of treated patients. This peripheral neuropathy is characterized by a glove-and-stocking distribution sensory loss, paresthesia, and dysesthesia, which can be triggered and aggravated by exposure to cold [3]. To prevent or attenuate this oxaliplatin-induced neuropathic pain, various strategies and drugs have been proposed such as "stop and go" strategy, Ca/Mg infusion, glutathione, and duloxetine. Recently, the American Society of Clinical Organization guidelines [4] and the Journal of the American Medical Association [5] recommended duloxetine, which is a well-established anticonvulsant and analgesic drug, to mitigate oxaliplatin-induced pain. However, even duloxetine has been reported to cause side effects, such as dizziness and headache, demonstrating the need for the development of alternative strategies [6].

For the past several years, our group has focused on understanding the underlying mechanism of oxaliplatin-induced neuropathic pain and on finding an effective treatment method. The effects of well-known analgesic drugs such as morphine [7], gabapentin [8], and duloxetine [9] have been assessed along with herbal medicines [10–12], acupuncture [8,13], and bee venom acupuncture (BVA) [7,14–16]. Bee venom (BV) is composed of peptides, enzymes, amines, and non-peptide components that have a variety of pharmaceutical properties [17]. Subcutaneous injection of BV at acupoints, BVA, is a widely used method in Korean medicine for the treatment of different kinds of pain such as musculoskeletal [18,19] and arthritis pain [20]. In our previous studies, BVA significantly attenuated cold and mechanical allodynia induced by oxaliplatin. Moreover, BVA induced an additive effect when simultaneously injected with morphine by increasing the action time in mice injected with a chemotherapeutic agent [8]. Furthermore, three weeks of treatment with BVA in patients with chemotherapy-induced neuropathic pain also resulted in positive effects [21], implying the efficacy of BVA against oxaliplatin-induced neuropathic pain.

The underlying mechanism of oxaliplatin-induced neuropathic pain remains unclear; however, oxaliplatin is known to directly affect the dorsal root ganglia (DRG) neurons, whereas in the central nervous system, its direct effect is smaller because of the limited permeability of oxaliplatin through the blood–brain barrier (BBB) [22]. Upon excitation, DRG neurons can transmit sensory signals such as pain to the spinal cord by generating action potentials [23]. The excitability of a neuronal cell depends upon various factors, but ion channels play a critical role. Oxaliplatin is reported to induce an immediate effect on the axonal excitability rather than cause structural changes, suggesting that ion channels in DRG neurons may be involved [24]. Indeed, abnormalities in the functions of voltage-gated potassium ion and calcium ion (K_V and Ca_V, respectively) channels have been reported [25]; however, sodium ion (Na_V) channels may play a major role in oxaliplatin-induced neuropathic pain, as these channels determine the occurrence and development of neuropathic pain in primary sensory neurons [26–28]. In addition, sodium channel blockers such as carbamazepine significantly attenuated oxaliplatin-induced neuropathic pain in clinical trials [29,30].

In the past decade, a number of studies have investigated the effect of BVA against chemotherapy-induced neuropathic pain, and different mechanisms of action have been proposed [31,32]; however, most of them focused on the spinal level. Therefore, its effect on the peripheral nervous system remains unclear. Moreover, to date, no studies have assessed its direct effect on acutely dissociated DRG neurons.

Thus, first, we aimed to assess the effect of oxaliplatin on voltage-dependent Na^+ currents in acutely dissociated myelinated and unmyelinated DRG neurons in this study. Second, we confirmed that different doses of BVA administered at ST36 could significantly attenuate oxaliplatin-induced neuropathic pain in rats. Finally, we analyzed the possible mechanism of BVA in decreasing the pain transmission by conducting whole-cell current patch-clamp experiments in DRG neurons.

2. Results

2.1. *Single Oxaliplatin Administration Induced Cold and Mechanical Allodynia in Rats*

A single intraperitoneal injection of oxaliplatin (6 mg/kg) elicited cold and mechanical allodynia (Figure 1). Cold and mechanical allodynia were measured by applying an acetone drop and von Frey filament (bending force of 0.4 g) on the mid-plantar hind paw, respectively. Before the injection of oxaliplatin or 5% glucose (control), rats in both groups showed no cold or mechanical hypersensitivity (pre-injection). However, four days after oxaliplatin injection, both cold ($p < 0.05$) and mechanical ($p < 0.01$) allodynia were significantly induced compared to the control group (post-injection).

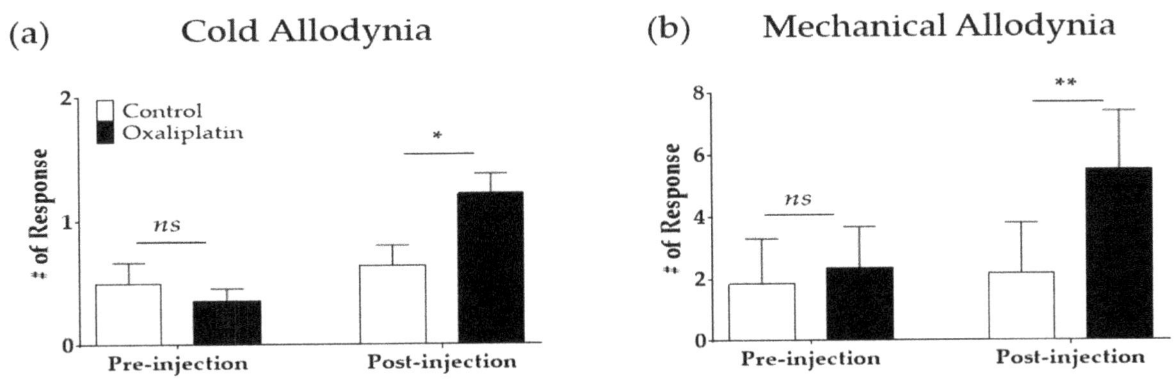

Figure 1. Single intraperitoneal injection of 6 mg/kg of oxaliplatin induced cold (**a**) and mechanical (**b**) allodynia in rats. The acetone and von Frey tests were used to assess cold and mechanical allodynia, respectively. Pre-injection: prior to the injection of oxaliplatin or 5% glucose (control). Post-injection: four days after the administration of oxaliplatin or 5% glucose. Control: $n = 6$, Oxaliplatin: $n = 7$. *ns*: Not significant, * $p < 0.05$, ** $p < 0.01$, vs. Control with two-way ANOVA followed by Sidak's post-test for multiple comparisons.

2.2. Oxaliplatin Modulates Voltage-Dependent Na^+ Currents in A- but Not C-fiber DRG Neurons

To observe the effect of oxaliplatin on the function of voltage-dependent Na^+ currents, a depolarization step from − 60 to + 50 mV at 10 mV increments with a duration of 150 ms was injected in acutely dissociated A- and C-fiber DRG neurons (Figure 2a,d and Figure 2b,e, respectively). Representative images of changes in inward Na^+ currents before (control) and after (oxaliplatin) treatment with oxaliplatin 100 µL in A- and C-fibers are shown (Figures 2a and 2b, respectively). The peak current–voltage (I–V) curves are shown in Figure 2d,e. An artificial external recording solution was used as a control. Oxaliplatin treatment (100 µM) affected the inward Na^+ currents in A-fibers but not in C-fiber neurons. Inward Na^+ currents were observed at −30 mV in oxaliplatin-treated cells, whereas the 10 µM-treated cells did not show a significant change. When the step voltage was increased to −20 mV, both 10 and 100 µM showed significant differences compared to the control group (*** $p < 0.001$). These results show that oxaliplatin shifted the voltage-dependence of sodium conductance toward negative membrane potentials in A-fiber neurons. This effect of oxaliplatin could not be reversed even at prolonged washout times, as reported in another study [33]. In contrast to A-fiber sensory neurons, the function of the voltage-dependent sodium channel in C-fiber neurons remained unaffected after 100 µM of oxaliplatin at all voltages. To identify the type of neurons, the size of neurons and response to capsaicin application have been observed after each experiment. Capsaicin, the pungent component of chili pepper, is known to induce dose-dependent inward Na^+ currents after its application [34], and 1 µM of capsaicin was selected as C-fiber neurons showed the highest response rate. Representative traces of C-fiber neuron responding to 1 µM of capsaicin treatment are shown in Figure 2c.

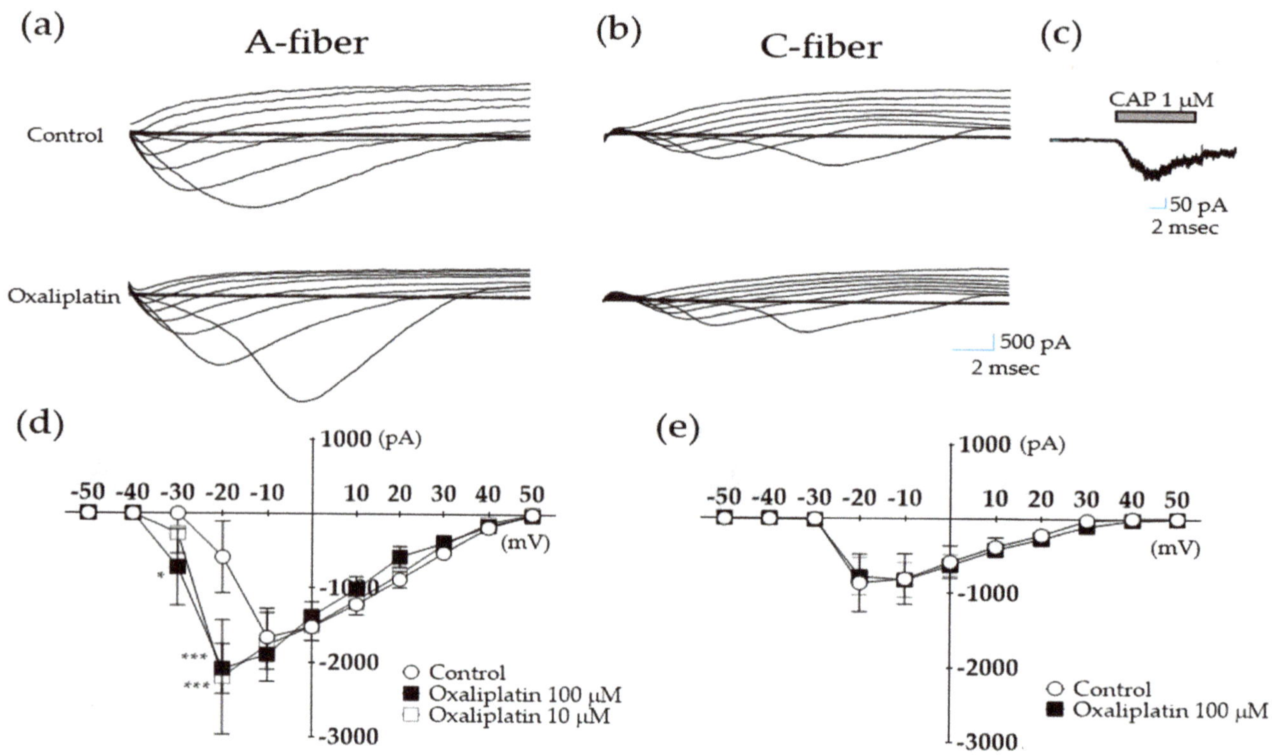

Figure 2. Effect of oxaliplatin on A- (**a**,**d**) and C- (**b**,**e**) fiber voltage-gated Na^+ currents. Traces of inward Na^+ currents recorded during depolarizing voltage steps from −60 to +50 mV at 10 mV increments with duration of 150 ms, before (control) and after the addition of either 10 or 100 μM of oxaliplatin to the external solution. Capsaicin (CAP, 1 μM) was used to identify A- and C-fiber neurons (**c**). Figure 2d: Control (external solution); $n = 11$, Oxaliplatin 100 μM; $n = 11$, Oxaliplatin 10 μM; $n = 4$. Figure 2e: Control (external solution); $n = 5$, Oxaliplatin 100 μM; $n = 5$. * $p < 0.05$, *** $p < 0.001$, vs. Control with two-way analysis of variance followed by Sidak's post-test for multiple comparisons.

2.3. Oxaliplatin Lowers the Current Threshold for Action Potential Generation in A-Fiber DRG Neurons

As we have observed, oxaliplatin could modulate the inward Na^+ currents in the previous experiments. Consequently, the current patch-clamp recording method was used to assess the effect of oxaliplatin on the excitability of A-fiber neurons. Step currents of 10 pA increments for 30 ms were injected to induce action potentials in A-fiber DRG neurons (Figure 3). The results show that the resting membrane potential did not change following oxaliplatin treatment, whereas the threshold for action potential initiation (−28.45 ± 2.44 mV (control) vs. −35.78 ± 2.03 mV (oxaliplatin); $p < 0.05$) and the amount of current needed to generate an action potential (115 ± 7.63 pA (control) vs. 74.28 ± 12.12 pA (oxaliplatin); $p < 0.05$) significantly decreased. Representative action potential traces recorded from A-fiber neurons before and after oxaliplatin treatment are shown in Figure 3d,e. Before the administration of oxaliplatin, DRG neurons showed subthreshold responses to 60–100 pA, and an action potential was generated after 110 pA injection (current threshold for this neuron). However, after oxaliplatin application, 60–100 pA current injection evoked an action potential (Figure 3e).

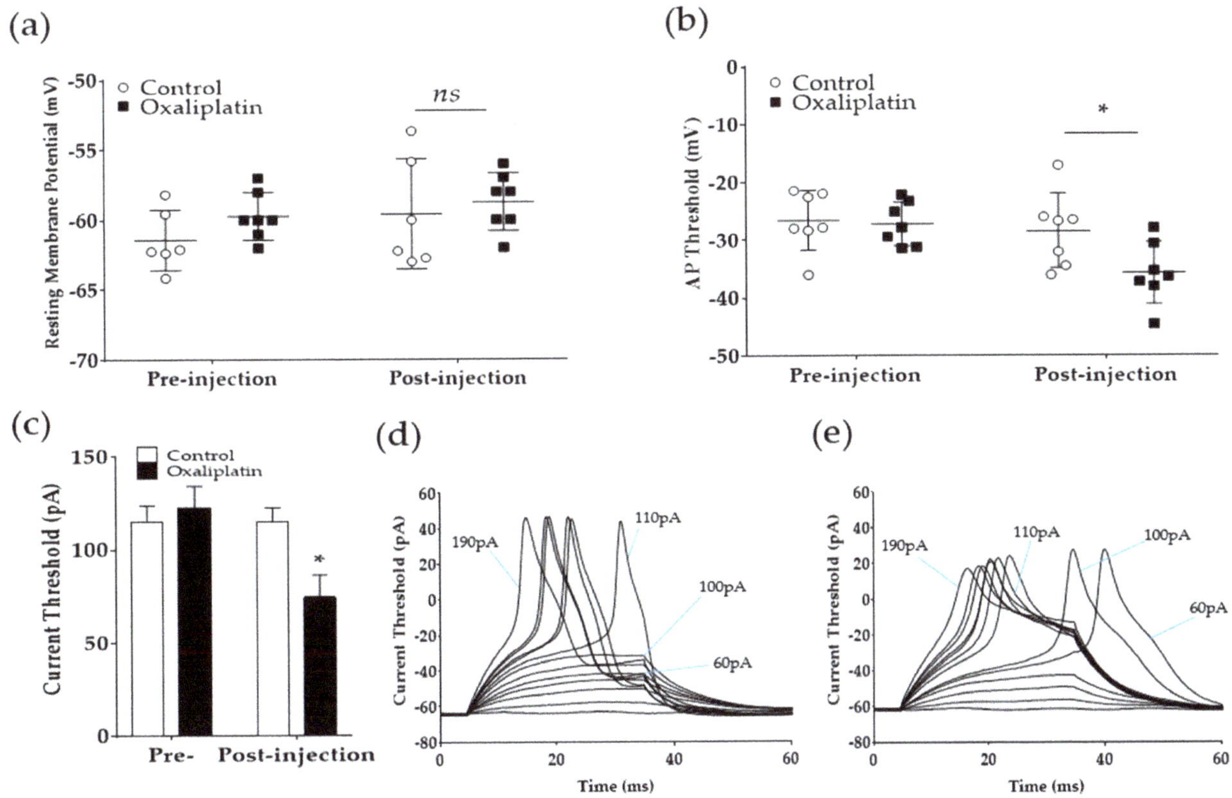

Figure 3. Effect of oxaliplatin on the resting membrane potential and action potential generation in A-fiber DRG neurons. In current patch-clamp analysis, the resting membrane potential was recorded. Action potentials were evoked using depolarizing step current injections of 10 pA from a set holding membrane potential of −60 mV. Resting membrane potential (**a**) and action potential threshold (**b**) in A-fiber DRG neurons before (pre-injection) and after (post-injection) the treatment of external solution or oxaliplatin (100 μM). Averaged current threshold for all cells tested (**c**). Representative traces of action potential generation after current injection before (**d**) and after oxaliplatin administration (**e**). Control (external solution): $n = 6$–7, oxaliplatin (100 μM): $n = 7$. *ns*: Not significant, * $p < 0.05$ vs. Control with two-way analysis of variance followed by Sidak's post-test for multiple comparisons.

2.4. Anti-Allodynic Effects of BVA against Oxaliplatin-Induced Cold and Mechanical Allodynia

On day four, following the oxaliplatin injection, when the cold and mechanical allodynia were significantly induced, two different doses of BVA (0.1 and 1 mg/kg) or phosphate-buffered saline (PBS, control) were subcutaneously injected in the right leg of the rats (ST36, Figure 4). The site of injection was chosen as in our previous study, and a significant effect was shown compared to other sites [35]. Cold (Figure 4a,c) and mechanical (Figure 4b,d) allodynia induced by oxaliplatin injection (pre-injection) were significantly alleviated 30 min after the treatment with 1 mg/kg of BV compared to control (post-injection; $p < 0.01$ and $p < 0.001$ for cold and mechanical allodynia, respectively). However, 0.1 mg/kg of BV was effective against mechanical allodynia ($p < 0.05$) but not cold allodynia. Furthermore, to verify whether the anti-allodynic effect of BVA is acupoint specific, 1 mg/kg of BVA was administered at ST36 and LI11 (Figure 4c,d). In addition, the syringe used to treat with BVA was briefly (3 s) inserted in ST36 (oxaliplatin + sham (ST36)) to demonstrate that the effect of BVA was not induced by syringe application. The results show that only BVA at ST36 possess significant analgesic effect against cold and mechanical allodynia induced by oxaliplatin, whereas animals in other three group failed to show any sign of alleviation. BVA administered at ST36 in naïve rats did not induced any significant behavioral change compared to PBS-injected animals (Supplementary Materials Figure S1).

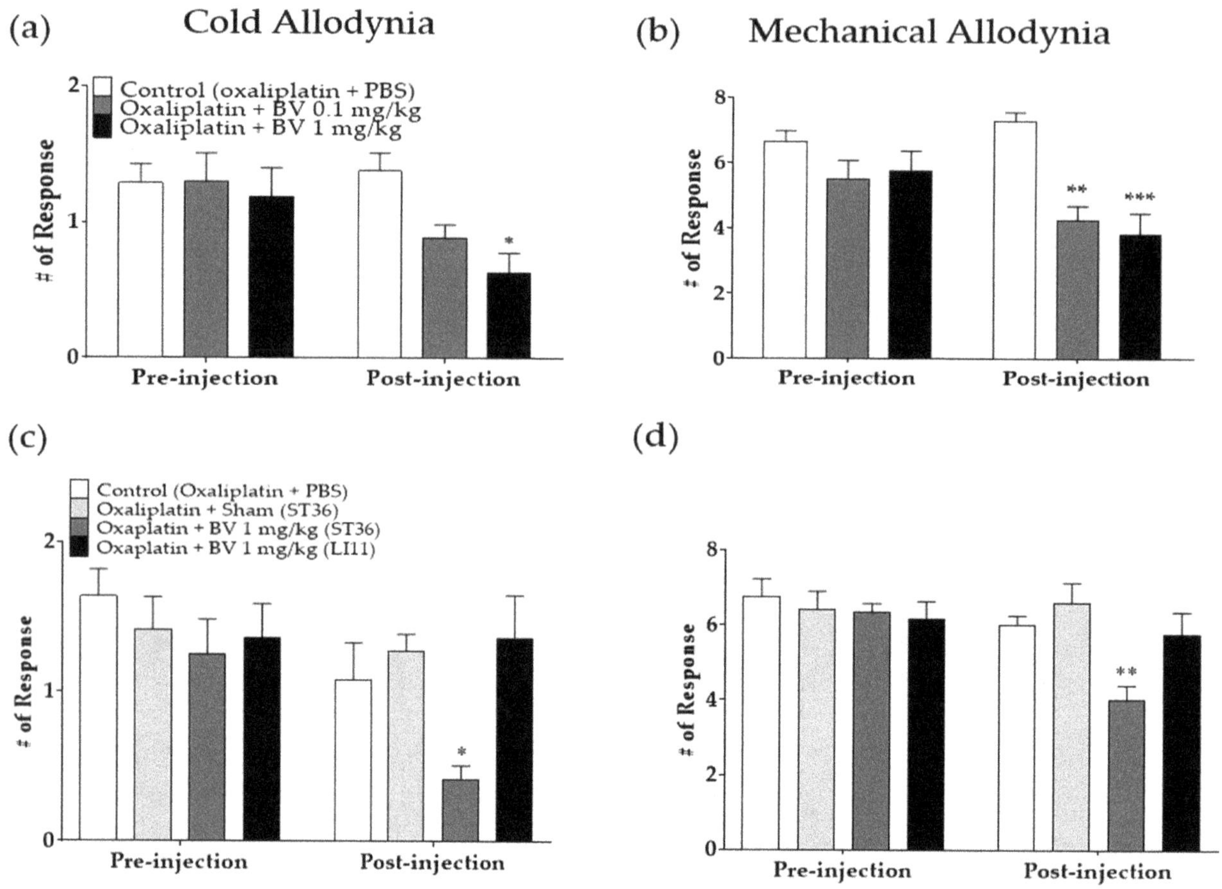

Figure 4. Single subcutaneous administration of bee venom acupuncture (BVA) at ST36 decreased cold (**a**,**c**) and mechanical (**b**,**d**) allodynia induced by oxaliplatin in rats. Cold and mechanical allodynia were assessed using acetone and von Frey tests, respectively. In all groups, behavioral assessments were conducted four days after the injection of 6 mg/kg of oxaliplatin (pre-injection), when significant allodynic signs were observed in rats and 30 min after the administration of phosphate-buffered saline (PBS) or 0.1 or 1 mg/kg of BVA or sham (brief syringe insertion) (post-injection). Control: $n = 7$, BV 0.1 mg/kg: $n = 10$, BV 1 mg/kg: $n = 10$ (**a**,**b**), Control: $n = 6$, Sham: $n = 6$, BV ST36: $n = 6$, BV LI11: $n = 6$ (**c**,**d**). * $p < 0.05$, ** $p < 0.01$, *** $p < 0.001$ vs. Control with two-way analysis of variance followed by Sidak's post-test for multiple comparisons.

2.5. BVA Increases the Action Potential and Current Threshold in Acutely Dissociated DRG Neurons

As BVA significantly attenuated cold and mechanical allodynia in vivo, in our next experiments, we applied BV to acutely dissociated A-fiber DRG neurons to observe whether it can increase the lowered action potential threshold after oxaliplatin treatment. The current patch-clamp technique was used for this experiment. Application of 0.1 μg/mL of BV significantly increased the lowered action potential threshold of A-fiber DRG neurons after oxaliplatin injection (−35.52 ± 1.75 mV (control) vs. −25.86 ± 2.20 (oxaliplatin); $p < 0.05$) (Figure 5a). Furthermore, the currents needed to evoke action potential significantly increased after the BV treatment (74 ± 7.48 pA (control) vs. 115 ± 11.33 pA (oxaliplatin); $p < 0.05$) (Figure 5b). Representative traces from DRG neuronal cells show that after oxaliplatin treatment, 90 to 110 pA current injection evoked an action potential (Figure 5c), whereas after BV application, the current threshold needed to generate action potential increased to 120 pA (Figure 5d).

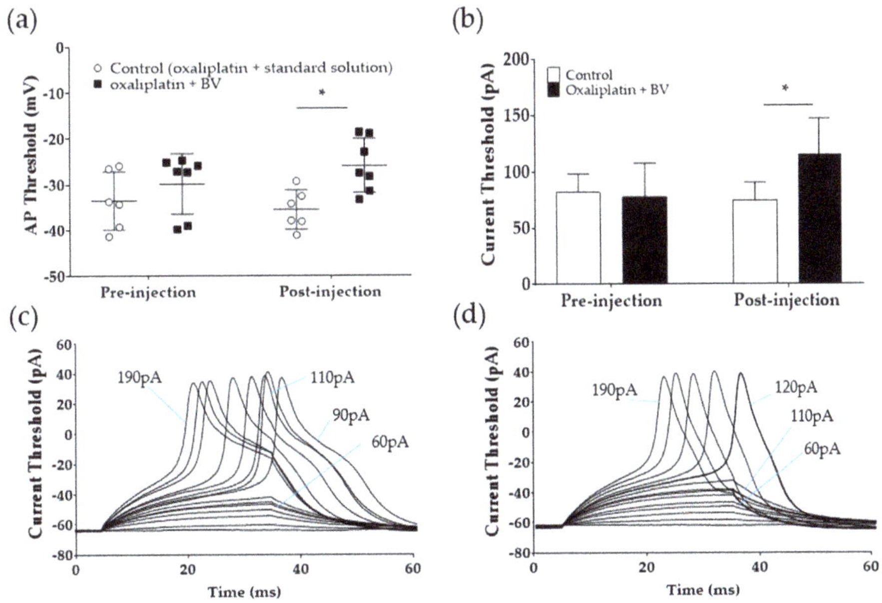

Figure 5. Effect of oxaliplatin on the current threshold for action potential generation in DRG neurons. Action potentials were evoked by using depolarizing step current injections of 10 pA from a set holding membrane potential of −60 mV. Action potential (**a**) and current threshold (**b**) in A-fiber DRG neurons before (pre-injection) and after (post-injection) the treatment of external solution or BV (0.1 μg/mL). Averaged current threshold for all cells tested (**b**). Representative traces of action potential generation after current injection before (**c**) and after 0.1 mg/kg BV administration (**d**). Control (external solution): $n = 5$, BV (0.1 μg/mL): $n = 8$. * $p < 0.05$ vs. Control with two-way analysis of variance followed by Sidak's post-test for multiple comparisons.

3. Discussion

In this study, first, by conducting both behavioral tests and voltage and current patch-clamp experiments, we showed that a single intraperitoneal oxaliplatin injection (6 mg/kg) can induce cold and mechanical allodynia in rats and modulate voltage-dependent Na^+ currents in acutely dissociated A- but not C-fiber DRG neurons. The action potential threshold also decreased. Second, we demonstrated that subcutaneous administration of BVA at the right hind leg (0.1 and 1 mg/kg, ST36) could attenuate both cold and mechanical allodynia in a dose-dependent manner in rats. Finally, we demonstrated that 0.1 μg/mL BV could decrease the pain signal transmission to the spinal cord by increasing the lowered action potential threshold following oxaliplatin (100 μM) treatment in myelinated DRG neurons.

In the present study, cold and mechanical allodynia were induced by a single injection of oxaliplatin. It has been reported that intraperitoneal injection of 6 mg/kg of oxaliplatin can mimic the acute allodynia observed in humans [36]. Moreover, other studies demonstrated that oxaliplatin treatment can cause rapidly developing pain signs in more than 85% of the patients, with peaks in the first 24–48 h after the injection [3]. The cause of this acute toxicity is not clearly understood, but alteration in Na_V channels that leads to peripheral-nerve hyperexcitability is suggested to be the cause [37].

Recently, many studies have observed the effect of BVA on different types of diseases [38]. However, to date, this is the first study to evaluate its effect on acutely dissociated DRG neurons after chemotherapeutic agent administration. Previous studies have mostly focused on its action on the spinal cord [7,32,35]. Conversely, understanding the effect of BVA on the DRG is important as the major site affected by oxaliplatin appears to be the DRG [39]. Postmortem histopathological analysis in humans showed that platinum levels were highest in the DRG and lowest in the area protected by the BBB [40] implying the importance of DRG in oxaliplatin-induced neuropathic pain.

DRG contain cell bodies of myelinated and unmyelinated sensory neurons (i.e., A- and C-fibers, respectively). To clarify which fiber type is affected by oxaliplatin, we assessed changes in voltage-dependent inward Na^+ currents in both A- and C-fibers. Compared to the control, 100 μM of oxaliplatin application induced a negative shift in Na^+ current activation (i.e., −30 vs. −20 mV (control)), whereas no difference was observed in C-fibers, showing that A- but not C-fiber DRG neurons are affected by oxaliplatin. These results corroborate two other studies conducted on human and animal nerves [33,41]. They showed that the function of A- but not C-fibers was affected by oxaliplatin, suggesting that A-fibers play a critical role in the transmission of oxaliplatin-induced pain. Although the specific subtype of A-fiber neurons was not elucidated in our study, it has been reported that Aδ-fibers, which are the thinnest myelinated fibers, may play an important role in oxaliplatin-induced neuropathic pain. Aδ-fibers are involved in the transduction of paresthesia (tickling or tingling sensations in the skin, whether distal or perioral), which is one of the most frequent symptoms of oxaliplatin-treated patients [42] as well as in cold pain [43].

In our subsequent experiments conducted using the whole-cell current patch-clamp technique, oxaliplatin significantly lowered the action potential threshold in A-fiber neurons, showing that an action potential could easily be generated after oxaliplatin administration. Accordingly, the current needed to generate the action potential also decreased. On the contrary, the resting membrane potential remained unchanged following oxaliplatin injection. These results show that membrane potential can be modulated at the depolarization level, and Na_V channels may be involved, as it was reported to modify the action potential threshold. Previously, Ruth et al. [41] reported that voltage-gated sodium channel 1.6 ($Na_V1.6$) is involved in oxaliplatin-induced neuropathic pain. In their experiments, $SCN8A^{med/med}$ mice, which lacked the function of $Na_V1.6$, showed no sign of cold allodynia. Deuis et al. [44] also demonstrated that intraplantar injection of μ-conotoxin (GIIIA, 10 μM), which is able to inhibit $Na_V1.6$, achieved near-complete reversal of oxaliplatin-induced cold allodynia. $Na_V1.6$ is a tetrodotoxin-sensitive Na_V channel expressed by both myelinated and unmyelinated DRG neurons. In A-fibers, they are located at the node of Ranvier, whereas they are expressed in a continuous fashion along the axon of unmyelinated C-fibers [45].

In the present study, the role K_V channels was been investigated. Other studies have suggested a critical role of K_V channels in oxaliplatin-induced pain as 4-aminopyridine, which is a classic antagonist of K_V channels, showed similar effect to oxaliplatin in rodents [25]. Furthermore, Mannelli et al. [46] reported that single subcutaneous administration of hydrogen sulfide donors could reduce the hypersensitivity to cold noxious stimuli in a chronic animal model of oxaliplatin-induced neuropathic pain. They were shown to possess longer inhibitory effect compared to duloxetine and pregabalin, and the effect of hydrogen sulfide donors were shown to be mediated by K_V7 channels, as its blocker nullified its analgesic effect. However, Benoit et al. [47] reported that the effect of oxaliplatin on Na_V channel appears to be greater than that on K_V channel. In addition, by measuring the compound action potential in rat sural, vagal, and peroneal nerves, Adelsberger et al. [33] reported that oxaliplatin did not block K^+ conductance but altered the activation and inactivation behavior of Na^+ channels. They further stated that the lengthening of action potential caused by oxaliplatin injection might be due to the slowdown of Na^+ channel inactivation kinetics but not from the blockade of K^+ channels. Thus, the prolonged repolarization phase seen in this study (Figure 3d) might also be due to the slowdown of Na_V channel inactivation kinetics, but future studies are needed to understand the precise role of Na_V and K_V channels in increase in the duration of action potential induced by oxaliplatin.

In this study, the dose-dependent relationship of BV was not measured as cells became easily unstable when BV at doses higher than 0.1 μg/mL (i.e., 0.3 and 1 μg/mL) was applied (data not shown). As mentioned previously, the effect of BV on acutely associated DRG neurons has never been observed before; however, the cytotoxic effect of BV has been analyzed in cultured cells. By using a 3-(4,5-dimethylthiazol-2-yl)-2,5-diphenyltetrazolium bromide cytotoxicity assay, rat brain cortical neurons showed cellular cytotoxicity with a 24 h treatment of 0.8 to 3 μg/mL BV, whereas 0.2 or 0.4 μg/mL BV did not show any cellular toxicity [48]. In the human lung carcinoma cell line NCI-H1299, 1 μg/mL of BV showed cytotoxic effects after 12 h of treatment. However, there may be a difference in the properties between acutely dissociated neurons and cultured cells. Conducting experiments on acutely dissociated animal DRG may have more clinical relevance than those on cultured cells, as differences in electrophysiological properties were observed, such as changes in the action potential size and reduced voltage-gated Na^+ currents along with its corresponding mRNA expression [49].

4. Conclusions

In conclusion, our study demonstrated that BVA injection could attenuate oxaliplatin-induced neuropathic pain by increasing the lowered action potential threshold. Future studies are needed to elucidate the action of BVA on the peripheral nervous system. The action of BVA on the function of various ion channels present in the DRG, such as potassium and calcium ion channels, should be investigated.

5. Materials and Methods

5.1. Animals

Sprague-Dawley (SD) rats (post-natal 10-18 days (for electrophysiological studies) and 6 weeks old (for behavioral tests)) were obtained from the supplier (DBL, Chungbuk, Korea) and housed in an specific pathogen free (SPF) animal center. Animals were randomly caged with a temperature of 23 ± 2 °C, humidity of 65% ± 5%, with food and water ad libitum, and a fixed 12 h light/dark cycle. All experimental protocols were approved by the Kyung Hee University Animal Care and Use Committee (KHUASP(SE)-20-147) on 12 May 2020.

5.2. Administration of Drugs

Oxaliplatin (Sigma Aldrich, St. Louis, MO, USA) was dissolved in 5% glucose solution at a concentration of 2 mg/mL. Oxaliplatin was administered intraperitoneally at a dose of 6 mg/kg. Capsaicin (Sigma Aldrich, St. Louis, MO, USA) was dissolved in ethanol at a concentration of 1 μM. BV was manufactured by Jayeonsaeng TJ (Gyeonggi-Do, Korea), controlled by regular high-performance liquid chromatography (HPLC) analysis (SNU National Instrumentation Center for Environmental Management, Seoul, Korea) [35]. BV was dissolved in PBS at a concentration of 1 mg/mL. BVA was subcutaneously injected into acupoint ST36 (right hind leg) or LI11 (located at the depression medial to the extensor carpi radialis, at the lateral end of the cubital crease) at doses of 0.1 or 1 mg/kg. A BD ultra-fine II short needle insulin syringe −31G (Becton, Dickinson, and company, NJ, USA) was used to inject BVA subcutaneously. In a previous study, 0.1 or 1 mg/kg of BVA was reported to be an effective concentration causing no side effects. Acupoint ST36 was chosen as it was shown to be effective compared to other sites in our previous studies [35].

5.3. Behavioral Tests

Behavioral tests were conducted as described in our previous studies [7,9]. Briefly, for acclimation, mice were caged in an inverted clear plastic cage (12 × 8 × 6 cm) on a metal mesh floor for 30 min prior to the measurements. Cold allodynia was assessed by gently applying a drop of acetone (10 μL, Daejung Chemical Ltd., Gyeonggi-do, Korea) to the mid-plantar skin (avoiding the base of the tori) of both hind paws (three times). The frequencies of brisk withdrawal, licking, and shaking of the hind paw were counted for 30 s as a sign of pain. Thus, "# of Response" in Figures 1a and 4a,c indicates the average number of responses to 10 μL of acetone drop counted for 30 s.

Mechanical allodynia was assessed using the von Frey filament (Linton Instrumentation, Norfolk, U.K.) test. Mice were placed on the same wire mesh floor covered with a clear plastic box as mentioned above, and a von Frey filament with a bending force of 0.4 g (3.61 log scale) was applied to the point of bending ten times to the mid plantar skin of each hind paw. Stimulation was applied at intervals of 3 s, and lifting the paw was counted as a sign of pain. The "# of Response" in Figures 1b and 4b,d represent the average number of paw-lifting instances to multiple von Frey filament stimulation (10 times).

5.4. *Acute Dissociation of DRG Neurons*

DRG neurons were dissociated using procedures previously described elsewhere [50]. Briefly, in deeply anesthetized (urethane, Sigma Aldrich, St. Louis, MO, USA) SD rats, the lumbar 4–6 DRG were separated from the surrounding tissue and immediately placed into a Petri dish containing 4 °C of artificial cerebrospinal fluid (ACSF), which was composed of the following (in mM): 125 NaCl, 3 KCl, 1.2 KH_2PO_4, 1.2 $MgSO_4$, 25 $NaHCO_3$, 10 glucose, and 2 $CaCl_2$, and bubbled with 95% O_2–5% CO_2. After removing excess connective tissues, the DRG was incubated for 30–45 min at 31 °C in an ACSF solution containing protease (type 2S trypsin, 5 to 6 mg/mL at 1310 U/mg; Sigma Aldrich). After protease treatment, the ganglion was placed in enzyme-free ACSF for 1–2 h at room temperature. The ganglia were mechanically dispersed using fire-polished Pasteur pipettes in a glass-bottom perfusion chamber filled with an artificial external recording solution containing (in mM): 150 NaCl, 5 KCl, 1 $MgCl_2$, 2 $CaCl_2$ 10 N-2-hydroxyethylpiperazine-N'-2-ethanesulfonic acid (HEPES); 10 glucose (pH was adjusted to 7.4 with Tris base).

5.5. *Whole Cell Voltage and Current Patch-Clamp*

For voltage and current patch-clamp recordings, isolated neurons were visualized using a phase contrast microscope (Eclipse Ti; Nikon, Tokyo, Japan). Recordings were performed using a Multiclamp 700B (Molecular Devices, Sunnyvale, CA, USA) and pClamp 9 software (Molecular Devices). Recording electrodes were back-filled with an intracellular solution containing the following (in mM): 10 NaCl, 130 K-gluconate, 11 EGTA, 1 $CaCl_2$, 2 $MgCl_2$, and 10 HEPES. Immediately before recording, 2 mM Na-ATP and Na-GTP were added to the pipette solution. The pH was adjusted to 7.3 using 1N KOH. During the experiments, the pipette solution was kept from light and chilled (8–12 °C). The osmolarities of the pipette solutions were adjusted to 260 and 267 mOsm. All experiments were conducted at room temperature (21–23 °C).

5.6. *Statistical Analysis*

All data are presented as mean ± standard error of the mean (SEM). Electrophysiological data were analyzed offline using the pClamp 9 software. Currents were sampled at 10 kHz with 3 kHz filtering. Statistical analysis and graphic works were performed using Prism 7.0 (GraphPad software, La Jolla, CA, USA). Two-way ANOVA followed by Sidak's post-test for multiple comparisons was used for statistical analysis. In all cases, $p < 0.05$ was considered significant.

Author Contributions: Conceptualization, W.K.; methodology, J.H.L., E.Y., W.K., and Y.-H.J.; resources, J.G., W.K., and Y.-H.J.; data curation, J.H.L., J.G., and W.K.; writing—original draft preparation, J.H.L. and W.K.; writing—review and editing, W.K. and Y.-H.J.; visualization, W.K.; supervision, W.K. and Y.-H.J.; project administration, W.K. and Y.-H.J.; funding acquisition, W.K. All authors have read and agreed to the published version of the manuscript.

References

1. André, T.; Boni, C.; Mounedji-Boudiaf, L.; Navarro, M.; Tabernero, J.; Hickish, T.; Topham, C.; Zaninelli, M.; Clingan, P.; Bridgewater, J. Oxaliplatin, fluorouracil, and leucovorin as adjuvant treatment for colon cancer. *N. Engl. J. Med.* **2004**, *350*, 2343–2351. [CrossRef] [PubMed]
2. Bray, F.; Ferlay, J.; Soerjomataram, I.; Siegel, R.L.; Torre, L.A.; Jemal, A. Global cancer statistics 2018: Globocan estimates of incidence and mortality worldwide for 36 cancers in 185 countries. *CA A Cancer J. Clin.* **2018**, *68*, 394–424. [CrossRef] [PubMed]

3. Cersosimo, R.J. Oxaliplatin-associated neuropathy: A review. *Ann. Pharmacother.* **2005**, *39*, 128–135. [CrossRef] [PubMed]
4. Hershman, D.L.; Lacchetti, C.; Dworkin, R.H.; Lavoie Smith, E.M.; Bleeker, J.; Cavaletti, G.; Chauhan, C.; Gavin, P.; Lavino, A.; Lustberg, M.B. Prevention and management of chemotherapy-induced peripheral neuropathy in survivors of adult cancers: American society of clinical oncology clinical practice guideline. *J. Clin. Oncol.* **2014**, *32*, 1941–1967. [CrossRef]
5. Smith, E.M.L.; Pang, H.; Cirrincione, C.; Fleishman, S.; Paskett, E.D.; Ahles, T.; Bressler, L.R.; Fadul, C.E.; Knox, C.; Le-Lindqwister, N. Effect of duloxetine on pain, function, and quality of life among patients with chemotherapy-induced painful peripheral neuropathy: A randomized clinical trial. *JAMA* **2013**, *309*, 1359–1367. [CrossRef]
6. Farshchian, N.; Alavi, A.; Heydarheydari, S.; Moradian, N. Comparative study of the effects of venlafaxine and duloxetine on chemotherapy-induced peripheral neuropathy. *Cancer Chemother. Pharmacol.* **2018**, *82*, 787–793. [CrossRef]
7. Kim, W.; Kim, M.J.; Go, D.; Min, B.-I.; Na, H.S.; Kim, S.K. Combined effects of bee venom acupuncture and morphine on oxaliplatin-induced neuropathic pain in mice. *Toxins* **2016**, *8*, 33. [CrossRef]
8. Kim, M.J.; Lee, J.H.; Jang, J.U.; Quan, F.S.; Kim, S.K.; Kim, W. The efficacy of combination treatment of gabapentin and electro-acupuncture on paclitaxel-induced neuropathic pain. *Korean J. Physiol. Pharmacol.* **2017**, *21*, 657–666. [CrossRef]
9. Kim, W.; Chung, Y.; Choi, S.; Min, B.-I.; Kim, S.K. Duloxetine protects against oxaliplatin-induced neuropathic pain and spinal neuron hyperexcitability in rodents. *Int. J. Mol. Sci.* **2017**, *18*, 2626. [CrossRef]
10. Chae, H.K.; Kim, W.; Kim, S.K. Phytochemicals of cinnamomi cortex: Cinnamic acid, but not cinnamaldehyde, attenuates oxaliplatin-induced cold and mechanical hypersensitivity in rats. *Nutrients* **2019**, *11*, 432. [CrossRef]
11. Kim, C.; Lee, J.H.; Kim, W.; Li, D.; Kim, Y.; Lee, K.; Kim, S.K. The suppressive effects of cinnamomi cortex and its phytocompound coumarin on oxaliplatin-induced neuropathic cold allodynia in rats. *Molecules* **2016**, *21*, 1253. [CrossRef] [PubMed]
12. Jung, Y.; Lee, J.H.; Kim, W.; Yoon, S.H.; Kim, S.K. Anti-allodynic effect of buja in a rat model of oxaliplatin-induced peripheral neuropathy via spinal astrocytes and pro-inflammatory cytokines suppression. *BMC Complementary Altern. Med.* **2017**, *17*, 1–8. [CrossRef] [PubMed]
13. Lee, J.H.; Go, D.; Kim, W.; Lee, G.; Bae, H.; Quan, F.S.; Kim, S.K. Involvement of spinal muscarinic and serotonergic receptors in the anti-allodynic effect of electroacupuncture in rats with oxaliplatin-induced neuropathic pain. *Korean J. Physiol. Pharmacol.* **2016**, *20*, 407–414. [CrossRef] [PubMed]
14. Li, D.; Lee, Y.; Kim, W.; Lee, K.; Bae, H.; Kim, S.K. Analgesic effects of bee venom derived phospholipase a2 in a mouse model of oxaliplatin-induced neuropathic pain. *Toxins* **2015**, *7*, 2422–2434. [CrossRef]
15. Li, D.; Kim, W.; Shin, D.; Jung, Y.; Bae, H.; Kim, S.K. Preventive effects of bee venom derived phospholipase a2 on oxaliplatin-induced neuropathic pain in mice. *Toxins* **2016**, *8*, 27. [CrossRef]
16. Choi, S.; Chae, H.K.; Heo, H.; Hahm, D.-H.; Kim, W.; Kim, S.K. Analgesic effect of melittin on oxaliplatin-induced peripheral neuropathy in rats. *Toxins* **2019**, *11*, 396. [CrossRef]
17. Son, D.J.; Lee, J.W.; Lee, Y.H.; Song, H.S.; Lee, C.K.; Hong, J.T. Therapeutic application of anti-arthritis, pain-releasing, and anti-cancer effects of bee venom and its constituent compounds. *Pharmacol. Ther.* **2007**, *115*, 246–270. [CrossRef]
18. Lee, M.S.; Pittler, M.H.; Shin, B.-C.; Kong, J.C.; Ernst, E. Bee venom acupuncture for musculoskeletal pain: A review. *J. Pain* **2008**, *9*, 289–297. [CrossRef]
19. Shin, B.-C.; Kong, J.C.; Park, T.-Y.; Yang, C.-Y.; Kang, K.-W.; Choi, S.-m. Bee venom acupuncture for chronic low back pain: A randomised, sham-controlled, triple-blind clinical trial. *Eur. J. Integr. Med.* **2012**, *4*, e271–e280. [CrossRef]
20. Lee, J.-D.; Park, H.-J.; Chae, Y.; Lim, S. An overview of bee venom acupuncture in the treatment of arthritis. *Evid. -Based Complementary Altern. Med.* **2005**, *2*, 397319. [CrossRef]
21. Yoon, J.; Jeon, J.-H.; Lee, Y.-W.; Cho, C.-K.; Kwon, K.-R.; Shin, J.-E.; Sagar, S.; Wong, R.; Yoo, H.-S. Sweet bee venom pharmacopuncture for chemotherapy-induced peripheral neuropathy. *J. Acupunct. Meridian Stud.* **2012**, *5*, 156–165. [CrossRef] [PubMed]

22. Jacobs, S.; McCully, C.L.; Murphy, R.F.; Bacher, J.; Balis, F.M.; Fox, E. Extracellular fluid concentrations of cisplatin, carboplatin, and oxaliplatin in brain, muscle, and blood measured using microdialysis in nonhuman primates. *Cancer Chemother. Pharmacol.* **2010**, *65*, 817–824. [CrossRef]
23. Hains, B.C.; Saab, C.Y.; Waxman, S.G. Changes in electrophysiological properties and sodium channel nav1. 3 expression in thalamic neurons after spinal cord injury. *Brain* **2005**, *128*, 2359–2371. [CrossRef] [PubMed]
24. Park, S.; Krishnan, A.; Lin, C.; Goldstein, D.; Friedlander, M.; Kiernan, M. Mechanisms underlying chemotherapy-induced neurotoxicity and the potential for neuroprotective strategies. *Curr. Med. Chem.* **2008**, *15*, 3081–3094. [CrossRef] [PubMed]
25. Kagiava, A.; Tsingotjidou, A.; Emmanouilides, C.; Theophilidis, G. The effects of oxaliplatin, an anticancer drug, on potassium channels of the peripheral myelinated nerve fibres of the adult rat. *Neurotoxicology* **2008**, *29*, 1100–1106. [CrossRef]
26. Cummins, T.R.; Sheets, P.L.; Waxman, S.G. The roles of sodium channels in nociception: Implications for mechanisms of pain. *Pain* **2007**, *131*, 243–257. [CrossRef]
27. Kim, W. Effect of oxaliplatin on voltage-gated sodium channels in peripheral neuropathic pain. *Processes* **2020**, *8*, 680. [CrossRef]
28. Rogers, M.; Tang, L.; Madge, D.J.; Stevens, E.B. *The Role of Sodium Channels in Neuropathic Pain, Seminars in Cell & Developmental Biology*; Elsevier: Amsterdam, The Netherlands, 2006; pp. 571–581.
29. Eckel, F.; Schmelz, R.; Adelsberger, H.; Erdmann, J.; Quasthoff, S.; Lersch, C. Prevention of oxaliplatin-induced neuropathy by carbamazepine. A pilot study. *Dtsch. Med. Wochenschr. (1946)* **2002**, *127*, 78–82. [CrossRef]
30. Gamelin, E.; Gamelin, L.; Bossi, L.; Quasthoff, S. Clinical aspects and molecular basis of oxaliplatin neurotoxicity: Current management and development of preventive measures. *Semin. Oncol.* **2002**, *29*, 21–33. [CrossRef]
31. Lim, B.-S.; Moon, H.J.; Li, D.X.; Gil, M.; Min, J.K.; Lee, G.; Bae, H.; Kim, S.K.; Min, B.-I. Effect of bee venom acupuncture on oxaliplatin-induced cold allodynia in rats. *Evid.-Based Complementary Altern. Med.* **2013**, *2013*, 369324. [CrossRef]
32. Lee, J.-H.; Li, D.X.; Yoon, H.; Go, D.; Quan, F.S.; Min, B.-I.; Kim, S.K. Serotonergic mechanism of the relieving effect of bee venom acupuncture on oxaliplatin-induced neuropathic cold allodynia in rats. *BMC Complementary Altern. Med.* **2014**, *14*, 471. [CrossRef] [PubMed]
33. Adelsberger, H.; Quasthoff, S.; Grosskreutz, J.; Lepier, A.; Eckel, F.; Lersch, C. The chemotherapeutic oxaliplatin alters voltage-gated na+ channel kinetics on rat sensory neurons. *Eur. J. Pharmacol.* **2000**, *406*, 25–32. [CrossRef]
34. Frot, M.; Feine, J.S.; Bushnell, M.C. Sex differences in pain perception and anxiety. A psychophysical study with topical capsaicin. *Pain* **2004**, *108*, 230–236. [CrossRef] [PubMed]
35. Choi, J.; Jeon, C.; Lee, J.H.; Jang, J.U.; Quan, F.S.; Lee, K.; Kim, W.; Kim, S.K. Suppressive effects of bee venom acupuncture on paclitaxel-induced neuropathic pain in rats: Mediation by spinal α2-adrenergic receptor. *Toxins* **2017**, *9*, 351. [CrossRef] [PubMed]
36. Soulie, P.; Bensmaine, A.; Garrino, C.; Chollet, P.; Brain, E.; Fereres, M.; Jasmin, C.; Musset, M.; Misset, J.; Cvitkovic, E. Oxaliplatin/cisplatin (l-ohp/cddp) combination in heavily pretreated ovarian cancer. *Eur. J. Cancer* **1997**, *33*, 1400–1406. [CrossRef]
37. Wilson, R.H.; Lehky, T.; Thomas, R.R.; Quinn, M.G.; Floeter, M.K.; Grem, J.L. Acute oxaliplatin-induced peripheral nerve hyperexcitability. *J. Clin. Oncol.* **2002**, *20*, 1767–1774. [CrossRef]
38. Zhang, S.; Liu, Y.; Ye, Y.; Wang, X.-R.; Lin, L.-T.; Xiao, L.-Y.; Zhou, P.; Shi, G.-X.; Liu, C.-Z. Bee venom therapy: Potential mechanisms and therapeutic applications. *Toxicon* **2018**, *148*, 64–73. [CrossRef]
39. Cavaletti, G.; Tredici, G.; Petruccioli, M.; Donde, E.; Tredici, P.; Marmiroli, P.; Minoia, C.; Ronchi, A.; Bayssas, M.; Etienne, G.G. Effects of different schedules of oxaliplatin treatment on the peripheral nervous system of the rat. *Eur. J. Cancer* **2001**, *37*, 2457–2463. [CrossRef]
40. Gregg, R.W.; Molepo, J.M.; Monpetit, V.; Mikael, N.Z.; Redmond, D.; Gadia, M.; Stewart, D.J. Cisplatin neurotoxicity: The relationship between dosage, time, and platinum concentration in neurologic tissues, and morphologic evidence of toxicity. *J. Clin. Oncol.* **1992**, *10*, 795–803. [CrossRef]
41. Sittl, R.; Lampert, A.; Huth, T.; Schuy, E.T.; Link, A.S.; Fleckenstein, J.; Alzheimer, C.; Grafe, P.; Carr, R.W. Anticancer drug oxaliplatin induces acute cooling-aggravated neuropathy via sodium channel subtype nav1. 6-resurgent and persistent current. *Proc. Natl. Acad. Sci. USA* **2012**, *109*, 6704–6709. [CrossRef]

42. Heide, R.; Bostock, H.; Ventzel, L.; Grafe, P.; Bergmans, J.; Fuglsang-Frederiksen, A.; Finnerup, N.B.; Tankisi, H. Axonal excitability changes and acute symptoms of oxaliplatin treatment: In vivo evidence for slowed sodium channel inactivation. *Clin. Neurophysiol.* **2018**, *129*, 694–706. [CrossRef] [PubMed]
43. Horowitz, S.H. The diagnostic workup of patients with neuropathic pain. *Anesthesiol. Clin.* **2007**, *25*, 699–708. [CrossRef] [PubMed]
44. Deuis, J.R.; Zimmermann, K.; Romanovsky, A.A.; Possani, L.D.; Cabot, P.J.; Lewis, R.J.; Vetter, I. An animal model of oxaliplatin-induced cold allodynia reveals a crucial role for nav1. 6 in peripheral pain pathways. *PAIN®* **2013**, *154*, 1749–1757. [CrossRef] [PubMed]
45. Bennett, D.L.; Clark, A.J.; Huang, J.; Waxman, S.G.; Dib-Hajj, S.D. The role of voltage-gated sodium channels in pain signaling. *Physiol. Rev.* **2019**, *99*, 1079–1151. [CrossRef] [PubMed]
46. Mannelli, L.D.C.; Lucarini, E.; Micheli, L.; Mosca, I.; Ambrosino, P.; Soldovieri, M.V.; Martelli, A.; Testai, L.; Taglialatela, M.; Calderone, V. Effects of natural and synthetic isothiocyanate-based h2s-releasers against chemotherapy-induced neuropathic pain: Role of kv7 potassium channels. *Neuropharmacology* **2017**, *121*, 49–59. [CrossRef] [PubMed]
47. Benoit, E.; Brienza, S.; Dubois, J. Oxaliplatin, an anticancer agent that affects both na^+ and k^+ channels in frog peripheral myelinated axons. *Gen. Physiol. Biophys.* **2006**, *25*, 263.
48. Lee, E.J.; Kim, B.J.; Jeong, J.E.; Chung, H.L.; Yang, E.K.; Kim, W.T. Bee venom exerts neuroprotective effects on neuronal cells and astrocytes under hypoxic conditions through mapk signaling pathways. *Neonatal Med.* **2016**, *23*, 43–52. [CrossRef]
49. Song, Y.; Zhang, M.; Tao, X.; Xu, Z.; Zheng, Y.; Zhu, M.; Zhang, L.; Qiao, J.; Gao, L. Difference of acute dissociation and 1-day culture on the electrophysiological properties of rat dorsal root ganglion neurons. *J. Physiol. Biochem.* **2018**, *74*, 207–221. [CrossRef]
50. Lee, G.; Yang, E.; Kim, S.; Park, C.-S.; Park, Y.S.; Jin, Y.-H. Parapheromones suppress chemotherapy side effects. *J. Pharmacol. Exp. Ther.* **2018**, *367*, 215–221. [CrossRef]

2

Identification of Acupoint Indication from Reverse Inference: Data Mining of Randomized Controlled Clinical Trials

Ye-Chae Hwang [1,†], In-Seon Lee [1,†], Yeonhee Ryu [2], Ye-Seul Lee [3,*] and Younbyoung Chae [1,*]

1 Acupuncture & Meridian Science Research Center, College of Korean Medicine, Kyung Hee University, Seoul 02447, Korea; mma3206@khu.ac.kr (Y.-C.H.); inseon.lee@khu.ac.kr (I.-S.L.)
2 KM Fundamental Research Division, Korea Institute of Oriental Medicine, Daejeon 34054, Korea; yhryu@kiom.re.kr
3 Department of Anatomy and Acupoint, College of Korean Medicine, Gachon University, Seongnam 13306, Korea
* Correspondence: yeseulee@gachon.ac.kr (Y.-S.L.); ybchae@khu.ac.kr (Y.C.)
† Both equally contributed to this study as co-first authors.

Abstract: The specificity of acupoint indication (i.e., reverse inference—diseases for which an acupoint could be used) might differ from the specificity of acupoint selection (i.e., forward inference—acupoints used for a disease). In this study, we explore acupoint specificity through reverse inferences from the dataset of prescribed acupoints for a certain disease in clinical trials. We searched acupuncture treatment regimens in randomized controlled trials included in the Cochrane Database of Systematic Reviews. For forward inference, the acupoints prescribed for each disease were quantified. For reverse inference, diseases for each acupoint were quantified. Data were normalized using Z-scores. Bayes factor correction was performed to adjust for the prior probability of diseases. The specificities of acupoint selections in 30 diseases were determined using forward inference. The specificities of acupoint indications regarding 49 acupoints were identified using reverse inference and then subjected to Bayes factor correction. Two types of acupoint indications were identified for 24 acupoints: regional and distal. Our approach suggests that the specificity of acupoint indication can be inferred from clinical data using reverse inference. Acupoint indication will improve our understanding of acupoint specificity and will lead to the establishment of a new model of analysis and educational resources for acupoint characteristics.

Keywords: acupoint indication; acupoint specificity; Bayesian modeling; data mining; clinical trials

1. Introduction

The action of acupuncture can be explained by various levels of neuromodulations by means of local, segmental, and general effects (descending analgesia and central regulation) [1,2]. Many neuroimaging studies have shown common brain activations and deactivation patterns following acupuncture stimulations [3]. However, it has been difficult to reveal the point specificities on clinical significances using these approaches [4,5]. Clinical acupoint selection involves three basic principles: (1) local acupoints near the area where symptoms occur, (2) distant acupoints from the symptom location along the meridian, and (3) distant acupoints based on symptom differentiation, regardless of symptom location [6–8]. Recent studies have investigated these principles through the novel paradigm of data mining, using a number of available datasets related to traditional medicine. The associations between symptom differentiations and acupuncture prescriptions are relatively clear in classical textbooks, although the associations from these classical textbooks are not likely to be prominent in clinical practice [9,10]. Previous studies have identified selections of acupoints for various diseases such as lumbar disc herniation, dysmenorrhea, rheumatoid arthritis, and visceral pain [11–14]. However, these findings do not directly reveal the specificity of acupoint indication; they only indicate which acupoints can be selected specifically for a particular disease [15].

In clinical practice, it is essential to identify which acupoints are specifically associated with a particular disease. However, selecting an acupoint to treat a particular disease does not always imply that the selected acupoint has specific indications for that disease [15]. Thus, indications for the selected acupoints may not always match the target disease for which the acupoints were selected. This crucial point is often missed in both education and clinical practice, which often leads to errors in logic. To clarify this relationship, we suggested two-directional relationships between diseases and acupoints: forward inference and reverse inference. Forward inference analysis identifies the specificity of acupoint selection by analyzing the probability that an acupoint would be selected for a given disease: P (Acupoint | Disease). In contrast, reverse inference analysis identifies the specificity of acupoint indication by analyzing the probability of a given disease based on the selected acupoint: P (Disease | Acupoint). In our previous study, we proposed that the specificity of acupoint selection might differ from the specificity of acupoint indication. For example, BL23, GB30, and GV3 showed strong forward inferences to lumbar herniated intervertebral disc, while lumbar herniated intervertebral disc showed a high reverse inference score for acupoint BL23 [15].

Implementation of forward and reverse inferences, based on a large database, is needed to clarify the associations between diseases and acupoints. The Cochrane Database of Systematic Reviews (CDSR) identifies, appraises, and synthesizes all empirical evidence that meets prespecified eligibility criteria for efficacy [16]. Therefore, we hypothesized that we could identify the specificity of acupoint indication by analyzing relationships between prescribed acupoints and diseases using CDSR data. We also applied data mining techniques and Bayes factor (BF) correction to CDSR data. Data mining can reveal associations between diseases and acupoints [1,15]. Bayes factor correction has been suggested as a way to avoid logical errors and fallacies in forward and reverse inference analyses [17–20]. Bayes factor correction can help define the specificities of acupoint indications by correcting the odds of the prior probability or the odds of the diseases presented in the data. By eliminating the prior probability of diseases, the substance of reverse inference can be formalized to determine the specificities of acupoint indications.

In the current study, we searched acupuncture regimens in randomized controlled trials included in the CDSR and then identified the specificities of acupoint selections and acupoint indications. We explored the specificity of acupoint selections using forward inference and the specificity of acupoint indications using reverse inference based on clinical trial data.

2. Methods

2.1. Data Extraction Process

To extract acupoint information from randomized controlled clinical trials, we searched the Cochrane Library (www.cochranelibrary.com) using the keyword "acupuncture" in records titled Cochrane Reviews. To ensure a sufficient number of studies of each disease in the frequency analysis, studies involving more than three clinical trials with acupoint information were included. From the retrieved studies, the following features were included for analysis: all relevant diseases, interventions using needle-type acupuncture (manual and electroacupuncture), and all acupuncture regimens (both standardized and semistandardized). Studies were excluded from analysis if they involved interventions with non-needle type acupuncture (e.g., acupressure and laser acupuncture), interventions that were not acupuncture (e.g., moxibustion), or acupuncture trials using only a subset of body areas for treatment (e.g., ears, face, head, or feet). Therefore, a total of 49 CDSR records were retrieved from the Cochran Library, and 30 CDSR records met for our criteria. A total of 421 randomized clinical trials were included for this analysis of a total of 30 diseases (i.e., 63 studies for depression, 30 studies for dysmenorrhea, and 25 studies for lower back pain). To remove possible outliers and include only acupoints with sufficient numbers of prescriptions, acupoints were included if they were used more than 14 times across all studies, for a total of 49 acupoints. To explore the associations between diseases and acupoints, the frequencies of co-occurrences of the 49 acupoints and 30 diseases were extracted (Figure 1).

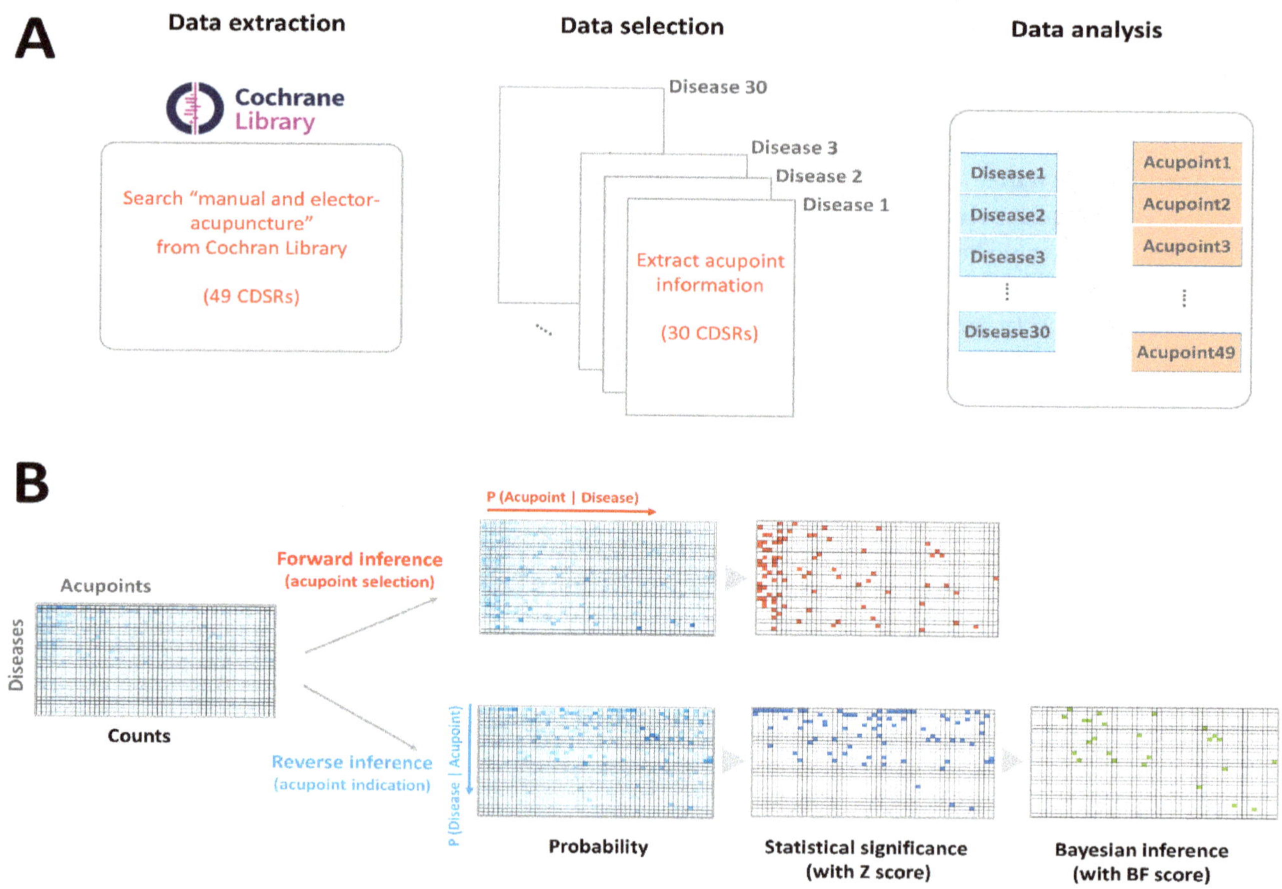

Figure 1. Data extraction and data analysis. (**A**): Data extraction procedures. The frequencies of the co-occurrences of the 49 acupoints and 30 diseases were extracted to explore the associations between diseases and acupoints. (**B**): Data analysis procedures. For forward inference, acupoints prescribed for each disease were quantified. For reverse inference, diseases for each acupoint were quantified. Probability values were Z-transformed to assess statistical significance for both forward and reverse inference ($Z > 1.96$). Bayes factor correction was applied to reverse inference to adjust for the odds of the prior probability of the disease. BF: Bayes factor

2.2. *Data Analysis of Acupoint Selection Using Forward Inference*

The specificity of acupoint selection can be inferred from observed data, with the probability of selecting one acupoint for a certain disease represented as P (Acupoint | Disease). The acupoint selection specificity was defined by forward inference (the probability that an acupoint would be selected for a given disease), calculated as the frequency of selection of that acupoint divided by the total number of acupoint selections. Probability values were Z-transformed for assessment of statistical significance ($Z > 1.96$).

2.3. *Data Analysis of Acupoint Indication Using Reverse Inference*

The specificity of an acupoint indication can be inferred from the observed data, with the probability of disease targeted by a certain acupoint represented as P (Disease | Acupoint). The acupoint indication specificity was defined by reverse inference (i.e., Bayesian inference, the probability that a given disease would be defined as the indication for a certain acupoint), calculated as the frequency selection of that disease divided by the total number of disease selections. Probability values were Z-transformed to assess statistical significance (Z > 1.96).

2.4. Bayes Factor Correction of Acupoint Indication

While conditional probability used in reverse inference helps clarify the probability of diseases in acupoint indications, it does not consider the prior odds of the diseases. To consider the prior probability of the diseases, Bayes factor correction was applied to the reverse inference results. According to Bayes' theorem, BF is the likelihood ratio of the marginal likelihood of one particular hypothesis to another. We investigated the relative strength of each hypothesis compared with the null hypothesis (e.g., H_α = disease K is highly treated by acupoint L in randomized controlled trials) by assessing BF (θ = data) as below (1).

$$BF_{\alpha N} = \frac{p(\theta|H_\alpha)}{p(\theta|H_N)} = \frac{p(D_k|A_l)}{1-p(D_k|A_l)} \Big/ \frac{p(D_k)}{1-p(D_k)} \quad (1)$$

To determine BF, the odds for the presence of disease when one acupoint is used were qualified by the odds of the prior probability of the disease (i.e., number of acupoints used for disease, the denominator). BF > 3 indicated substantial evidence in favor of the inference.

3. Results

3.1. Patterns of Acupoint Selection for 30 Diseases Using Forward Inference

Figure 2 lists the 49 most frequently prescribed acupoints in descending order of their probability values (p) for the 30 diseases. Among all diseases, the most frequently prescribed acupoints were SP6 (p = 0.082), ST36 (p = 0.068), LR3 (p = 0.066), and LI4 (p = 0.064). The most frequently selected acupoints were similar across the 30 diseases, whereas different patterns of selected acupoints were found for each disease.

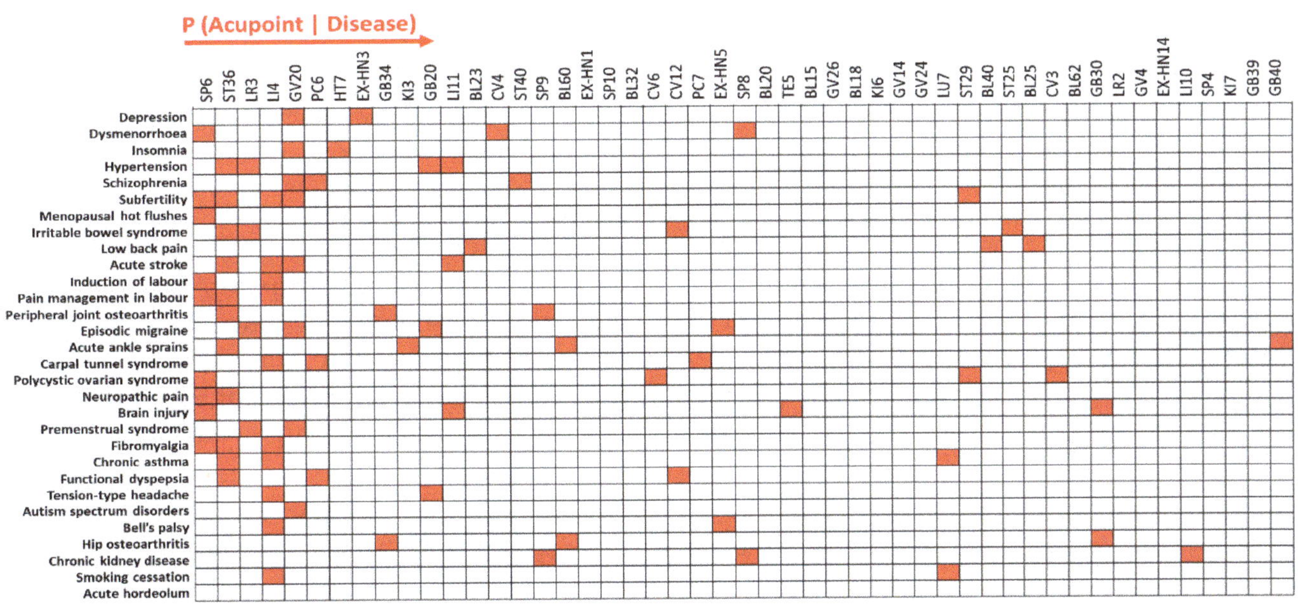

Figure 2. Patterns of acupoint selection for 30 diseases using forward inference. The most frequently selected acupoints were similar across the 30 diseases, while different patterns of selected acupoints were found for each disease. Z-scores indicate the frequency of each acupoint in each disease trial, compared to the overall acupoint selection pattern for that disease.

The Z-scores illustrate how frequently each acupoint was used in each disease trial compared to the overall acupoint selection pattern for that disease. The Z-scores of the 49 acupoints for the 30 diseases are depicted on a heatmap. For example, acupoints with a high Z-score (Z > 1.96) for the 3 main diseases are as follows: GV20 (Z = 3.82) and EX-HN3 (Z = 2.65) for depression; SP6 (Z = 4.29), CV4 (Z = 2.37), and SP8 (Z = 2.37) for dysmenorrhea; HT7 (Z = 3.55) and GV20 (Z = 1.98) for insomnia (Figure 2).

3.2. *Patterns of Acupoint Indications for 49 Acupoints Using Reverse Inference*

Figure 3 lists the 30 diseases in descending order of their overall trial frequencies for the 49 acupoints. Depression was the most prominent acupoint indication across the 49 acupoints, although different acupoint indications were also found for each acupoint.

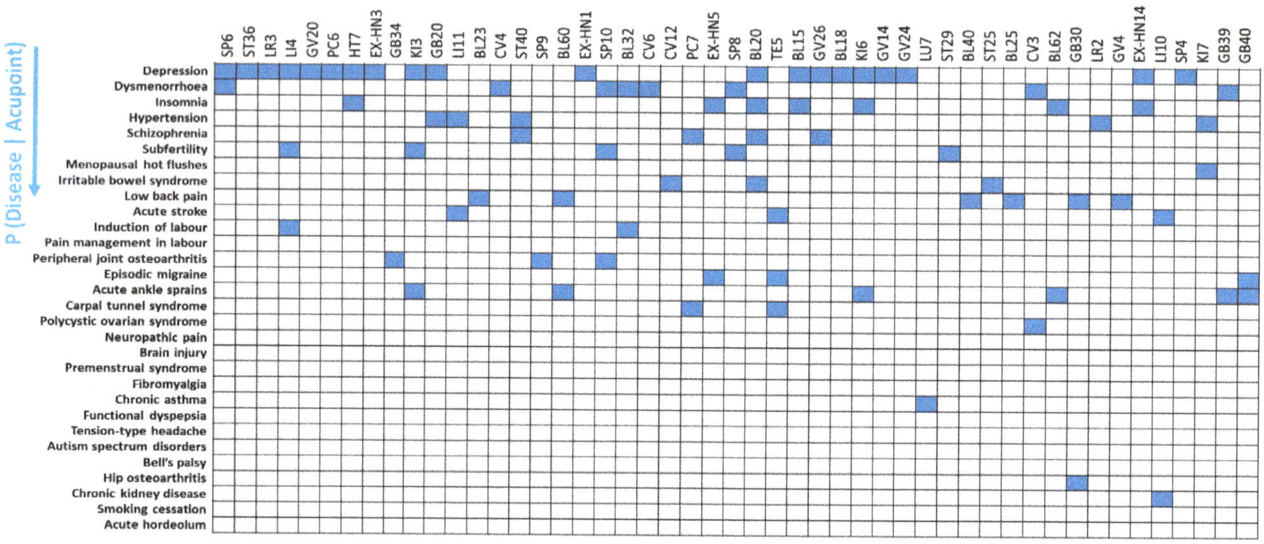

Figure 3. Patterns of acupoint indications for 49 acupoints using reverse inference. Depression was the most prominent indication across the 49 acupoints, while different acupoint indications were also found for each acupoint. Z-scores indicate the frequency at which each disease was treated by each acupoint compared to the indications for that acupoint.

The Z-scores illustrate how frequently each disease was treated by each acupoint, compared to the indications for that acupoint. The Z-scores of the 30 indications for the 49 acupoints are depicted on a heatmap. For example, diseases with a high Z-score (Z > 1.96) for the 4 main acupoints are as follows: depression (Z = 3.28) and dysmenorrhea (Z = 2.54) for SP6; depression (Z = 2.71) for ST36; depression (Z = 4.07) for LR3; depression (Z = 3.13), induction of labor (Z = 2.26), and subfertility (Z = 2.26) for LI4 (Figure 3).

3.3. *Specificity of Acupoint Indications Using Bayes Factor Correction*

The acupoint indications were more specific to each disease after correction with BF (BF > 3). Diseases with a high BF score (BF > 3) for acupoints are as follows: insomnia (BF = 3.69) for HT7; depression (BF = 6.36) for EX-HN3; peripheral joint osteoarthritis (BF = 7.60) for GB34; acute ankle sprains (BF = 5.39) for KI3 (Figure 4). The results indicate that few acupoint indications for diseases with greater prior probabilities, such as depression and dysmenorrhea, did not survive the BF correction.

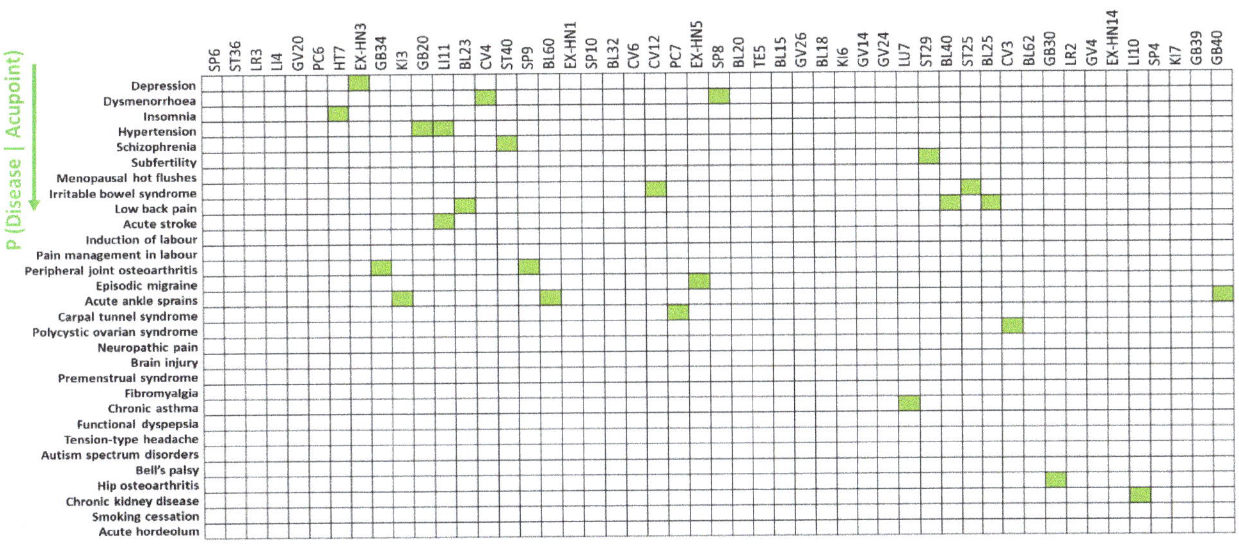

Figure 4. Specificity of acupoint indications using Bayes factor (BF) correction. The acupoint indications were more specific to the respective diseases after BF correction (BF > 3).

3.4. *Two Different Patterns of Acupoint Indications*

After BF correction, the acupoint indications were classified into two categories based on the distance between acupoint and disease area. Acupoints with regional indications were distributed in the head, back, abdomen, and ankle (type 1, $n = 17$). Acupoints with distal indications were mainly distributed in the upper/lower limbs (type 2, $n = 7$; Table 1). The acupoints were overlaid on a human body template (Figure 5).

Table 1. Classification of acupoint indications with strong inference (BF > 3).

Type I (Regional Acupoints, *n* = 17)	
BL23 (back)	Low back pain (BF = 10.12)
BL25 (back)	Low back pain (BF = 36.87)
BL60 (feet)	Acute ankle sprain (BF = 13.47)
CV3 (abdomen)	Polycystic ovarian syndrome (BF = 18.53)
CV4 (abdomen)	Dysmenorrhea (BF = 5.51)
CV12 (abdomen)	Irritable bowel syndrome (BF = 8.29)
EX-HN3 (head)	Depression (BF = 6.36)
EX-HN5 (head)	Episodic migraine (BF = 9.03)
GB20 (head)	Hypertension (BF = 3.94)
GB30 (lower limb)	Hip osteoarthritis (BF = 53.94)
GB34 (lower limb)	Peripheral joint osteoarthritis (BF = 7.60)
GB40 (feet)	Acute ankle sprain (BF = 38.50)
KI3 (feet)	Acute ankle sprain (BF = 5.39)
PC7 (upper limb)	Carpal tunnel syndrome (BF = 35.31)
SP9 (lower limb)	Peripheral joint osteoarthritis (BF = 9.39)
ST25 (abdomen)	Irritable bowel syndrome (BF = 33.16)
ST29 (abdomen)	Subfertility (BF = 27.09)
Type II (Distal Acupoints, *n* = 7)	
BL40 (lower limb)	Low back pain (BF = 32.26)
HT7 (upper limb)	Insomnia (BF = 3.68)
LI10 (upper limb)	Chronic kidney disease (BF = 105.3)
LI11 (upper limb)	Hypertension (BF = 6.60), Acute stroke (BF = 6.57)
LU7 (upper limb)	Chronic asthma (BF = 22.48)
SP8 (lower limb)	Dysmenorrhea (BF = 17.56)
ST40 (lower limb)	Schizophrenia (BF = 5.29)

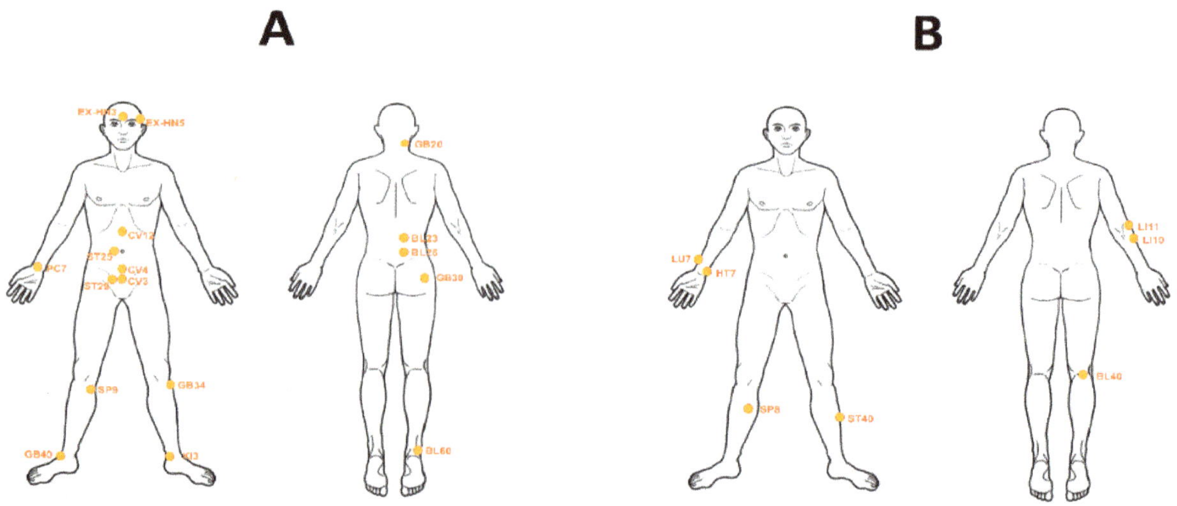

Figure 5. Two patterns of acupoint indications. (**A**) Type 1 includes acupoints with regional indications distributed in the head, back, abdomen, and ankle ($n = 17$; BL23, BL25, BL60, CV3, CV4, CV12, EX-HN3, EX-HN5, GB20, GB30, GB34, GB40, KI3, PC7, SP9, ST25, ST29). (**B**) Type 2 includes acupoints with distal indications distributed in the upper/lower limbs ($n = 7$; BL40, HT7, LI10, LI11, LU7, SP8, ST40).

4. Discussion

The findings of the present study revealed patterns of acupoint selection for 30 diseases, as well as patterns of acupoint indications for 49 acupoints, using clinical trial data from the CDSR. We demonstrated the specificity of acupoint selection for each disease using forward inference. We also demonstrated the specificity of acupoint indication using reverse inference. Considering the prior probabilities of diseases, acupoint indications were further refined with BF correction. Finally, we identified two types of acupoint indications for 24 acupoints: regional and distal. Identification of the specific patterns of acupoint indications through data mining from clinical trials will be useful for understanding the characteristics of acupoints in education and clinical practice.

The core set of acupoints can be widely used to treat a variety of diseases, whereas some acupoints are only used to treat specific diseases. In our previous study, we identified the commonality and specificity of acupoint selections based on virtual acupuncture treatments prescribed by practicing clinicians. We found that acupoints ST36, LI4, and LR3 were the most commonly prescribed across all diseases [21]. Mining of CDSR data also revealed that the main acupoints commonly used for a variety of pain management approaches were SP6, ST36, LI4, and LR3 [1]. Consistent with the findings of previous studies, we found that the core acupoints were widely used for all 30 diseases, regardless of disease type. In contrast, acupoints GV20 and EX-HN3 were specifically used for the treatment of depression, while acupoints CV4 and SP8 were specifically used for the treatment of dysmenorrhea (Figure 2). These findings support the common rule of acupoint selections, in which some acupoints are common among all diseases while other acupoints are specifically prescribed for the treatment of certain diseases.

Forward and reverse inference have been used in various areas of academic research. Notably, reverse inference has been used in neuroscience to assign a certain cognitive process to activation of a certain brain region, while forward inference has been used to evaluate cognitive theories based on different patterns of brain activation [18,20]. As forward and reverse inferences can link associations directly, they demonstrate causal relationships without possible logical errors. This study extends the concept of forward and reverse inference in terms of the relationship between acupoints and diseases using CDSR data. The specificity of acupoint indication is generally inferred from the specificity of acupoint selection. However, we demonstrated that forward inference alone can lead to errors in logic regarding the acupoint indication specificity and that the application of reverse inference can improve the acupoint specificity.

Previous studies have indicated that reverse inference should be approached with caution if the prior probability (i.e., the odds of the prior probability of the disease) remains unknown [19]. By implementing reverse inference, we found that depression and dysmenorrhea were specific indications for acupoint SP6, while depression, induction of labor, and subfertility were specific indications for acupoint LI4 (Figure 3). However, the total number of trials can influence the specificity of acupoint indications. For example, depression was an indication for many acupoints (e.g., SP6, ST36, LR3, LI4) in the reverse inference because the total number of studies on depression was greater than the number of studies on other diseases. To avoid possible fallacy following the distortion of data, BF correction was implemented when identifying the specificity of acupoint indications; this approach corrected the odds of the prior probability of the disease. Implementation of BF correction led to the identification of insomnia as the indication for acupoint HT7 while ruling out diseases with high frequency in the data (e.g., depression) and specific acupoints (e.g., EX-HN3) (Figure 4). This analysis demonstrated that reverse inference using BF correction is useful for inferring specificity of acupoint indications.

In the current study, two types of acupoint indications were identified: regional and distal. Both regional and distal acupoints were specifically linked with certain diseases. Among regional acupoints, low back pain was the indication for acupoint BL23 in the back, while acute ankle sprain was the indication for acupoint BL60 in the feet. Among distal acupoints, low back pain was the indication for BL40 in the lower limb, while insomnia was the indication for acupoint HT7 in the wrist (Figure 5). Classification of acupoint indications into regional and distal types is consistent with the approach used in previous studies, where both regional and distal acupoints were mainly used for pain management during acupuncture, based on data mining from clinical trials [1,8,11].

Two different strategies for acupoint prescription, including branch treatment and root treatment, are widely used in the context of traditional East Asian medicine [22]. Pattern identification can extract and synthesize patients' signs and symptoms and lead to making treatment decisions [23]. Acupuncture practitioners can choose the most appropriate acupoints based on the disease or symptoms (i.e., branch treatment) or on the results of pattern identification (i.e., root treatment) [21,24]. Although some clinical trials consider individualized treatment strategies, clinical trials are generally conducted to find out the efficacy of the acupuncture treatment on a certain disease. Furthermore, pattern identification can be varied across patients even though they have the same disease [25]. Only a limited number of studies provided the information of pattern identification from the CDSR. Thus, the present study only determined the acupoint indication based on the relationship between disease/symptoms and acupoints without considering pattern identification. The acupoint indication associated with pattern identification should be further studied in the future.

Our study had several limitations. First, it did not consider the effectiveness of the acupuncture treatment in each study. To include the effectiveness of acupoints, future studies with appropriate control groups will be needed to enable the extraction of the effectiveness of acupuncture treatment administered to a group of acupoints. Due to the limited number of included studies, we were not able to analyze the data considering the clinical effectiveness of needling at each point. More sufficient data will be needed to ensure the acupoint indications based on clinical significance in the future. Second, this study did not restrict methodological quality among the assessed studies. Insufficient evidence was available to reveal discrepancies between acupoints used in high-quality and low-quality studies. Future analyses should incorporate inclusion criteria to ensure the inclusion of studies with meaningful information. Finally, this study identified acupoint indications only from clinical trials. Additional analyses will be needed to clarify the associations between diseases and acupoints based on clinical data obtained in a real-world setting.

In summary, data mining, forward and reverse inference analyses, and BF correction of clinical trial data revealed the bidirectional specificity of acupoints for various diseases. We expect our approach to provide new information regarding the specificities of acupoint indications from clinical observations.

Author Contributions: Conceptualization, Y.-C.H., Y.R. and Y.C.; Methodology, Y.-C.H. and Y.-S.L.; Formal analysis, Y.-C.H. and I.-S.L.; Writing—original draft preparation, Y.-C.H. and Y.C.; Writing—review and editing, I-S.L. and Y.-S.L.; Supervision, Y.C. All authors have read and agreed to the published version of the manuscript.

References

1. Hwang, Y.C.; Lee, I.S.; Ryu, Y.; Lee, M.S.; Chae, Y. Exploring traditional acupuncture point selection patterns for pain control: Data mining of randomised controlled clinical trials. *Acupunct. Med.* **2020**, 964528420926173. [CrossRef] [PubMed]
2. White, A. Editorial Board of Acupuncture in M. Western medical acupuncture: A definition. *Acupunct. Med.* **2009**, *27*, 33–35. [CrossRef] [PubMed]
3. Chae, Y.; Chang, D.S.; Lee, S.H.; Jung, W.M.; Lee, I.S.; Jackson, S.; Kong, J.; Lee, H.; Park, H.J.; Lee, H.; et al. Inserting needles into the body: A meta-analysis of brain activity associated with acupuncture needle stimulation. *J. Pain* **2013**, *14*, 215–222. [CrossRef]
4. Jung, W.M.; Lee, I.S.; Lee, Y.S.; Kim, J.; Park, H.J.; Wallraven, C.; Chae, Y. Decoding spatial location of perceived pain to acupuncture needle using multivoxel pattern analysis. *Mol. Pain* **2019**, *15*, 1744806919877060. [CrossRef] [PubMed]
5. Lee, I.S.; Jung, W.M.; Park, H.J.; Chae, Y. Spatial Information of Somatosensory Stimuli in the Brain: Multivariate Pattern Analysis of Functional Magnetic Resonance Imaging Data. *Neural Plast.* **2020**, 8307580. [CrossRef]
6. Chen, Y.R.; Zhu, J.; Song, J.S.; She, Y.F. Discussion on point selection and compatibility of acupuncture formula. *Zhongguo Zhen Jiu* **2012**, *32*, 65–68. [PubMed]
7. Jung, W.M.; Lee, T.; Lee, I.S.; Kim, S.; Jang, H.; Kim, S.Y.; Park, H.J.; Chae, Y. Spatial Patterns of the Indications of Acupoints Using Data Mining in Classic Medical Text: A Possible Visualization of the Meridian System. *Evid. Based Complement. Altern. Med.* **2015**, *2015*, 457071. [CrossRef] [PubMed]
8. Lee, S.H.; Kim, C.E.; Lee, I.S.; Jung, W.M.; Kim, H.G.; Jang, H.; Kim, S.J.; Lee, H.; Park, H.J.; Chae, Y. Network analysis of acupuncture points used in the treatment of low back pain. *Evid. Based Complement. Altern. Med.* **2013**, *2013*, 402180. [CrossRef]
9. Alvim, D.T.; Ferreira, A.S. Inter-expert agreement and similarity analysis of traditional diagnoses and acupuncture prescriptions in textbook- and pragmatic-based practices. *Complement. Ther. Clin. Pract.* **2018**, *30*, 38–43. [CrossRef]
10. Lee, T.; Jung, W.M.; Lee, I.S.; Lee, Y.S.; Lee, H.; Park, H.J.; Kim, N.; Chae, Y. Data Mining of Acupoint Characteristics from the Classical Medical Text: DongUiBoGam of Korean Medicine. *Evid. Based Complement. Altern. Med.* **2014**, *2014*, 329563. [CrossRef]
11. Lee, I.S.; Cheon, S.; Park, J.Y. Central and Peripheral Mechanism of Acupuncture Analgesia on Visceral Pain: A Systematic Review. *Evid. Based Complement. Altern. Med.* **2019**, *2019*. [CrossRef] [PubMed]
12. Li, J.B.; Xiong, Q.L.; Qu, S.K.; Qi, F.; Zhang, L.; Wang, Q.; Bao, K.; Li, F.B. Discussion on the regular of acupoint selection of acupuncture and moxibustion for lumbar disc herniation during recent 10 years. *Zhongguo Zhen Jiu* **2013**, *33*, 668–672. [PubMed]
13. Yu, S.; Yang, J.; Ren, Y.; Chen, L.; Liang, F.; Hu, Y. Characteristics of acupoints selection of moxibustion for primary dysmenorrhea based on data mining technology. *Zhongguo Zhen Jiu* **2015**, *35*, 845–849. [PubMed]
14. Zhang, K.; Xu, Y.; Ding, S.; Hong, S.; Zhao, X.; Guo, Y. Literature study for acupoint selection rule of rheumatoid arthritis treated with acupuncture. *Zhongguo Zhen Jiu* **2017**, *37*, 221–224. [CrossRef] [PubMed]
15. Hwang, Y.C.; Lee, Y.S.; Ryu, Y.; Lee, I.S.; Chae, Y. Statistical inference of acupoint specificity: Forward and reverse inference. *Integr. Med. Res.* **2020**, *9*, 17–20. [CrossRef]
16. Smith, C.A.; Armour, M.; Lee, M.S.; Wang, L.Q.; Hay, P.J. Acupuncture for depression. *Cochrane Database Syst Rev.* **2018**, *3*. [CrossRef]
17. Heit, E. Brain imaging, forward inference, and theories of reasoning. *Front. Hum. Neurosci.* **2014**, *8*, 1056. [CrossRef]
18. Henson, R. Forward inference using functional neuroimaging: Dissociations versus associations. *Trends Cogn Sci.* **2006**, *10*, 64–69. [CrossRef]

19. Hutzler, F. Reverse inference is not a fallacy per se: Cognitive processes Can be inferred from functional imaging data. *Neuroimage* **2014**, *84*, 1061–1069. [CrossRef]
20. Poldrack, R.A. Can cognitive processes be inferred from neuroimaging data? *Trends Cogn Sci.* **2006**, *10*, 59–63. [CrossRef]
21. Lee, Y.S.; Ryu, Y.; Yoon, D.-E.; Kim, C.H.; Hong, G.; Hwang, Y.C.; Chae, Y. Commonality and specificity of acupuncture points selections. *Evid. Based Complement. Altern. Med.* **2020**, *2020*, 2948292. [CrossRef] [PubMed]
22. Lee, Y.S.; Ryu, Y.; Chae, Y. Acupoint selection based on pattern identification results or disease state. *Integr. Med. Res.* **2020**, *9*, 100405. [CrossRef]
23. Birch, S.; Alraek, T. Traditional East Asian medicine: How to understand and approach diagnostic findings and patterns in a modern scientific framework? *Chin. J. Integr. Med.* **2014**, *20*, 336–340. [CrossRef] [PubMed]
24. Kim, C.H.; Yoon, D.E.; Lee, Y.S.; Jung, W.; Kim, J.H.; Chae, Y. Revealing Associations between Diagnosis Patterns and Acupoint Prescriptions Using Medical Data Extracted from Case Reports. *J. Clin. Med.* **2019**, *8*, 1663. [CrossRef] [PubMed]
25. Kam, W.; Zhang, Z.J.; Baarnhielm, S. Traditional Chinese Medicine Explanatory Models of Depressive Disorders: A Qualitative Study. *Cult. Med. Psychiatry* **2019**, *43*, 387–403. [CrossRef]

3

Effect of Acupuncture on the p38 Signaling Pathway in Several Nervous System Diseases

Tzu-Hsuan Wei [1] and Ching-Liang Hsieh [1,2,3,*]

1 Department of Chinese Medicine, China Medical University Hospital, Taichung 40447, Taiwan; u102030015@cmu.edu.tw

2 Chinese Medicine Research Center, China Medical University, Taichung 40402, Taiwan

3 Graduate Institute of Acupuncture Science, College of Chinese Medicine, China Medical University, Taichung 40402, Taiwan

* Correspondence: clhsieh@mail.cmuh.org.tw

Abstract: Acupuncture is clinically used to treat various diseases and exerts positive local and systemic effects in several nervous system diseases. Advanced molecular and clinical studies have continually attempted to decipher the mechanisms underlying these effects of acupuncture. While a growing understanding of the pathophysiology underlying several nervous system diseases shows it to be related to inflammation and impair cell regeneration after ischemic events, the relationship between the therapeutic mechanism of acupuncture and the p38 MAPK signal pathway has yet to be elucidated. This review discusses the latest advancements in the identification of the effect of acupuncture on the p38 signaling pathway in several nervous system diseases. We electronically searched databases including PubMed, Embase, and the Cochrane Library from their inception to April 2020, using the following keywords alone or in various combinations: "acupuncture", "p38 MAPK pathway", "signaling", "stress response", "inflammation", "immune", "pain", "analgesic", "cerebral ischemic injury", "epilepsy", "Alzheimer's disease", "Parkinson's disease", "dementia", "degenerative", and "homeostasis". Manual acupuncture and electroacupuncture confer positive therapeutic effects by regulating proinflammatory cytokines, ion channels, scaffold proteins, and transcription factors including TRPV1/4, Na_V, BDNF, and NADMR1; consequently, p38 regulates various phenomena including cell communication, remodeling, regeneration, and gene expression. In this review article, we found the most common acupoints for the relief of nervous system disorders including GV20, GV14, ST36, ST37, and LI4. Acupuncture exhibits dual regulatory functions of activating or inhibiting different p38 MAPK pathways, contributing to an overall improvement of clinical symptoms and function in several nervous system diseases.

Keywords: acupuncture; p38 signaling pathway; nervous system diseases

1. Introduction

Acupuncture is a form of therapy that has been practiced for more than 3000 years in Asia [1,2]. Medical doctors practice acupuncture under the guidance of meridian theory, which was first recorded in detail in The Yellow Emperor's Classic of Internal Medicine [2]. To perform acupuncture, doctors use thin and sterile metal needles to penetrate specific stimulation points termed acupoints, and they manipulate the needle to achieve "de qi" status [2]. Both manual and electroacupuncture (EA) are used in medical practice. Acupuncture is generally a safe, easy to perform, [3–5] and economical procedure that provides another choice for those who are concerned about the adverse effects of routine managements such as drug prescription [6,7]. Occasional minor problems, such as needles left in patients by mistake, headaches, and drowsiness have been reported after acupuncture treatment; usually, these symptoms are self-resolved after a short rest [1,3,6,7]. Due to the limited number of controlled clinical trials that have been published, the efficacy of acupuncture as treatment for has been questioned [8].

Acupuncture is widely used to treat various diseases and exerts positive effects, including analgesia, at both local and systemic levels [3,8–12]; it improves consciousness and cognition [13–20], and it induces therapeutic effects in several nervous system diseases [8,13–20]. Advanced molecular and clinical studies have continually attempted to decipher the mechanisms underlying these effects of acupuncture [2,7,16,17,20–72]. The signal transduction pathways through which acupuncture treats nervous system diseases involves multiple signal pathways, including p38 mitogen-activated protein kinases (p38 MAPKs) [7,33–39], Raf/MAPK/extracellular signal-regulated kinases (ERK) 1/2 [27–32,39], Toll-like receptor 4 (TLR4)/ERK [40–43,59], phosphatidylinositol-4,5-bisphosphate 3-kinase (PI3K)/protein kinase B (Akt) [26,31,38,49], adenyl cyclase (AC)/cyclic-adenosine mono-phosphate (cAMP)/protein kinase A (PKA) [25,31,44,47,50–52], apoptosis signal-regulating kinase 1 (ASK1)-c-Jun amino-terminal kinases (JNK)/p38 [7,33–39,44,47,48,63], and downstream cAMP response element-binding protein (CREB), JNK [7,24,54–61,63], mammalian target of rapamycin (mTOR) [26,44–46], nuclear factor kappa-light-chain-enhancer of activated B cells (NF-κB) [41–44,47,62], and B-cell lymphoma 2 (Bcl-2)/ Bcl-2 associated X (Bax) balance [57,63–69]. While a growing understanding of the pathophysiology underlying several nervous system diseases shows that it is related to inflammation and the impairment of cell regeneration, the relationship between the therapeutic mechanism of acupuncture and the p38 MAPK signal pathway has yet to be elucidated. A reverse of the detrimental effect of cerebral ischemic or hemorrhagic injury involves the modulation of the ERK/JNK/p38 signal pathway, which leads to anti-apoptosis of the affected brain area. Improvements of Alzheimer's disease, vascular dementia, and Parkinson's disease involves depression or inactivation of the p38 MAPK pathway [32,69–79]. The inactivation of interleukin (IL) 1 β (IL-1β)/p38 in the frontal lobe and hippocampus has a positive effect on improving cognition and memory. Moreover, acupuncture exerts analgesic effects through the interference of both the ascending and descending pain signaling pathway. These findings continue to shed light on the pivot role of the p38 signaling pathway in several nervous system diseases. The common signal transduction pathways through which acupuncture treats nervous system diseases are summarized in Figure 1.

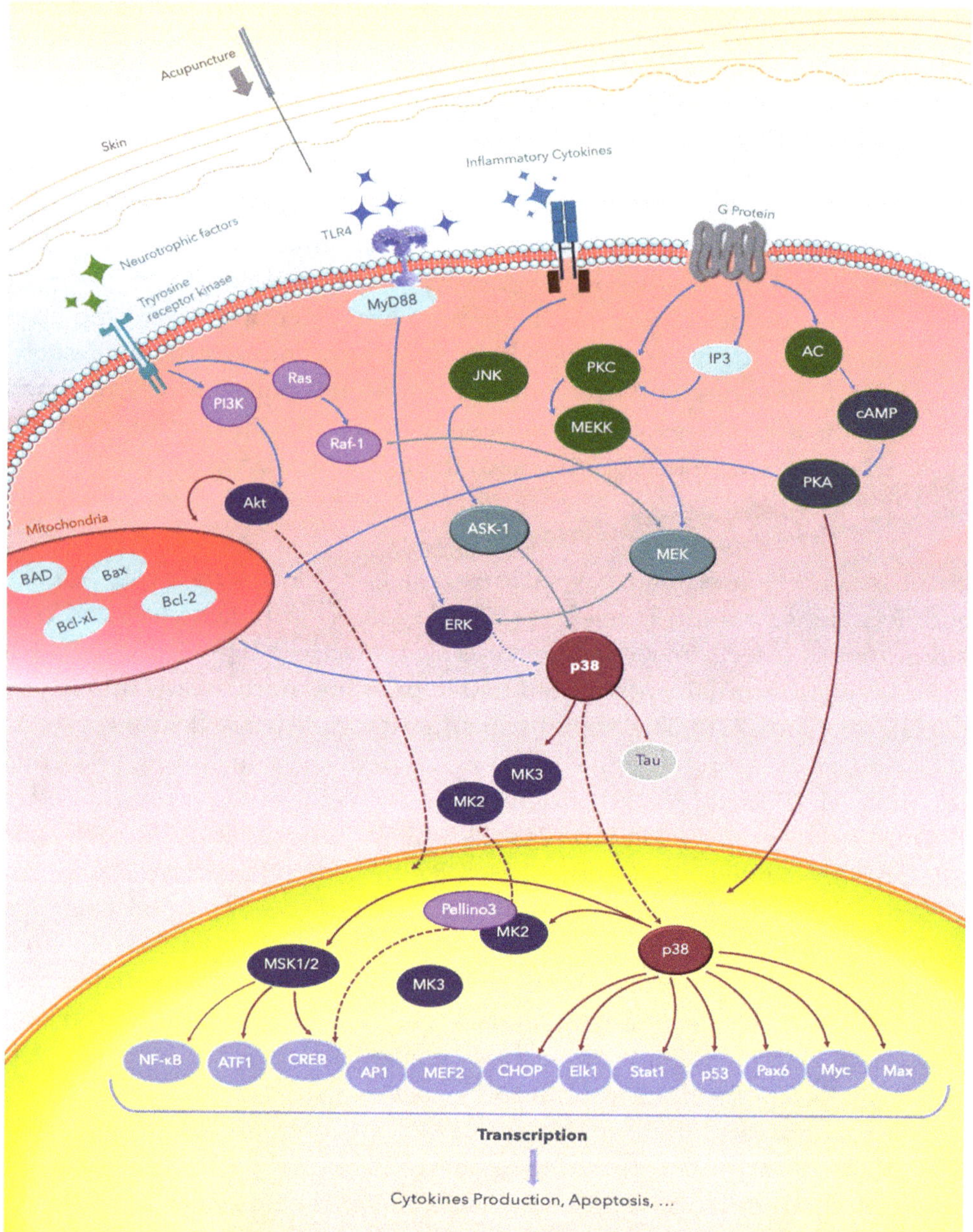

Figure 1. Summary of the signal transduction pathways through which acupuncture treats nervous system diseases. Acupuncture is applied on acupoints and results in de qi, evoking the excitation of cell membrane receptors, such as the Tyrosine receptor kinase and TLR/ligand, and subsequently producing signal transduction. AC: adenyl cyclase; Akt: protein kinase B; AMPK: AMP-activated protein kinase; ASK-1: apoptosis signal-regulating kinase 1; Bad: Bcl-2-associated death promoter; Bax: Bcl-2 associated X; Bcl-2: B-cell lymphoma 2; Bcl2-xl: B-cell lymphomaextralarge; cAMP: cyclic adenosine monophosphate; CREB: cAMP response element-binding protein; ERK: extracellular signal-regulated kinase; IP3: inositol triphosphate; JNK: c-Jun N-terminal kinases; Elk-1: erythroblast transformation specific (ETS) like-1 protein; Max: a transcription factor coded by the myc-associated factor X; MEF: myocyte-enhancing factor; MEK: MEK kinase; MEKK: MK kinase kinase; MSK: mitogen- and stress-activated protein kinase; Myc: a group of transcription factors coded by regulator genes and a proto-oncogene called Myc; MyD88: myeloid differentiation primary response 88; TLRs: Toll-like receptors; NF-κB: nuclear factor kappa B; Pax6: a paired-box protein encoded by the master gene Pax-6; PI3K: phosphatidylinositol-4,5-bisphosphate 3-kinase; PKA: protein kinase A; PKC: protein kinase C; ATF: activating transcription factor; AP-1: activator protein; CHOP: C/EBP homologous; Stat1: signal transducer and activator of transcription 1.

2. The p38 MAPKs

MAPKs are a large group of evolutionarily conserved proteins in the plant and animal kingdoms. MAPKs have been implicated in diverse cellular processes including cell survival, proliferation, differentiation, and migration.

Three major subfamilies of MAPK proteins have been defined: ERK, JNK, and the p38 MAPKs (Figure 2). The middle amino acid residue of the conserved Thr-Xxx-Tyr dual-phosphorylation domain (*dP-consensus*) designates a MAPK protein to its cognate subfamily, and the p38 MAPK subfamily bears the Thr-Gly-Tyr (TGY) dual-phosphorylation domain [77,78].

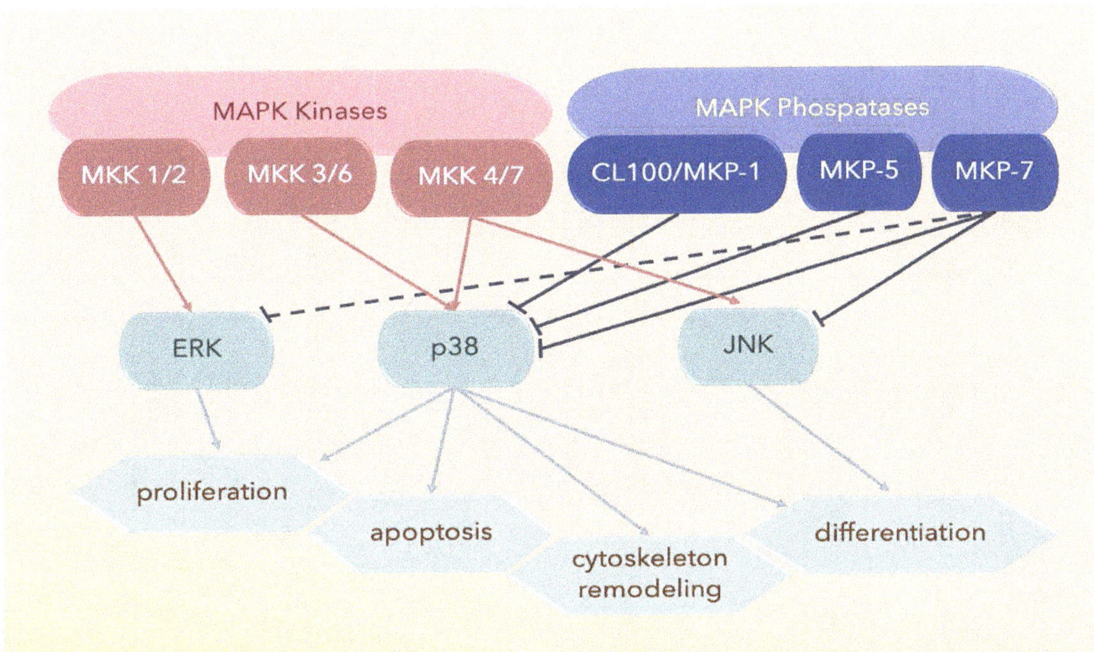

Figure 2. Three major subfamilies of mitogen-activated protein kinases (MAPKs) include extracellular signal-regulated kinases (ERKs), the c-Jun amino-terminal kinases (JNKs), and the p38 MAPKs. The solid lines ending with arrowheads denote activated proteins, solid lines with blunt ends denote deactivated proteins, and the dotted lines with blunt ends denote partially deactivated proteins.

The most extensively studied MAPK pathways are activated by dual-specificity serine-threonine/ tyrosine kinases (STK) termed MAPK kinases (MKKs, MAPKKs, or MAP2Ks), which are activated by MAPKK kinases (MAPKKKs or MAP3Ks). For the p38 MAPK pathway, MKK3 and MKK6 serve as MKKs, and the identified MAPKKKs include MAPKKK2, MAPKKK3, ASK-1, tumor progression locus-2 (Tpl2), and transforming growth factor-β-activated kinase 1 (TAK-1) of the non-canonical transforming growth factor-β (TGFβ) pathway. In general, ERK proteins are primarily activated by growth factors; JNKs are activated by stress-, differentiation-, and growth-related factors; and p38 is activated by stress-related factors [78–84].

The p38 MAPK family comprises p38α, p38β, p38γ, and p38δ (summarized in Table 1). Considering its central role in developmental programming, cellular adaptation to environmental stress, immune responses, inflammation, tissue regeneration, and tumorigenesis, this protein subfamily has gained increasing attention since its initial discovery. Recent studies using new genetic and pharmacological tools have provided essential information regarding the functions of p38 MAPKs in the pathogenesis of prevalent conditions associated with inflammation, diabetes, neurodegeneration, and cancer [78–99].

The subfamily p38α is reportedly a homolog of *Saccharomyces cerevisiae* Hog1, which is an important regulator of osmotic response [77,78,84,100–105]. Other p38 MAPK family members, sharing approximately 60% sequence similarity with p38α, were subsequently cloned and named p38β, p38γ, and p38δ [77,78,84,100–105].

Table 1. Members of the p38 mitogen-activated protein kinase (MAPK) subfamily.

p38 Subfamily	Other Names	Upstream	Location/Function	Dysfunction and Diseases
p38α	MAPK14, SAPK2a, CSBP	MKK3, MKK4, MKK6, MKK7	Ubiquitously expressed at significant levels in most cell types. Involved in the regulation of cell proliferation, differentiation, development, and response to stress [77,78,84,99].	Defective placental angiogenesis causing embryo death (mouse), symmetric synchronous cell cleavage (zebrafish), reduction in erythropoietin (Epo) production [99], leading to anemia, the impairment of glucogenesis (mice), and lipid-induced insulin-resistance (rat) [77,97].
p38β	MAPK 11	MKK3, MKK4, MKK6	Ubiquitously expressed; upregulated in the CNS and lungs, downregulated in the healthy heart [104–106].	No phenotype found [77].
p38γ	MAPK 13, ERK6, SAPK3 [1]	MKK3, MKK4, MKK6MKK7	Myoblast and skeletal muscle./ (1) Under stress conditions, they act on scaffold proteins targeting the plasma membrane cytoskeleton at sites of neuromuscular junctions and gap junctions [107]. (2) Recent studies indicate that the microbial metabolite imidazole propionate may contribute to the pathogenesis of type 2 diabetes via the activation of p38γ/p62/mTORC1 [89].	No phenotype found (mouse) [77]. Meiotic G2/M progression of oocytes (xenopus) [77,104,105].
p38δ	MAPK 12, SAPK4	MKK3, MKK4, MKK6, MKK7	Only expressed in the lungs, kidney, testis, spleen, pancreas, and small intestine in humans, rats, and mice, but not in other vertebrates; enriched in endocrine glands [107,108]./ (1) Regulates cytoplasmic microtubule dynamics, including tau protein [107]. (2) Upregulated in the liver in obese patients with NAFLD [89].	No phenotype found [77].

SAPK: stress-activated protein kinase; CNS: central nervous system; mTORC1: mammalian target of rapamycin complex 1 or mechanistic target of rapamycin complex 1; NAFLD: nonalcoholic fatty liver disease.

X-ray crystallographic studies have yielded structural insights into the mechanisms underlying the interaction between an MAPKK and an MAPK [103,107]. Both p38α and p38β are well-conserved at both the gene and protein levels and are important in eliciting innate immunity [77,78,84,101–105]. Some p38α and p38β physiological substrates are summarized in Figure 3; these include transcription factors, transcription factor kinases, cytoskeletal proteins, translational machinery components, and other proteins including metabolic enzymes, glycogen synthase, or cytosolic phospholipase A2 (cPLA2). The p38γ and p38δ MAPK isoforms can phosphorylate typical p38 MAPK substrates including transcription factors activating transcription factor 2 (ATF2), erythroblast transformation specific (ETS) like-1 protein (Elk-1), or stress-activated protein kinase (SAP1). However, they cannot phosphorylate MK2 or MK3, which are suitable substrates for the other two p38 MAPK isoforms [109–111].

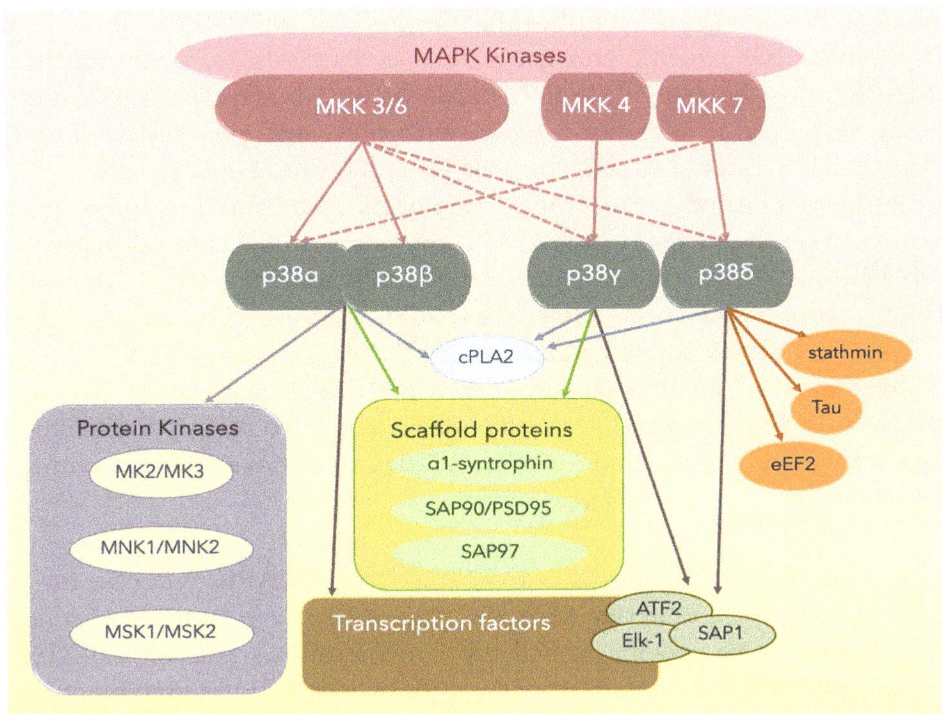

Figure 3. The four p38 MAPK isoforms are p38α, p38β, p38γ, and p38δ. Solid lines denote activated proteins, and dotted lines denote partially activated proteins. MNK: mitogen-activated protein kinase-interacting protein; MSK: mitogen- and stress-activated protein kinase; cPLA2: cytosolic phospholipase A2; ATF2: the activating transcription factor 2; Elk-1: the [erythroblast transformation specific (ETS)] like-1 protein; SAP1: stress-activated protein 1; PSD: postsynaptic density proteins; eEF2: eukaryotic elongation factor 2.

Of the MAPKs, p38γ has a unique short C-terminal sequence, KETXL, which is ideal for binding PDZ domains in proteins, thus accounting for the regulatory role of p38γ in the localization of cellular elements and interactions with cytoskeletal components. Under stress conditions, p38γ interacts with and activates various scaffold proteins including α1-syntrophin, SAP90/PSD95, and SAP97, which are generally targeted to the plasma membrane cytoskeleton at specialized sites, including the neuromuscular junction and gap junctions through protein–protein interactions [111].

With respect to p38δ, it potentially contributes to cytoskeletal regulation because it phosphorylates the cytoplasmic protein stathmin [110,111], which is a crucial regulator of microtubule dynamics and the cell cycle, by promoting the depolymerization of microtubules and/or preventing the polymerization of tubulin heterodimers [109,111]. Furthermore, eukaryotic elongation factor 2 (eEF2) kinase and microtubule-associated protein tau are substrates of p38δ [109,111]. The four p38 isoforms and the substrates are shown in Figure 3.

These four p38 MAPKs are encoded by different genes and display different histotypic expression patterns, with p38α being ubiquitously expressed at significant levels in most cell types, whereas the others potentially display more histotypic expression patterns. For example, p38β is expressed in the brain, p38γ is expressed in skeletal muscle (neuromuscular junction, gap junction), and p38δ is expressed in endocrine glands [108–115]. The genetic ablation of specific p38 MAPK family members has revealed functional redundancy in this protein subfamily. For example, the osmotic shock-induced phosphorylation of the stress-activated protein 97 (alternatively termed synapse-associated protein 97, SAP97; also known as discs large homolog 1 scaffold protein, hDLG1) is usually mediated by p38γ; however, in the absence of this kinase, other p38 MAPKs can perform this function.

3. MAPK Substrates, Signaling Pathways, and Functions

Nine members of the dual-specificity phosphatases specific for MAPKs, termed MKPs, have been reported. Each member has specific substrates, tissue distribution, and subcellular localization. For example, MAPK phosphatase 7 (MKP-7) binds to and inactivates p38α and p38β through dephosphorylation; however, it does not interact with p38γ and p38δ; MKP-5 and CL100/MKP-1 also bind to p38α and p38β, but not to p38γ or p38δ [115] (Figures 2 and 3).

Several studies have revealed a direct interaction of the N-terminal region of the MAPKK with a docking groove present on the surface of the MAPK distant from the catalytic active site. The second determinant of MAPKK specificity is the structure of the MAPK activation loop harboring the Thr-Xxx-Tyr dual-phosphorylation motif. The specificity of these interactions partly mediates the potential of an individual MAPKK to selectively activate a particular MAPK.

A recent study emphasized that dynamic changes are necessary for enzyme activity [116]. For instance, two MAPKs, ERK2 and p38, are differentially activated owing to differences in dynamism. A comparison of the dynamics of PKA and p38 revealed similarities in their dynamic properties.

3.1. *Dual Phosphorylation by MKKs*

In yeast, only a single MAPKK appears to activate each MAPK, whereas mammalian MAPK signaling modules include more than one MAPKK. The MAPKKs responsible for activating the p38 MAPK pathways appear to be specific to cell type and stimulus [105,107,114,116]. Brancho and Tanaka et al. investigated the mechanism underlying p38 activation in vivo by examining the effect of disruption of the murine *Mkk3*, *Mkk4*, and *Mkk6* genes on the p38 MAPK signaling pathway [100]; they found that Mkk3 and Mkk6 are essential for tumor necrosis factor (TNF)-mediated p38 activation. By contrast, ultraviolet (UV) radiation-induced p38 activation was mediated by Mkk3, Mkk4, and Mkk6. Furthermore, they reported that the role of Mkk4 in p38 MAPK activation in fibroblasts was largely redundant with those of Mkk3 and Mkk6. Mkk4 is a potentially important p38 MAPK activator in cells with low levels of Mkk3 and Mkk6. These data indicated that p38 MAPK was regulated by the coordinated and selective action of the three different protein kinases MKK3, MKK4, and MKK6 in response to cytokines and exposure to environmental stress. The inactivation of p38 MAPK was reportedly associated with defects in cell cycle arrest and increased tumorigenesis [117–123].

Several MAPKKKs have been implicated in the regulation of p38 MAPK signaling, including the mixed-lineage kinases (MLKs), apoptosis signal-regulating kinase 1 (ASK-1), TAK-1, and some members of the MAPK/ERK kinase kinase (MEKK) family. Low-molecular-weight guanosine-5′-triphosphate (GTP)-binding proteins of the Rho subfamily, including Ras-related C3 botulinum toxin substrate 1 (Rac1), the erythrocyte membrane glycoprotein Cd242, the nonlipid modified Ras-related protein (Rit), the transcription termination factor Rho, and heterotrimeric G-protein-coupled receptors (GPCRs) contribute to p38 activation upstream of MAPKKKs [124–135]. More recently, a new signaling pathway, different from TAK1, that involves the inhibitor of nuclear factor kappa-B kinase (IκBK), NFκB/p105, and Tpl2 stimulating MKK3/6, and downstream p38 was established in macrophages [135–139]. The p38 MAPK pathways are shown in Figure 4.

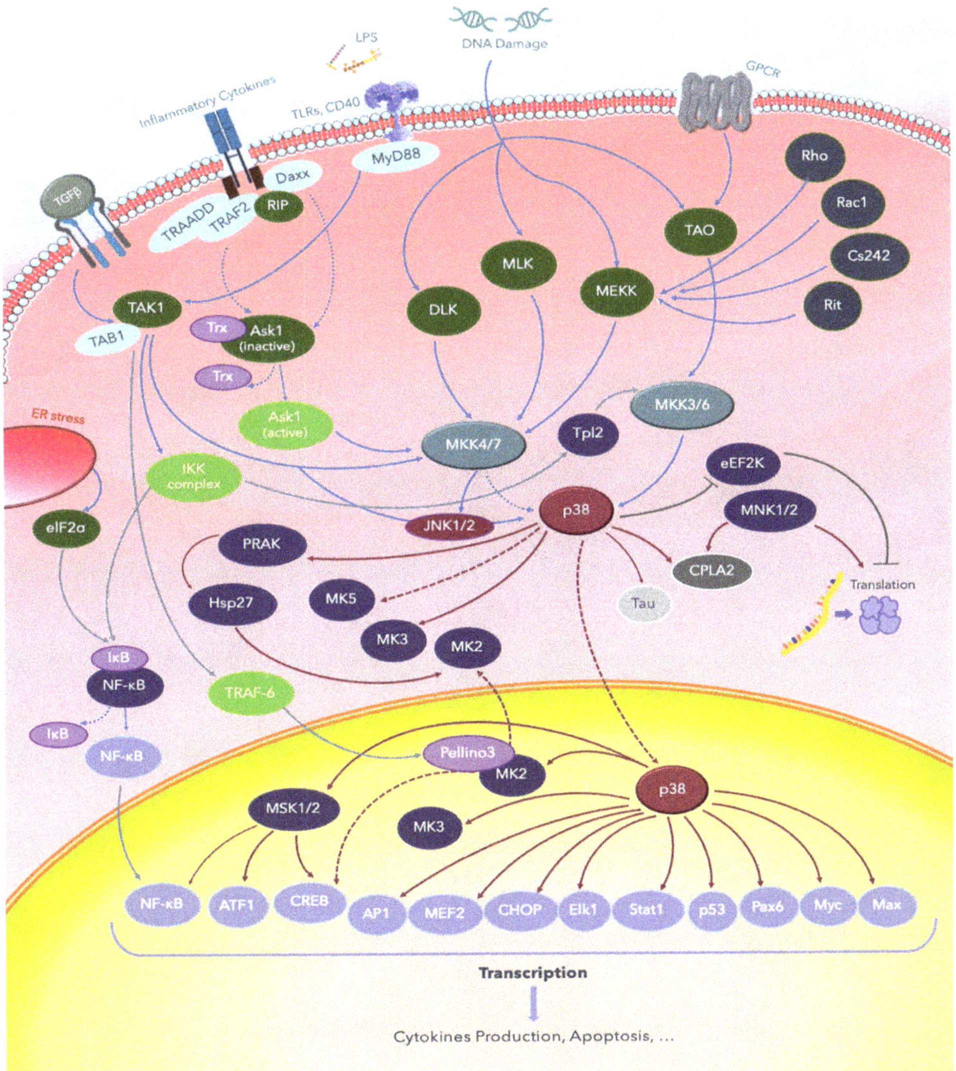

Figure 4. The p38 MAPK signaling pathways. Solid lines indicate signaling pathways and the proteins involved in them; dotted lines indicate the regulatory mechanisms reported in several studies, and lines with blunt ends indicate pathways inhibiting or deactivating downstream substrates. LPS: lipopolysaccharide; TGFβ: growth factor beta; TLRs: Toll-like receptors; CD40: cluster of differentiation 40 receptors; GPCRs: G-protein-coupled receptors; elF2a: eukaryotic translation initiation factor 2A; ER: endoplasmic reticulum; NF-κB: nuclear factor kappa B; TAB1: TGF-beta-activated kinase1; TRADD: tumor necrosis factor receptor type 1-associated DEATH domain protein; TRAF: tumor necrosis factor receptor (TNFR)-associated factor; Daxx: death domain-associated protein; RIP: receptor-interacting protein kinases; MyD88: myeloid differentiation primary response 88; PRAK: p38-regulated and -activated kinase; Hsp: heat shock proteins; DLK: dual leucine zipper kinase; MLK: mixed-lineage protein kinase; MEKK: MEKK kinase; MEK: MEK kinase; MKK: MK kinase; MNK: mitogen-activated protein kinase-interacting protein; TAO: thousand and one amino acids; eEF2K: eukaryotic elongation factor 2 kinase; cPLA2, cytosolic phospholipase A2; ATF: activating transcription factor; MSK: mitogen- and stress-activated protein kinase; CREB: cAMP response element–binding protein; AP-1: activator protein 1; MEF: myocyte enhancing factor; CHOP: C/EBP homologous protein, a member of the CCAAT/enhancer-binding proteins; Elk-1: erythroblast transformation specific (ETS) like-1 protein; Stat1: signal transducer and activator of transcription 1; Pax6: a paired-box protein encoded by the master gene Pax-6; Myc: a group of transcription factors coded by a regulator genes and proto-oncogene called Myc; Max: a transcription factor coded by the myc-associated factor X.

3.2. Autophosphorylation

MKK-independent activation is achieved through autophosphorylation and activation of p38α after interaction with TGFβ-activated kinase 1 (TAB1), which appears to activate p38α via the 5′ AMP-activated protein kinase (AMPK) in ischemic heart tissue (Figure 5). TAB1 sequesters p38α in the cytosol, thus potentially preventing some MKK-activated p38α functions. However, this mechanism does not contribute to p38 MAPK activation in fibroblasts or epithelial cells under the same conditions [134].

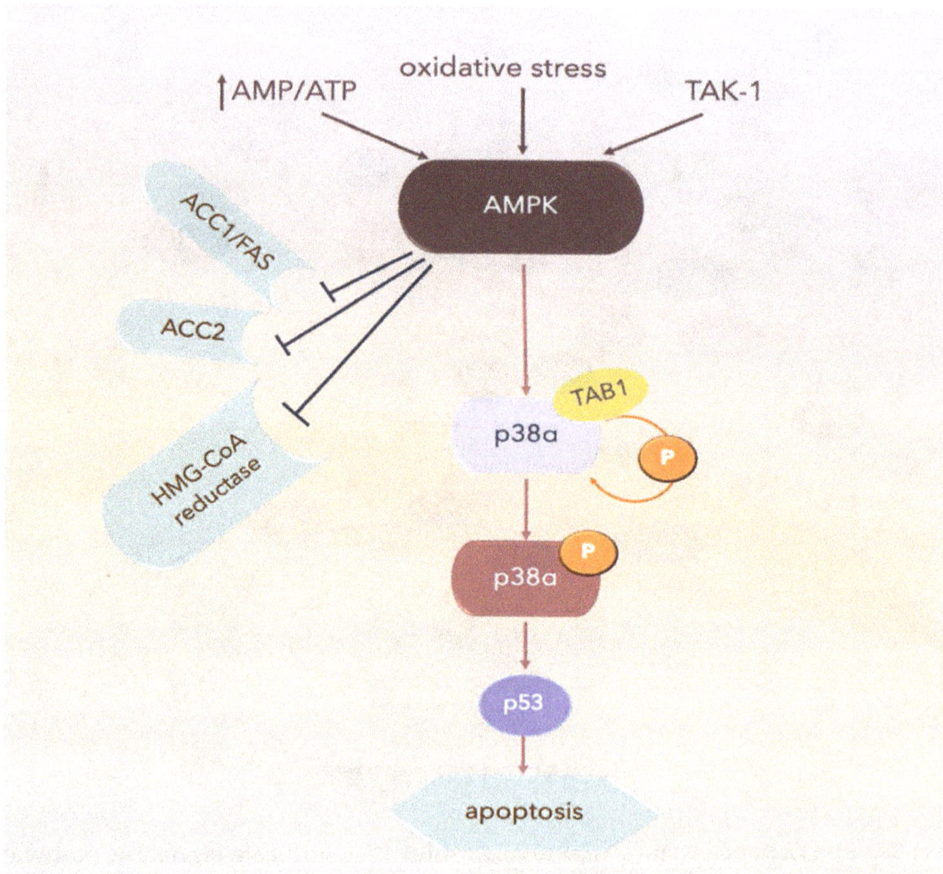

Figure 5. AMPK-activated-p38α pathways in ischemic heart tissue. Arrow: activated; TAK-1: transforming growth factor-β-activated kinase 1; AMPK: 5′ AMP-activated protein kinase; P: phospho-; AMP: adenosine mono-phosphate; ATP: adenosine tri-phosphate; AMP/ATP: AMP/ATP ratio; ACC1: Acetyl-CoA carboxylase 1; Fas signal pathway, Fas and Fas Ligand (FasL) regulate cell death; HMG-CoA reductase: a rate-controlling enzyme of the mevalonate pathway responsible for cholesterol and other isoprenoid biosynthesis.

Another MKK-independent mechanism underlying p38α activation has been observed in T-cell stimulation, wherein p38α is activated by T-cell antigen receptor (TCR)-mediated stimulation through p38α phosphorylation on a noncanonical activating residue, Tyr323. This activated p38α alters its structural conformation, phosphorylating third-party substrates and its TGY motif [115].

4. TRPV1 and the p38 Pathway

Transient receptor potential vanilloid receptors (TRPVs) are mechanosensitive channels highly associated with nervous system functions including pain, memory, and mechanical sensations. Furthermore, capsaicin receptor TRPV1 is a key regulator of pain and inflammation and is upregulated in microglia in the brain, especially in the anterior cingulate cortex [138–140]. The stimulation of microglial TRPV1 induces cortical microglial activation and indirectly enhances glutamatergic neuronal transmission by promoting the shedding of extracellular microglial microvesicles (release of vesicles in the extracellular space [141]). Moreover, in the cortex of mice with neuropathic pain, TRPV1 affects the intrinsic electrical properties of neurons and synaptic strength [142,143]. This signal transduction can be inhibited by the p38 MAPK inhibitor SB203580. Thus, p38 MAPK is a downstream TRPV1 activator whose phosphorylation plays an essential role in microglial microvesicle shedding by activating P2X purinoceptor 7 (P2X7) ATP receptor [138–143]. Whereas TRPV1 mediates communication between microglia and neurons, inhibition of the phosphorylation of its downstream p38 MAPK inhibits sphingosine metabolism [140–143].

Furthermore, several studies have examined biomarkers of nerve damage, including astrocytic marker glial fibrillary acidic protein (GFAP), microglial marker ionized calcium-binding adapter molecule 1 (Iba-1), S100 calcium-binding protein B (S100B), and the receptor for advanced glycation end-products (RAGE), revealing marked upregulation of these molecules in the dorsal root ganglion (DRG) and spinal cord dorsal horn (SCDH) of Complete Freund's adjuvant (CFA)-treated mice. This inflammatory effect was reversed through electroacupuncture, which achieved an equivalent result to that of TRV1 gene deletion [143].

5. Brain-Derived Neurotrophic Factor and p38 Pathways

Microglia cells are resident macrophages in the central nervous system (CNS) with a small soma with thin and branched processes. In the case of neural injury, their processes rapidly migrate toward the site of injury. In peripheral nerve injury, spinal cord microglia are activated. Spinal P2X4 receptors (P2X4Rs), phosphorylated p38 MAPK (p-p38-MAPK), and brain-derived neurotrophic factor (BDNF) are upregulated in spared nerve injury (SNI) rats [144]. BDNF signals to neurons in spinal lamina I and increases intracellular chloride concentration, thereby counteracting gamma-aminobutyric acid (GABA)- and glycine-mediated inhibition in these cells. The disinhibition unmasks innocuous inputs to lamina I neurons and facilitates their responses to noxious inputs [145]. In other studies, BDNF/TrkB was reported to promote inflammation in spinal cord injury through the p38 signaling pathway in the murine model [40,146]. Moreover, an upregulation of BDNF expression was observed in rats when applying electroacupuncture (EA) to acupoints GV20 and GV14, which later revealed that EA counteract caspase-3-dependent neuronal apoptosis by activating the Raf-1/MEK1/2/ERK1/2/p90RSK/Bad signaling pathway [147].

These results suggest that increasing the expression of BDNF synthesis, the downregulation of P2X4Rs, and the inhibition of p38 phosphorylation might account for the therapeutic effects induced by acupuncture in nerves injury.

6. Acupuncture and the Effects of Electric Fields on Nerve Regeneration

Previous in vitro and a few in vivo studies have reported positive nerve growth-promoting effects of electric fields where the cathode was placed toward the distal end of the injured nerve stumps [148–154]. Chen et al. reported that regenerated nerves in the electrical stimulation group may have a more mature ultrastructure compared with those in the control group [155]. Furthermore, they reported low regeneration success in patients receiving electrical stimulation relative to controls [155].

Together with several previous clinical studies [155–158], these studies show that patients with nerve anastomosis should not receive any electrical stimulation for rehabilitation until their reconnected nerve stumps have grown into a more mature stage of regeneration. One of the mechanisms underlying electroacupuncture (EA) is the relief of acute pain through the release of opiates to activate μ-, δ-, and κ-opioid receptors; furthermore, it can regulate persistent pain by activating μ- and δ-opioid receptors [25]. These findings explain the application of EA in treating neuropathic pain when pharmacotherapeutic approaches are ineffective.

Furthermore, the analgesic effect of low-frequency (2 Hz) EA is exerted on the noradrenergic descending pathway, involving the modulation of spinal GABAergic nerves ($GABA_A$). Administering EA at 2 Hz at acupoint ST36-37 reportedly relieved neuropathic pain through long-term depression (LTD) of the C-fiber [159]. This phenomenon could be blocked by N-methyl-D-aspartate (NMDA) and an opioid receptor antagonist. By contrast, high-frequency (100 Hz) EA induces long-term potentiation (LTP) of endogenous GABAergic ($GABA_B$) and the serotonergic inhibitory systems through modulation of μ-opioid and 5-hydroxytryptamine 1 (5-HT1) receptors [25,160]. Other studies have reported that delivering EA at acupoints GV14 and GV20 exerts neuroprotective effects by activating CREB, BDNF [161], and α7 nicotinic acetylcholine receptor (α7 nAChR) [162] while simultaneously reducing S100B-mediated neurotoxicity [163]. Moreover, EA at acupoint ST36 can evoke excitatory signals in either the peripheral nervous system or CNS in vivo [163].

7. Inflammatory and Neuropathic Pain

7.1. *Inflammatory Pain*

Protein kinase C (PKC) is rapidly activated by heat or bradykinin and translocates, assisted by scaffolding proteins, from intracellular compartments to the plasma membrane. In rat DRG, the TRPV1 signaling pathways involve the phosphatidylinositol 3-kinases (PI3K), PKC, and calmodulin-dependent protein kinase II (CaMKII) [143,163]. The p38α MAPK was first recognized for its role in inflammation where it regulates the biosynthesis of proinflammatory cytokines IL-1 and TNFα [77,78,98–105,115,164–169]. After noxious stimulation, activated p38 (phospho-p38) is increased in the spinal cord and DRG neurons and continues to propagate pain signaling by phosphorylating transcription factors and proinflammatory cytokines including TNF-α [168,169]. Inflammation is induced through the activation of these cytokines, followed by their interactions with their cognate receptors and via the small GTPases (e.g., Rac1 and CDC42), leading to p38 activation [169].

7.2. *Neuropathic Pain*

In contrast to physiological pain, pathological pain does not depend on the presence of tissue-damaging stimuli. Neuropathic pain can be agonizing, potentially persisting over long periods, and it is often resistant to known painkillers. Increasing evidence indicates that spinal microglia react and undergo a series of changes that directly influence the establishment of painful peripheral neuropathy [168–170]. After nerve damage, purinergic P2X4 receptors (nonselective cation channels activated by extracellular ATP) are upregulated in spinal microglia in a manner dependent on transcription factors interferon regulatory factor 8 and 5 (IRF8 and IRF5), both of which are expressed in microglia after peripheral nerve injury [171,172]. Furthermore, in spinal microglia, the response to extracellular stimuli results in signal transduction through intracellular signaling cascades involving p38 and ERK. Inhibition of the function or expression of these microglial molecules suppresses the aberrant excitability of dorsal horn neurons and neuropathic pain [172].

Since MAPKs significantly contribute to the development of hyperalgesia, the inhibition of any of the three pathways, namely the ERK, p38, and JNK pathways, can rescue inflammatory or neuropathic pain. Several studies have reported that 2- and 15-Hz EA can downregulate cerebral TRPV4 expression and attenuate chronic constriction injury (CCI)-induced neuropathic pain in an animal model [173–179]. Furthermore, Huang et al. reported that EA modulates both excitatory and inhibitory neurotransmitters to relieve neuropathic pain in the higher brain regions [175]. The hippocampus plays an integral role in the transition from acute to chronic pain in the limbic system by activating NMDA receptors and subsequently prolonging acute nociceptive stimuli that continue activating the descending pathways of pain (Figure 6).

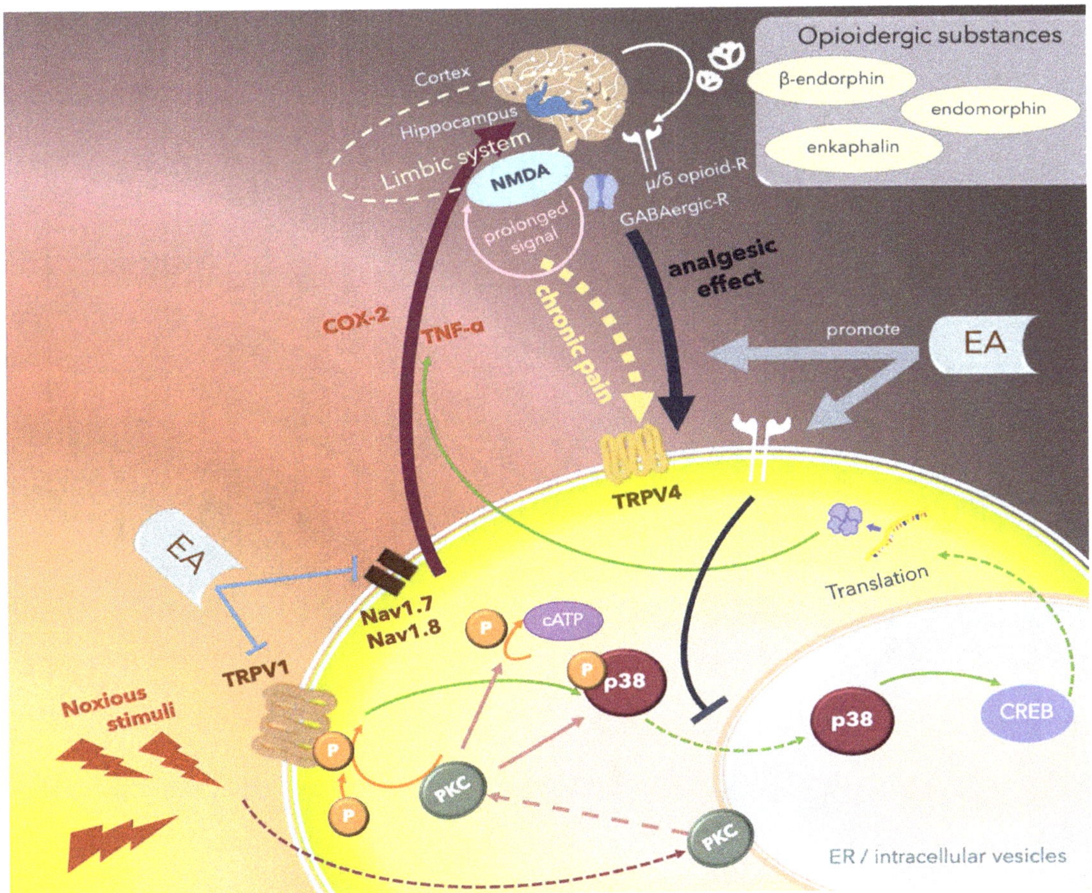

Figure 6. Schematic of the potential mechanism underlying the electroacupuncture (EA)-mediated analgesic effect. Noxious stimuli including heat or proinflammatory cytokines are transduced by the transient receptor potential vanilloid 1 (TRPV1) into the cells, thus phosphorylating and activating p38, which translocates from the cytosol to the nucleus and promotes transcription by affecting cAMP response element-binding protein (CREB), thus upregulating specific proteins including inflammatory cytokines or inducing apoptosis. These noxious stimuli can also directly activate protein kinase C (PKC). Nociception regulation by TRPV1 and $Na_V1.7/1.8$ receptor stimulation in the peripheral nerves propagates the signal through the ascending pathway and upregulates proinflammatory cytokines including cyclooxygenase-2 (COX-2) and tumor necrosis factor-α (TNFα) in the central nervous system, and the signal is then perceived as "pain". Chronic pain re-emerges when nociceptive signals cause prolonged stimulation through hippocampal N-methyl-D-aspartate receptor (NMDA) receptors and some other areas of the limbic system, and the signals are transmitted through the descending pathway, stimulating TRPV4 and triggering pain. Endogenic analgesic mechanisms involve the release of opioidergic substances that bind to γ-aminobutyric acidergic (GABAergic) receptors and μ- or δ-opioid receptors that act locally in the central nervous system and inhibit the descending pain pathway. EA exerts therapeutic effects by inhibiting the ascending pain pathway and intracellular p38-mediated inflammatory pathway by stimulating peripheral opioid receptors. Furthermore, EA promotes endogenic analgesic mechanisms, thus exerting immediate local analgesic effects and rescuing CNS-induced chronic pain.

7.3. Post-Operation Pain

Presurgical sham-, low-, and high-frequency EA treatments were reported to significantly reduce the postoperative patient-controlled analgesia morphine requirement; moreover, both low- and high-frequency EA decreased opioid-related side effects including nausea and dizziness throughout the first postoperative day [176,177]. Among these studies, ST36 and LI4 were the most frequent acupoints manipulated to achieve analgesic effects [summarized in Table 2].

Table 2. The effect of acupuncture on inflammatory and neuropathic pain.

Study	Model	Intervention	Acupoints	Evaluation	Result
Hsu et al., (2014) [173]	SD rats	CCI-induced neuropathic pain; EA, 2- and 15-Hz, 20 min	Ipsilateral ST36-ST37 of the affected limb	Behavioral responses to stimuli; expression of TRPV1/4 in the cerebral cortex and lumbar spinal cord	EA relieved neuropathic pain; downregulation of cerebral TRPV4 expression.
Jiang et al., (2018) [174]	SD rats	CCI-induced neuropathic pain; EA, 2- and 15-Hz, 20 min	Bilateral L4-L6 Hua Tuo Jia Ji (EX-B2)	$GABA_A$, A1R, TRPV1/4, and mGluR3 in the DRG	EA reduced the pain response, upregulating the $GABA_A$ receptor in the spinal cord.
Huang et al., (2019) [175]	SD rats	CCI-induced neuropathic pain; EA, 2-, 15- and 50-Hz, 20 min	GV20, GV14	Expression of the $GABA_A$ receptor and the level of glutamate in the hippocampus and periaqueductal gray (PAG) area.	EA reduced the pain response; suppressed hippocampal $GABA_A$ receptors; decreased thalamic glutamate levels.
Lin et al., (2002) [176]	Human	Preoperative EA, 2- (low) or 100- (high) Hz, 20 min	Bilateral ST36	Postoperative pain and opioid-related side effects	Both low- and high-frequency EA reduced postoperative analgesic requirements and associated side effects.
Wang et al., (1997) [177]	Human	Postoperative TAES, 2- (low) or 100- (high) Hz, 30 min	Bilateral LI4	Postoperative pain and opioid-related side effects	Both low- and high-frequency EA reduced postoperative analgesic requirements and associated side effects.
Chen et al. (2011) [178]	CD1 mice	EA, 2-Hz, 20 min	Bilateral ST36	Behavioral responses in the paw and ASIC3 overexpression in DRG neurons.	Rescued mechanical hyperalgesia and an ASIC3 downregulation.
Chen et al. (2012) [179]	ICR mice	EA, 2-Hz, 15 min	Bilateral ST36	Behavioral responses in the paw and TRPV1/4 overexpression in DRG neurons.	TRPV1 and TRPV4 upregulation in DRG neurons was attenuated by EA.
Huang et al. (2013) [180]	ICR mice	EA, 2-Hz, 15 min	Bilateral ST36	Behavioral responses in the paw and the overexpression of Na_V1 in DRG neurons.	EA attenuated inflammatory pain by suppressing Na_V1 overexpression.
Wu et al. (2014) [181]	ICR mice	MA, 60 min	Ipsilateral ST36 of the inflamed limb	Behavioral responses in paw; the overexpression of TRPV1/4, ASIC3, and CWP components in the anatomical layers of ST36.	MA induced analgesia, with high TRPV1 and CWP overexpression at ST36 upon MA.

Table 2. *Cont.*

Study	Model	Intervention	Acupoints	Evaluation	Result
Lu et al. (2016) [182]	C57/B6 mice	EA, 2-Hz, 15 min	Ipsilateral and contralateral ST36-ST37 of the inflamed limb	Behavioral responses in the paw; Na_V and TRPV1 overexpression in DRG neurons.	Hyperalgesia was suppressed through ipsilateral and contralateral EA. Na_V and TRPV1 were suppressed through EA.
Liao et al. (2017) [143]	C57/B6 mice	EA, 2-Hz, 15 min	Bilateral ST36	Behavioral responses in the paw and the expression of Na_V, GFAP, Iba-1, S100B, RAGE, and TRPV1 in DRG neurons.	EA attenuated inflammatory pain by suppressing Nav1.8 through S100B, TRPV1, opioid, and adenosine pathways.
Liao et al. (2017) [183]	C57/B6 mice	EA, 2-Hz, 15 min	Bilateral ST36	Behavioral responses in the paw and the expression of GFAP, S100B, RAGE, PKCε, ERK, NF-κB, and COX-2 in DRG neurons.	EA attenuated inflammatory pain by suppressing opioid and adenosine pathways.
Yang et al. (2017) [184]	C57/B6 mice	EA, 2-Hz, 15 min	Bilateral ST36	Behavioral responses in the paw and the expression of TRPV1, PKA, PKC, PI3K, ERK1/2, p38, JNK, Akt, mTOR, CREB, NF-κB, Na_V1.7/1.8, GFAP, S100B, and RAGE in DRG neurons.	EA significantly reduced chronic inflammatory pain by downregulating the TRPV1 pathway from the peripheral DRG neurons to the central spinal cord.
Yen et al. (2019) [185]	C57/B6 mice	EA, 2-Hz, 15 min	Bilateral LI4	Behavioral responses in the paw and the expression of TRPV1 and ERK1/2 in the prefrontal cortex, the hypothalamus, the PAG area, and DRG neurons.	Pain alleviation immediately after EA; the expression of TRPV1-associated molecules was attenuated by EA in the prefrontal cortex, the hypothalamus, the PAG area, and DRG.
Hsu et al. (2019) [186]	C57/B6 mice	EA, 2-Hz, 15 min	Bilateral ST36	Behavioral responses in the paw and the expression of TLR2, PI3K, ERK1/2, p38, JNK, Akt, mTOR, CREB, NF-κB, and Na_V1.7/1.8 in the thalamus.	EA attenuated inflammatory pain via TLR2 signaling.

Table 2. *Cont.*

Study	Model	Intervention	Acupoints	Evaluation	Result
Yang et al. (2009) [187]	Patients with CTS	MA, 30 min/session, 2 session a week, 8 session in total	Affected side(s), PC6, PC7	Motor and sensory NCS; designed symptomatic questionnaire.	Short-term acupuncture was as effective as short-term low-dose steroid for mild-to-moderate CTS.
Yang et al. (2011) [188]	Patients with CTS	MA, 30 min/session, 2 session a week, 8 session in total	Affected side(s), PC6, PC7	NCS; global symptom score.	Acupuncture had superior efficacy to steroid treatment not only in terms of objective changes in nerve conduction but also in terms of subjective symptom assessment in long-term follow-up.
Yang et al. (2011) [189]	Patients with chronic migraine (CM)	MA, 30 min/session, 2 session a week, 24 session in total	Bilateral BL2, GB20, EX-HN5, EX-HN3 (acupoints relate to the trigeminal and cervical dermatomes)	Changes in headache events, MIDAS scores, HADS scores, BDI-II scores, reduction of medication.	Acupuncture was similarly effective or more effective than prophylactic drug treatment with less side effects in migraine.

A1R: adenosine A1 receptor; ASIC3: acid-sensing ion channel; BDI-II: Beck Depression Inventory-II; CCI: chronic constriction injury; CWP components: components of calcium wave propagation, including pannexin 1, connexin 43, P2Y1, and P2Y2, which can activate a release of ATP after mechanical stimulation of nonneural cells such as subepithelial fibroblasts; $GABA_A$: γ-aminobutyric acid A; GFAP: glial fibrillary acidic protein, an astrocytic marker; HADS: hospital anxiety and depression scale; Iba-1: ionized calcium-binding adaptor molecule 1, a microglia/macrophage specific protein (marker); MA: manual acupuncture; MIDAS: Migraine Disability Assessment; mGluR3: metabotropic glutamate receptor 3; Na_Vs: voltage-gated sodium channels; NCS: nerve conduction study; RAGE: receptor for advanced glycation end-products; TAES: transcutaneous acupoint electrical stimulation; 100B: calcium-binding protein B.

Furthermore, overexpression of the voltage-gated sodium channel (Na_V), TRPV1, and acid-sensing ion channel 3 (ASIC3) in DRG neurons in response to proinflammatory cytokines is a key component of inflammatory pain [179–192]. Low-frequency (2-Hz) EA at acupoint ST36 can reduce inflammatory pain by attenuating ASIC3 overexpression in peripheral DRG neurons. ASIC3 downregulation potentially prolongs the clinical benefits of EA. Goldman et al. reported that acupuncture stimulates adenosine A1 receptor and induces adenosine release, thus relieving inflammation and neuropathic pain, which was not observed in mice lacking adenosine A1 receptors [193]. These results suggest that the opioid and adenosine pathways potentially contribute to analgesia in both manual acupuncture and EA.

7.4. Migraine

Migraine is a complex disorder; each episode begins with prodromes and aura (transient focal neurological symptoms). The origin of recurrent headache accompanied by visual or sensory symptoms is speculated to involve the hypothalamus, brain stem, and cortex. Current theories suggest that migraine is a neurovascular disorder involving cortical spreading depression, neurogenic inflammation, and vasodilation [194,195]. Owing to the disease itself or its genetic underpinnings, the brains of individuals who experience migraine are altered structurally and functionally; these molecular, anatomical, and functional abnormalities provide a neuronal substrate for extreme sensitivity to fluctuations in homeostasis, decreased adaptability, and recurrent headaches [194].

A randomized controlled trial investigated the efficacy and tolerability of acupuncture in comparison with topiramate treatment in chronic migraine prophylaxis. The effectiveness of acupuncture was similar to or greater than that of prophylactic pharmacotherapy, with fewer side effects in migraine [194]. The selected acupoints were bilateral BL2, GB20, EX-HN5, and EX-HN3, which are all associated with the trigeminal and cervical dermatomes. Although different combinations of peripheral effects, spinal/supraspinal mechanisms, and cortical and psychological mechanisms potentially contribute to the clinical effects of acupuncture, several other studies have reported that acupuncture potentially exerts curative effects not only through local analgesia but also through anti-inflammation, neuropeptide regulation, cytoskeleton remodeling, cell repair, and improvement in overall homeostasis.

7.5. Transcutaneous Electrical Nerve Stimulation Versus EA

The difference between transcutaneous electrical nerve stimulation (TENS) and EA is that TENS involves the application of the cathode at the affected area rather than at acupoints. Furthermore, TENS is used to reduce mechanical hyperalgesia in knee joint inflammatory pain [196,197], although its effectiveness is only sustained for a short time (several days) [198,199]. The analgesic effect of low-frequency TENS and EA can be attenuated using μ-opioid receptor blockers, thus indicating the involvement of peripheral opiate release in the underlying mechanism [196]; furthermore, the blockade of β-endorphin and corticotropin-releasing factor also reduces EA-induced analgesia.

7.6. Hypothesis Regarding the Long-Term Effect of Acupuncture

Although proinflammatory cytokines are regulated at different levels, the role of the p38α MAPK pathway in posttranscriptional regulation has received increasing attention. Numerous p38 MAPK–regulated mRNAs often contain an adenylate-uridylate-rich element (termed AU-rich element or ARE) in the 3′ untranslated region (3′UTR) [200,201]. The regulation of mRNA stability is particularly important for the expression of proteins involved in inflammatory response. These elements target mRNAs for rapid decay. The decay of ARE-containing reporter mRNAs is blocked upon p38 MAPK activation. Numerous ARE-containing endogenous mRNAs of inflammatory proteins are destabilized upon p38 inhibition. Some studies have reported a common mechanism underlying gene regulation via the p38α MAPK pathway for posttranscriptional regulation by the ARE.

These results are consistent with those of several previous animal and clinical studies reporting that EA improves analgesia during the acute phase posttraumatic healing and pain after major surgery [176,177]. Numerous prospective randomized controlled trials on carpal tunnel syndrome (CTS) have reported that acupuncture at acupoints PC7 and PC6 is as effective and safe as steroid treatment of mild-to-moderate CTS, both in the acute phase and throughout the 1-year follow-up period [187,188]. Based on the analgesic mechanisms of acupuncture and EA, which attenuate the p–p38 signaling pathway, the long-term effect of acupuncture or EA may result from neural modulation through posttranscriptional regulation. The potential mechanism underlying EA-mediated analgesic effects is depicted in Figure 6. The underlying mechanisms and the primary results of these studies are summarized in Table 2.

8. Cerebral Ischemia

During a cerebral ischemia (CI) event, hypoxia is induced in the brain, followed by the upregulation of various cytokines and potentially neurotoxic molecules. Nitric oxide reportedly influences cerebral oxygen vasoreactivity during severe hypoxia [202]. Both manual acupuncture and EA can increase cerebral blood flow [13,14]. Furthermore, 2- and 15-Hz EA at acupoint ST36 increased cerebral blood fluid (CBF) in rats with and without CI [14]. Per the traditional Chinese medicine theory, the Governor Vessel (or the Governor Meridian) directly communicates with the brain. In a previous study, EA at acupoints GV20 and GV14 before artificial mild cerebral ischemia–reperfusion (I/R) injury in an animal model exerted a neuroprotective effect against reperfusion injury [165]. Another neuroprotective mechanism of EA involves the downregulation of astrocytic S100B, which in turn deactivates p38 MAPK and its downstream substrate NF-κB. These effects subsequently reduce oxidative/nitrative stress and inhibit the TNF-α/tumor necrosis factor receptor type 1-associated DEATH domain protein (TRADD)/ Fas-associated protein with death domain (FADD)/cleaved caspase-8/cleaved caspase-3 apoptotic pathway in the ischemic cortical penumbra after reperfusion [89,201–207]. Both 5- and 25-Hz EA at acupoints GV20 and GV16 effectively downregulated reactive astrocytosis to exert neuroprotective effects against cerebral infarction-induced neuronal apoptosis, probably by activating the p38 MAPK/CREB signaling pathway [203].

Heat shock proteins (Hsp) significantly contribute to cellular regenerative processes in injured tissues because Hsp is upregulated during stem cell differentiation; however, the depletion or inhibition of Hsp70/Hsc70 impairs this process [206]. Hsp27 and Hsp70 reportedly contribute to intracellular protein repair after acute CI [206–211]. The dual phosphorylation of p38 MAPK was increased through early ischemia in an in vitro study wherein Hsp27 served as a terminal substrate of the p38 MAPK cascade. A later study indicated that among the p38 MAPKs, p38γ is the principal isoform responsible for the phosphorylation of HSF1 at Ser326 (S326) in cells (phosphorylation at S326 is a hallmark for HSF1 activation) [212], thus contributing to mitotic progression. A protease–mass spectrometry approach unexpectedly revealed that p38 MAPK also catalyzes the phosphorylation of HSF1 at S303/307, which is a repressive posttranslational modification [212,213]. Hsp70 bound MK2 to regulate MK2–p38MAPK interaction in the stem cells, and the essential regions required for Hsp70–MK2 interaction have been identified [206,209–213]. Taken together, Hsp can regulate cell differentiation by interacting with MK2 to stabilize p38 MAPK.

Another study administered 2 Hz EA the GV20 and ST36 acupoints in rat models of cerebral I/R injury and observed lowered peak levels of adrenocorticotrophic hormone and HSP70, suggesting that EA may inhibit excessive stress, reduce inflammation, and promote neural repair, thus facilitating healing in ischemic stroke [211]. The mechanisms and main results of the identified articles are summarized in Table 3.

Table 3. The p38 signaling pathway in cerebral ischemic stroke.

Study	Model	Intervention	Acupoints	Evaluation	Result
Bäcker et al., (2003) [13]	Healthy human	MA; manipulation as either high frequency (4–8 Hz) and low amplitude (Hf–La) or low frequency (1–2 Hz) and high amplitude (Lf–Ha).	Right LI4	Cerebral blood flow velocity (CBFV) in both middle cerebral arteries, arterial blood pressure (BP), heart rate (HR).	(1) Lf–Ha stimulation was perceived as more intense and markedly increased the CBFV in the right hemisphere; (2) Hf–La stimulation slightly decreased BP and HR; (3) Lf–Ha stimulation induced an initial pressor response (increase of BP, decrease of HR) and a more marked long-term BP reduction.
Hsieh et al., (2006) [14]	SD rats	EA, 2-Hz, 15 min	Both ST36	The levels of nitric oxide in the peripheral blood and amounts of calcitonin gene-related peptide (CGRP) in the cerebral cortex and thalamus. L-N (G)-nitro arginine methyl ester (L-NAME) was used to measure the changes in CBF.	Both 2- and 15-Hz EA increased CBF in rats with and without CI.
Cheng et al. (2014) [147]	SD rats	EA, 2-Hz, 25 min once daily for 2 consecutive days.	GV20, GV14	Cerebral infarct area, caspase-3, BDNF, pRaf-1, MEK1/2, ERK1/2, p90RSK, and Bad.	EA significantly reduced the cerebral infarct area, caspase-3 protein expression levels, and apoptosis in the ischemic cortex. BDNF, phospho-Raf-1 (pRaf-1), phospho-MEK1/2 (pMEK1/2), phospho-ERK1/2 (pERK1/2), phospho-90 kDa ribosomal S6 kinase (pp90RSK), and phospho-Bad (pBad) were markedly upregulated, and neuronal nuclear antigen (NeuN) expression was restored.
Cheng et al. (2014) [161]	SD rats	EA, 2-Hz, 15 min once daily for 6 consecutive days.	GV20, GV14	Cerebral infarct area, GFAP, S100B, NF-κB, p50, p38 MAPK, TNF-α, and iNOS.	EA significantly reduced the cerebral infarct area and downregulated astrocytic S100B expression and decreased p-p38 NF-kB.

Table 3. *Cont.*

Study	Model	Intervention	Acupoints	Evaluation	Result
Cheng et al. (2015) [203]	SD rats	EA, 5- or 25-Hz, 30 min once daily for 7 consecutive days.	GV20, GV16	Cerebral infarct area, GFAP, Bax, Bcl-xL, Smac/DIABLO, p-p38, and CREB.	Both 5- and 25-Hz EA effectively downregulated reactive astrocytosis to exert neuroprotective effects against cerebral infarction, most likely by activating the p38 MAPK/CREB signaling pathway.
Xu et al. (2014) [208]	SD rats	EA, 2-Hz, 20 min once a day.	GV20, ST36	Hsp70 and TNF-α peripheral serum.	Lowered peak levels of adrenocorticotrophic hormone and Hsp70.
Kuo et al. (2016) [15]	SD rats	Electrostimulation, 2-Hz, 20 min once daily for 7 consecutive days.	Both ears	Brain nicotinic acetylcholine receptors.	Two-hertz ES for ameliorated learning and memory impairment.

GFAP: glial fibrillary acidic protein; iNOS: inducible nitric oxide synthase; MA: manual acupuncture; Smac/DIABLO: second mitochondrial-derived activator of caspase/direct inhibitor of apoptosis protein-binding protein with low isoelectric point.

9. Epilepsy and Seizure

Epilepsy is characterized by an abnormal electric discharge of the brain, especially in the hippocampus. Epilepsy is usually associated with neuronal loss, astrocyte proliferation, mossy fiber sprouting, and synaptic reorganization in the hippocampus [40,214–219]. Pharmacological treatment approaches, including those employing Western medicine and Chinese herbal medicine, have been attempted to treat or prevent the harmful effect of seizures. For example, *Uncaria rhynchophylla* is a herb used in traditional Chinese medicine for epilepsy management; its therapeutic effect was reportedly associated with attenuated mossy fiber sprouting, astrocyte proliferation, S100B protein overexpression, and increased hippocampal neuronal survival [219].

Acupuncture has been applied for clinically managing epilepsy. Previous studies have reported that auricular acupuncture positively influences drug-resistant epilepsy patients, potentially through vagus nerve stimulation, attenuating the hyperactive hippocampus, regulating inflammatory cytokine pathways, protecting the hippocampus from apoptosis, and ameliorating the sprouting of mossy fibers in the hippocampus [40,218,220,221]. Several antiepileptic mechanisms have been proposed, including the downregulation of JNK or ERK1/2 and pro-inflammatory factors (IL-1β, IL-6, TNF-α) in the cerebral cortex and hippocampus [216]. Another study suggested that auricular EA and EA at ST36-ST37 achieved therapeutic effects by reducing hippocampal hyperactivity and the transient receptor potential cation channel subfamily A member 1 (TRPA1), PKCε, PKCα, and pERK1/2 signaling pathways [40]. Moreover, auricular EA with EA at ST36–ST37 exerted long-term (6-week observation in the study) beneficial effects by reducing the anti-inflammatory response in numerous cyclooxygenase-2 (COX-2) immunoreactive cells and hippocampal COX-2 levels [218].

Acupuncture exerts antiepileptic effects by inducing anatomical changes and changes in neurotransmitter, inflammatory cytokine, and transcription factor levels. Regarding studies to date, the related mechanisms primarily involve the suppression of TRPA1/pERK and TLR4/ERK pathways and activation of the PI3K/Akt pathway. Although some studies have reported the inactivation of the TLR4 pathway, accompanied by a reduction in pCaMKIIα, pERK, pp38, pJNK, and pNFκB levels [40], the role of p38 and its association with the aforementioned signaling pathways remain unclear. These mechanisms and the primary results of the aforementioned studies are summarized in Table 4.

Table 4. The effect of acupuncture on epileptic seizures.

Study	Model	Intervention	Acupoints	Evaluation	Result
Kim et al., (2008) [215]	ICR mice	MA, 20 min/day, for 2 days	Bilateral HT8	Hippocampal expression of c-Fos, c-Jun, and GAD-67 (CA1 and CA3 areas).	Reduced severity of epileptic seizures and the rate of neuronal death; downregulation of c-Fos and c-Jun; upregulation of GAD-67.
Kim et al. (2012) [216]	C57BL/6 mice	MA, 20 min/day, for 2 days	Bilateral HT8	Neuronal survival, microglial and astrocyte activation, and hippocampal mRNA expression of IL-1β and TNF-α.	Inhibition of hippocampal cell death and suppression of KA-induced inflammatory events.
Bae et al. (2013) [217]	C57BL/6 mice	MA, 20 min/day, for 3 days	Bilateral HT8	Neuronal survival and hippocampal astrocyte activation.	Acupuncture altered hippocampal protein expression to promote neuronal survival.
Liu et al. (2014) [218]	SD rats	EA, 2 Hz, 30 min/day for 7 consecutive days.	Bilateral ST-36-ST37 and ears	Changes in mossy fibers sprouting in the hippocampus.	Amelioration of mossy fibers sprouting in the hippocampus.

Table 4. *Cont.*

Study	Model	Intervention	Acupoints	Evaluation	Result
Lin et al., (2014) [220]	SD rats	EA, 2 Hz, 20 min/day, 3 days/week for 6 weeks	Bilateral ears, ST36, ST37	EEG and EMG changes; hippocampal TRPA1, TRPV4, PKCα, PKCε, and pERK1/2 expression.	EA reduced hippocampal hyperactivity accompanied by alterations in the TRPA1, PKCε, PKCα, and pERK1/2 signaling pathways.
Liao et al., (2017) [221]	SD rats	EA, 2 Hz, 20 min/day, 3 days/week for 6 weeks	Bilateral ears, ST36, ST37	EEG and EMG changes; hippocampal COX-2 levels.	Attenuated COX-2 and COX-2 immunoreactive cells in the hippocampal CA1 region after epileptic seizures.
Liao et al. (2018) [40]	SD rats	EA, 2 Hz, 20 min/day, 3 days/week for 6 weeks	Bilateral ears	Brain TLR4, CaMKIIα, ERK, JNK, and NF-κB expression.	Auricular EA controlled epileptic seizures by regulating the TLR4 signaling pathway.

GAD-67: glutamate decarboxylase-67; c-Fos, c-Jun: proto-oncogenes that are expressed within some neurons following depolarization, the two form the AP-1 early response transcription factor that regulates gene expression in response to extracellular stimuli; KA: kainic acid; EEG: electroencephalogram; EMG: electromyogram; PKC: protein kinase C; TRPA1: transient receptor potential cation channel subfamily A member 1; TRPV: transient receptor potential vanilloid receptors; pERK: phosphor-extracellular signal-regulated kinases; COX-2: cyclooxygenase-2; TLR4: Toll-like receptor 4; CaMKIIα: calmodulin-dependent protein kinase II alpha.

10. Motion Sickness

External noxious stimulation alters intracellular signal transduction pathways in primary afferents, potentially contributing to pain hypersensitivity. This pathway proceeds via TRPVs, especially TRPV1 and TRPV4, leading to the rapid phosphorylation of p38 MAPK in the afferent neurons and the induction of hyperalgesia. Recent studies have revealed that thermal stimulation may not be the only trigger for TRPV activation [222,223]. Kaolin consumption was quantified as a behavioral response of an emetic reflex (pica behavior) in a murine model. A previous study reported that TRPV1 levels were significantly increased upon stimulation of motion sickness, and EA at PC6 acupoints attenuated hypothalamic TRPV1 levels and exerted an antiemetic effect [222]. The acupoint PC6 is well-known for its therapeutic effect, especially in relieving nausea and vomiting. This study revealed that the mechanism underlying the reduction of motion sickness potentially involves the TRPV1 pathway [222].

11. Degenerative Nerve Diseases

Microglia, the endogenous macrophages of the CNS, monitor their territory through a constant movement of their elaborated thin processes and responses to local stressors and immune disruptions. Clinical studies and preclinical animal models have implicated the dysregulation and overproduction of proinflammatory cytokines from activated microglia in the CNS as contributors to the pathophysiology of chronic neurodegenerative disorders including Alzheimer's disease [16], Parkinson's disease, and multiple sclerosis and acute neurodegenerative conditions including traumatic brain injury and stroke. The p38α MAPK pathway helps increase the microglial production of proinflammatory cytokines induced by diverse stressors [16,17,223]. These results indicate the feasibility of targeting p38α MAPK to modulate the production of pro-inflammatory cytokines by the CNS.

Few studies have focused on the effects of androgens on neuroinflammation. Yang et al. investigated the neuroprotective role of androgens (including testosterone and its metabolite dihydrotestosterone, DHT) in lipopolysaccharide (LPS)-induced neuroinflammation, neuronal damage, and behavioral dysfunction [18]. DHT potentially inhibits the LPS-induced release of proinflammatory factors in primary microglia by suppressing the TLR4-mediated NF-κB and p38 signaling pathways, thus protecting neurons from inflammatory damage induced by activated microglia.

Sodium ferulate is used in traditional Chinese medicine (such as the root of *Ligusticum chuanxiong* and *Angelica sinensis*) and is speculated to help treat cardiovascular and cerebrovascular diseases by preventing thrombosis. Furthermore, sodium ferulate prevents Aβ-induced MKK3/MKK6-p38-Hsp27 signaling and reduces apoptosis in the rat hippocampus [17].

11.1. Alzheimer's Disease

The pathological hallmarks of Alzheimer's disease (AD) are the accumulation of extracellular plaques and intracellular neurofibrillary tangles that are composed of filaments of β-amyloid polymers and the neuronal microtubule-associated protein Tau, respectively. Elevated β-amyloid levels in an AD brain are speculated to induce microglial activation and the consequent release of proinflammatory cytokines induced by the p38 MAPK pathway, potentially contributing to AD pathogenesis together with other disorders including neuronal injury, trauma, ischemia, and the accumulation of oxidants associated with brain aging [16,18,224].

Since more than half of the phosphorylation sites in paired helical filament–Tau are serine and threonine residues followed by proline, members of the MAPK family, especially p38α, potentially play an important role in phosphorylating Tau [16]. Considering that aberrantly activated JNK and p38 MAPKs are reportedly associated with cells containing filamentous Tau in some neurodegenerative diseases, these kinases may contribute to Tau hyperphosphorylation. Moreover, the p38 MAPK activator, MKK6, is active in neurodegenerative diseases, indicating a potential contribution to Tau hyperphosphorylation in these diseases. Recent studies have reported that Tau is a suitable in vitro substrate for p38 isoforms p38δ and p38γ, and its phosphorylation by these two enzymes reduces its ability to promote microtubule assembly [18,225–228]. Moreover, p38γ overexpression in neuroblastoma induces Tau phosphorylation, which is associated with a reduction in Tau that is associated with the cytoskeleton and an increase in soluble Tau. Furthermore, p38δ is the major Tau kinase in neuroblastoma in response to osmotic shock [227]. This evidence indicates that p38 MAPKs potentially regulate Tau hyperphosphorylation in neurodegenerative diseases and are potentially suitable therapeutic targets for those diseases.

Other studies have focused on the receptor for advanced glycation end products (RAGE), a multiligand member of the immunoglobulin superfamily of cell surface molecules, which serves as a receptor for Aβ on neurons, microglia, astrocytes, and endothelial cells of blood vessels. RAGE is upregulated in brain regions affected by AD. A murine transgenic model revealed that RAGE is a potential therapeutic target for AD [229].

Several studies have reported that EA and manual acupuncture have a therapeutic effect on AD. For example, EA at acupoint GV20 suppresses Aβ generation [228]. Stimulation at acupoints GV14 and BL23 downregulates beta-secretase 1, which is an enzyme that is responsible for Aβ generation in AD and increases hippocampal ATP levels in AD mice [230]. Low-frequency (2-Hz) EA at acupoint GV20 and bilateral acupoints KI3 and ST36 for 15 min once daily for 12 sessions was reported to significantly downregulate p-p38 MAPK and IL-1β mRNA expression in the hippocampus and the frontal lobe [65]. Other studies have reported that EA at GV20 reversed behavioral deficit and LTP impairment, possibly through the N-methyl-D-aspartate receptor 1 (NMDA-R1) and TRPV1 pathway, thus reversing NR1- (one of the NMDA receptor subunits) and TRPV1-mediated neurotoxicity in vascular dementia [208,209]. This implies that 2-Hz EA can rescue p38 MAPK signal transduction, resulting in anti-apoptotic and anti-inflammatory effects that reduce Aβ deposits in the brain and improve learning and memory in AD patients [20].

11.2. Parkinson's Disease

Parkinson's disease is a neurodegenerative disorder that causes severe motor impairment owing to loss of dopaminergic neurons in the substantia nigra pars compacta (SNpc). Several studies have focused on PD pathophysiology and reported potential therapeutic targets for PD.

One of the direct neuroprotective effects is exerted by the protein deglycase DJ-1, which inhibits ASK1 through the nuclear sequestration of death domain–associated protein (Daxx) [230–232].

DJ-1 is speculated to scavenge reactive oxidative species (ROS) and subsequently attenuate oxidative stress, thereby reducing cellular ROS burden [233,234]. Furthermore, DJ-1 interacts with p38-regulated/activated kinase (PRAK/MK5) under cellular oxidative stress to facilitate nuclear localization of DJ-1 [235]. Thus, DJ-1 co-localizes with PRAK in the nuclei of NIH3T3 cells. Since DJ-1 lacks both nuclear localization and nuclear export signals, PRAK may be a crucial factor assisting DJ-1 in regulating the cellular localization of Daxx and in ASK1 signaling and concomitant cell death [236].

A recent study reported that EA at acupoint KI3 reduced the excitotoxicity of dopaminergic neurons by regulating the NMDA receptor function and thus may potentially serve as a novel therapeutic approach for PD [237]. The levels of pNR1 and pNR2B, phosphorylated PKA, PKC, α-Ca2+/CaMKII, pERK, and CREB were also reduced following EA [237].

12. Fibromyalgia

Fibromyalgia is a common chronic pain syndrome characterized by chronic widespread mechanical pain. TRPV1 and TRPV4 are believed to play a crucial role in the pathophysiology of fibromyalgia. EA at 2 Hz at bilateral ST36 acupoints was reported to reduce long-lasting mechanical hyperalgesia by downregulating TRPV4, p-p38, p-JNK, and pCREB in the peripheral nervous system and CNS [238,239].

Taken together, acupuncture exerts anti-inflammation, anti-apoptosis, and neuroprotection effects via modulating proinflammatory cytokines, increasing the levels of neurotrophic factors and modulating signaling pathways, such as p38 MAPKs, Raf/MAPK/ERK1/2, TLR4/ERK, PI3K/AKT, AC/cAMP/PKA, ASK1–JNK/p38, and downstream CREB, JNK, m-TOR, NF-κB, and Bcl-2/Bax balance. EA relieves acute pain through inhibiting the TRPV1 signaling and PI3K/PKC/CaMKII pathway. EA also promote the release of opiates to activate μ-, δ-, and κ-opioid receptors, therefore producing immediate and persistent analgesic effects. Furthermore, EA can downregulate TRPV1-mediated inflammation and the release of proinflammatory cytokines, GFAP, Iba-1, and S100B by inhibiting the phosphorylation of p38 MAPK, therefore inhibiting microglial activation that triggers nerve damage and pain. Combining acupuncture to the treatment of a cerebral ischemic/hemorrhagic event can have a positive effect; an upregulation of BDNF synthesis, downregulation of P2X4Rs, and inhibition of p38 phosphorylation leads to the activation of the Raf-1/MEK1/2/ERK1/2/p90RSK/Bad signaling pathway, which contributes to the downregulation of caspase-3-dependent neuronal apoptosis. Acupuncture also inhibits the TNF-α/TRADD/FADD/cleaved caspase-8/cleaved caspase-3 apoptotic pathway in the ischemic cortical penumbra after reperfusion. In the case of treating epilepsy and seizure, several antiepileptic mechanisms have been proposed, including the downregulation of JNK or ERK1/2 and proinflammatory factors (IL-1β, IL-6, TNF-α) in the cerebral cortex and hippocampus. Auricular EA can reduce hippocampal hyperactivity through TRPA1 and PKCε/PKCα/pERK1/2 signaling pathways. Furthermore, acupuncture can regulate p38γ and p38δ and reduce Tau hyperphosphorylation in neurodegenerative diseases. Acupuncture also exhibits a therapeutic effect that was reported to involve the regulation of DJ-1, ASK1, Daxx, phosphorylated PKA, PKC, α-Ca2+/CaMKII, pERK, and CREB. Acupuncture exerts curative effects in migraine through local analgesia, anti-inflammation, neuropeptide regulation, cytoskeleton remodeling, cell repair, and improvement in overall homeostasis. Furthermore, the downregulation of TRPV4, p-p38, p-JNK, and pCREB in the peripheral nervous system and CNS may account for the therapeutic effect of acupuncture in fibromyalgia.

This literature review based on the results of previous studies where we electronically searched databases including PubMed, Embase, and the Cochrane Library from their inception to April 2020, using the following keywords alone or in various combinations: "acupuncture", "p38 MAPK pathway", "signaling", "stress response", "inflammation", "immune", "pain", "analgesic", "cerebral ischemic injury", "epilepsy", "Alzheimer's disease", "Parkinson's disease", "dementia", "degenerative", and "homeostasis". The schematic explanation of the searching process is presented as Appendix A.

13. Conclusions

Among the aforementioned cell pathways, the p38 MAPK signaling pathway plays a role in the therapeutic effect of acupuncture in several nervous system diseases. EA inhibits the ascending pain pathway and intracellular p38-mediated inflammatory pathway by stimulating peripheral opioid receptors. Furthermore, EA promotes endogenic analgesic mechanisms, thus exerting immediate local analgesic effects and rescuing CNS-induced chronic pain. Acupuncture also counteracts p38 MAPK signal transduction, reduces Aβ deposits in the brain, and improves learning and memory in AD patients.

Acupuncture exhibits a dual regulatory function through the activation or inhibition of different p38 MAPK pathways and contributes to an overall improvement of clinical symptoms and physiological functions in several nervous system diseases. The p38 MAPK pathway potentially induces both protective and inhibitory effects in highly similar systems. Further studies are required to identify and characterize the various substrates of these kinases involved in cell differentiation/cell repair, neurotoxicity, and neurodegeneration, thus potentially furthering the current understanding of the mechanism underlying acupuncture in treating these diseases.

Author Contributions: Data curation, T.-H.W.; writing—original draft preparation, T.-H.W.; review and editing, C.-L.H. All authors have read and agreed to the published version of the manuscript.

Abbreviations

A1R	adenosine A1 receptor
α7 nAChR	α7 nicotinic acetylcholine receptor
AC	adenyl cyclase
ACC1	acetyl-CoA carboxylase (ACC) 1 is a biotin-dependent enzyme that catalyzes the irreversible carboxylation of acetyl-CoA to produce malonyl-CoA
AD	Alzheimer's disease
Akt (PKB)	protein kinase B (PKB) is also known as Akt
Alk5	TGFβ type I receptor kinase
AMP	adenosine mono-phosphate
AMPK	5′ AMP-activated protein kinase
AP-1	activator protein 1
ARE	AU-rich elements
ASIC3	acid-sensing ion channel 3
ASK-1	apoptosis signal-regulating kinase 1
ATF	activating transcription factor
ATP	adenosine tri-phosphate
BACE1	beta-secretase 1, an enzyme responsible for Aβ generation in Alzheimer's disease
Bad	BCL2 associated agonist of cell death; a protein involved in initiating apoptosis.
Bax	Bcl-2 associated X
Bac-2	B-cell lymphoma 2
BDNF	brain-derived neurotrophic factor
CaMKII	calmodulin-dependent protein kinase II
CCI	chronic constriction injury
Cd242	The 40- to 42-kiloDalton red cell membrane glycoprotein bearing the ICAM-4 antigen named by the LW blood system.
CFA-treated	Complete Freund's adjuvant injections produced significant mechanical and thermal hyperalgesia in mice.
c-Fos	A proto-oncogene that is expressed within some neurons following depolarization.
CHOP	C/EBP homologous protein; belongs to the family of CCAAT/enhancer-binding proteins (C/EBPs) and is involved in the regulation of genes that encode proteins involved in proliferation
c-Jun	A proto-oncogene that with c-Fos forms the AP-1 early response transcription factor that regulates gene expression in response to extracellular stimuli.

CL100	The human CL100 gene is induced in skin fibroblasts in response to oxidative/heat stress and growth factors. The CL100 gene encodes a dual specificity (Tyr/Thr) protein phosphatase that specifically inactivates MAPKs.
CLCA3A2	chloride channel accessory 3A2
CLIC3	chloride intracellular channel 3
Cot (Tp2)	cancer Osaka thyroid oncogene (=Tpl-2)
COX-2	cyclooxygenase-2
cPLA2	cytosolic phospholipase A2
CREB	cAMP response element-binding protein
CRF	corticotropin-releasing factor
CWP	components of calcium wave propagation
DLK (MAP3K12)	dual leucine zipper kinase, also known as MAP3K12
DJ-1	a protein deglycase
DLG1 (SAP97)	discs large homolog 1 scaffold protein
Daxx	the death-associated protein
DHT	dihydrotestosterone
DRG	dorsal root ganglion
EA	electroacupuncture
elF2a	eukaryotic translation initiation factor 2A; functions by a separate mechanism in eukaryotic translation
eEF2	eukaryotic elongation factor 2
eEF2K	eukaryotic elongation factor 2 kinase
elF2α	a subunit of the heterotrimeric eIF2 complex
Elk-1	erythroblast transformation specific (ETS) like-1 protein
ERK	extracellular signal–regulated kinases
ETS	erythroblast transformation specific protein, or E26 transformation-specific, or E-twenty-six transcription factors family
FADD	Fas-associated protein with death domain; also called MORT1
Fas pathway	Fas and Fas Ligand (FasL) are involved in the regulation of cell death.
GABA	gamma-aminobutyric acid
GFAP	glial fibrillary acidic protein; a marker of astrocytes
GPCRs	G-protein-coupled receptors
HMG-CoA Reductase	3-hydroxy-3-methyl-glutaryl-CoA reductase or HMGR is the rate-controlling enzyme of the mevalonate pathway, responsible for cholesterol and other isoprenoid biosynthesis.
Hsc70	heat shock cognate 70
Hsp	heat shock proteins
5-HT	5-hydroxytryptamine
Iba-1	ionized calcium–binding adapter molecule 1
IκB	inhibitor of nuclear factor kappa-B
IκB	inhibitor of nuclear factor kappa-B kinase
IKKs	I-kappa-B kinases
IL-1β	Interleukin 1 beta is a member of the interleukin 1 family of cytokines produced by activated macrophages.
IRF	interferon regulatory factor
JNK	c-Jun amino-terminal kinases
LTD	long-term depression; a term in neurophysiology describing an activity-dependent reduction in the efficacy of neuronal synapses lasting hours or longer following a long patterned stimulus.
LTP	long-term potentiation; a persistent strengthening of synapses based on recent patterns of activity. These are patterns of synaptic activity that produce a long-lasting increase in signal transmission between two neurons.
MA	manual acupuncture
MAPK	mitogen-activated protein kinase
MAPKK (MAP2K, MKK)	MAPK kinase
MAPKKK (MAP3K)	MAPKK kinase
Max	a transcription factor coded by the myc-associated factor X

MEF	myocyte enhancing factor
MEK (MKK)	MAPK/ERK kinase
MEKK	MEK kinase
mGluR3	metabotropic glutamate receptor 3
MKP	MAPK-phosphatase
MAPKAPK-2	mitogen-activated protein kinase-activated protein kinase 2
MLK	mixed-lineage protein kinase
MNK	mitogen activated protein kinase–interacting protein
Myc	A group of transcription factors coded by a regulator genes and proto-oncogenes called Myc
MyD88	myeloid differentiation primary response 88
MSK	mitogen and stress activated protein kinase
mTOR	mammalian target of rapamycin
Na_V	voltage-gated sodium channel
NFκB	nuclear factor-kappa-B
P105	The 105 kD protein is a Rel protein-specific transcription inhibitor encoded by the NFKB1 gene
PAG	periaqueductal gray area
NIH3Ts cells	A cell line derived from mouse embryonic fibroblasts.
NMDA	N-methyl-D-aspartate, an amino acid derivative
PKB	Protein kinase B; also known as Akt
NO	nitric oxide
NR1	NMDA receptor subunits includes NR1 and NR2Bi
Pax6	Paired-box protein Pax-6, also known as aniridia type II protein (AN2) or oculorhombin; a "master control" gene for the development of eyes and other sensory organs
P2RX7	P2X purinoceptor 7 is a protein belonging to the family of purinoceptors for ATP.
P2X4Rs	P2X4 receptors are a subtype of ionotropic ATP receptors
P2Y1, -2	human purinergic G protein-coupled receptors
PD	Parkinson's disease
Pellino	A group of proteins extremely well conserved during evolution; Pellinos interact with key mediators in TLR/IL-1R-induced signaling pathways.
PHF-tau	paired helical filament–tau protein
PI3K	phosphoinositide 3-kinases; also called phosphatidylinositol 3-kinases
PKC	protein kinase C
PSD	postsynaptic density protein
PRAK	p38-regulated and -activated kinase
Rac2	Ras-related C3 botulinum toxin substrate 2
RAF	rapidly accelerated fibrosarcoma-related oncogene
Raf1	v-raf-1 murine leukemia viral oncogene homolog 1
RAGE	The receptor for advanced glycation end products is a member of the immunoglobulin superfamily of cell surface molecules.
RCT study	randomized controlled trial study
Rel	A proto-oncogene protein encoded by the REL gene. It is a member of the NF-κB family of transcription factors and contains a Rel homology domain (RHD) at its N-terminus and two C-terminal transactivation domains.
Rho	Rho (ρ) factor is a protein that acts in bacterial cells to mediate termination of transcription at distinct sites, which mediates the dissociation of the RNA from the very stable ternary transcription complex.
Rit	Ras-like protein in tissues
RIP	receptor-interacting protein kinases; a class of serine/threonine protein kinases
ROS	reactive oxidative species
S100B	S100 calcium-binding protein B
SAP	stress-activated protein or synapse-associated protein; SAP90 [(synapse-associated protein 90 is also known as PSD-95 (postsynaptic density-95)]
SAPK	stress-activated protein kinase

Smac/DIABLO	second mitochondrial-derived activator of caspase/direct inhibitor of apoptosis protein-binding protein with low isoelectric point
SNpc	substantia nigra pars compacta
Stat1	signal transducer and activator of transcription 1
STK	serine-threonine/tyrosine kinases
TAES	transcutaneous acupoint electrical stimulation
TAK-1	transforming growth factor-β-activated kinase 1
TAO	thousand and one amino acids
TAB1	TGF-beta-activated kinase
TGFβ	transforming growth factor-β
TLR4	toll-like receptor 4
TNF	tumor necrosis factor
Tpl2	tumor progression locus 2, also known as COT or MAP3K8
TRADD	tumor necrosis factor receptor type 1-associated DEATH domain protein
TRAF6	tumor necrosis factor receptor (TNFR)-associated factor 6
TrkB	tyrosine kinase receptor B
TRPA1	transient receptor potential cation channel subfamily A member 1
TRPV	transient receptor potential vanilloid receptors
3′UTR	3′untranslated region

Appendix A

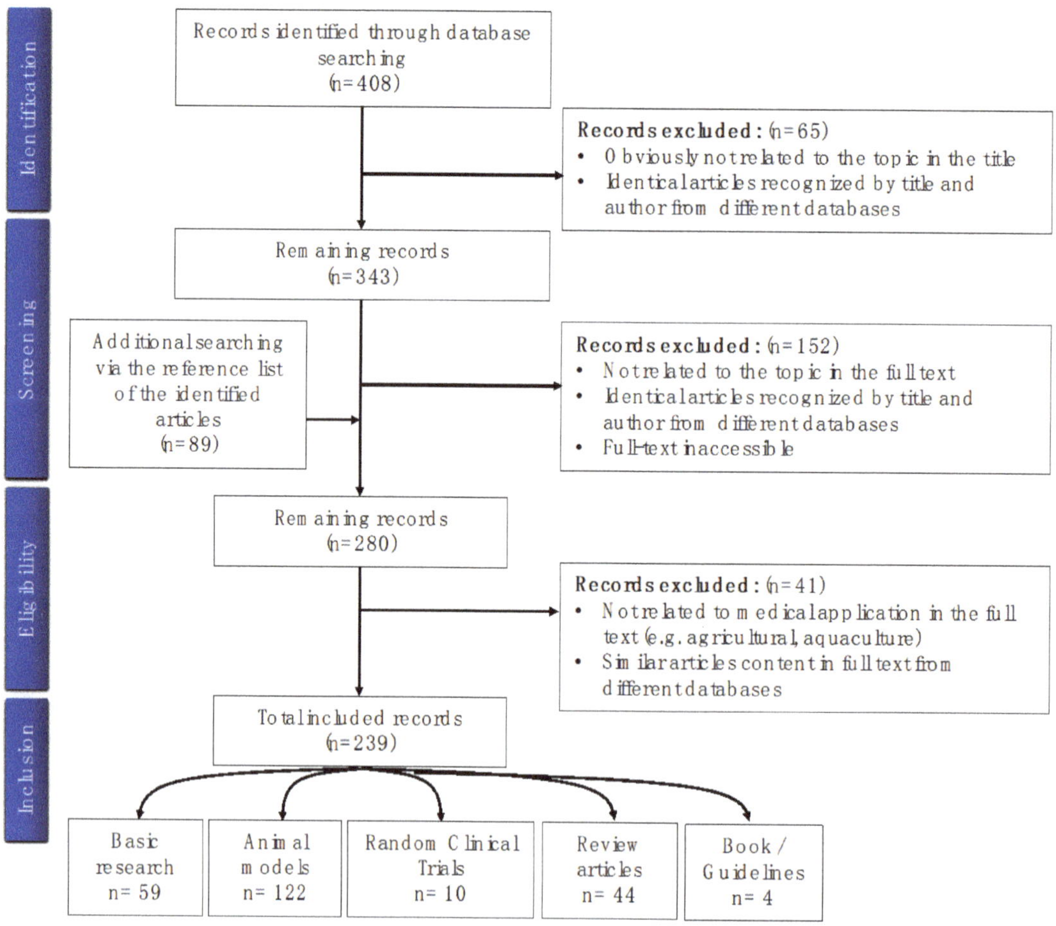

Figure A1. Schematic of the literature review search process.

References

1. Zhou, W.; Benharash, P. Effects and mechanisms of acupuncture based on the principle of meridians. *J. Acupunct. Meridian Stud.* **2014**, *7*, 190–193. [CrossRef] [PubMed]
2. Wang, B.; Wu, N.L.; Wu, A.Q. *The Yellow Emperor's Canon of Internal Medicine*, 1st ed.; China Science & Technology. Press: Beijing, China, 1997; 1999, 2nd edition.
3. Bannerman, R.H. *Acupuncture: The WHO View*; World Health Organization: Geneva, Switzerland, 1979; Volume 12, p. 27e8.
4. Park, J.; Sohn, Y.; White, A.R.; Lee, H. The safety of acupuncture during pregnancy: A systematic review. *Acupunct. Med.* **2014**, *32*, 257–266. [CrossRef] [PubMed]
5. Yang, C.; Hao, Z.; Zhang, L.L.; Guo, Q. Efficacy and safety of acupuncture in children: An overview of systematic reviews. *Pediatr. Res.* **2015**, *78*, 112–119. [CrossRef] [PubMed]
6. Fan, A.Y.; Miller, D.W.; Bolash, B.; Bauer, M.; McDonal, J.; Faggert, S.; He, H.; Li, Y.M.; Matecki, A.; Camardella, L.; et al. Acupuncture's role in solving the opioid epidemic: Evidence, cost-effectiveness, and care availability for acupuncture as a primary, nonpharmacologic method for pain relief and management–white paper. *J. Integr. Med.* **2017**, *15*, 411–425. [CrossRef]
7. Acupuncture: In Depth. National Center for Complementary and Alternative Medicine. Available online: https://nccih.nih.gov/health/acupuncture/introduction (accessed on 25 January 2020).
8. Hsieh, C.L. Acupuncture as treatment for nervous system diseases. *BioMed* **2012**, *2*, 51–57. [CrossRef]
9. He, X.R.; Wang, Q.; Li, P.P. Acupuncture and moxibustion for cancer-related fatigue: A systematic review and meta-analysis. *Asian Pac. J. Cancer Prev.* **2013**, *14*, 3067–3074. [CrossRef]
10. Cox, J.; Varatharajan, S.; Côté, P.; Optima Collaboration. Effectiveness of acupuncture therapies to manage musculoskeletal disorders of the extremities: A systematic review. *J. Orthop. Sports Phys. Ther.* **2016**, *46*, 409–429. [CrossRef]
11. Forde, J.C.; Jaffe, E.; Stone, B.V.; Te, A.E.; Espinosa, G.; Chughtai, B. The role of acupuncture in managing overactive bladder: A review of the literature. *Int. Urogynecol. J.* **2016**, *27*, 1645–1651. [CrossRef]
12. Yao, Q.; Li, S.; Liu, X.; Qin, Z.; Liu, Z. The effectiveness and safety of acupuncture for patients with chronic urticaria: A systematic review. *Biomed Res. Int.* **2016**, *2016*, 5191729. [CrossRef]
13. Bäcker, M.; Hammes, M.G.; Valet, M.; Deppe, M.; Valet, M.; Conrad, B.; Tölle, T.R.; Doboset, G. Different modes of manual acupuncture stimulation differentially modulate cerebral blood flow velocity, arterial blood pressure and heart rate in human subjects. [published correction appears in *Neurosci. Lett.* **2003**, *6*, 337, 117]. *Neurosci. Lett.* **2002**, *333*, 203–206. [CrossRef]
14. Hsieh, C.L.; Chang, Q.Y.; Lin, I.H.; Lin, J.G.; Liu, C.H.; Tang, N.Y.; Lane, H.Y. The study of electroacupuncture on cerebral blood flow in rats with and without cerebral ischemia. *Am. J. Chin. Med.* **2006**, *34*, 351–361. [CrossRef] [PubMed]
15. Kuo, C.; Lin, Y.; Tang, N.; Cheng, C.Y.; Hsieh, C.L. Electric stimulation of the ears ameliorated learning and memory impairment in rats with cerebral ischemia-reperfusion injury. *Sci. Rep.* **2016**, *6*, 20381. [CrossRef] [PubMed]
16. Bachstetter, A.D.; Xing, B. Microglial p38alpha MAPK is a key regulator of proinflammatory cytokine up-regulation induced by toll-like receptor (TLR) ligands or beta-amyloid (Abeta). *J. Neuroinflammation* **2011**, *8*, 79. [CrossRef] [PubMed]
17. Jin, Y.; Fan, Y. Effects of sodium ferulate on amyloid-beta-induced MKK3/MKK6-p38 MAPK-Hsp27 signal pathway and apoptosis in rat hippocampus. *Acta Pharm. Sin.* **2006**, *27*, 1309–1316. [CrossRef]
18. Yang, L.; Zhou, R. Neuroprotection by dihydrotestosterone in LPS-induced neuroinflammation. *Neurobiol. Dis.* **2020**, 104814. [CrossRef]
19. Yan, S.D.; Bierhaus, A. RAGE and Alzheimer's disease: A progression factor for amyloid-beta-induced cellular perturbation? *J. Alzheimers Dis* **2009**, *16*, 833–843. [CrossRef]
20. Tang, Y.; Xu, A.; Shao, S.; Zhou, Y.; Xiong, B.; Li, Z. Electroacupuncture ameliorates cognitive impairment by inhibiting the JNK signaling pathway in a mouse model of Alzheimer's disease. *Front. Aging Neurosci.* **2020**, *12*, 23. [CrossRef]
21. Wang, K.; Wu, H.; Wang, G.; Li, M.; Zhang, Z.; Gu, G. The effects of electroacupuncture on TH1/TH2 cytokine mRNA expression and mitogen-activated protein kinase signaling pathways in the splenic T cells of traumatized rats. *Anesth Analg.* **2009**, *109*, 1666–1673. [CrossRef]

22. Cheng, K.J. Neurobiological mechanisms of acupuncture for some common illnesses: A clinician's perspective. *J. Acupunct. Meridian Stud.* **2014**, *7*, 105–114. [CrossRef]
23. Xue, X.; You, Y.; Tao, J.; Ye, X.; Huang, J.; Yang, S.; Lin, Z.; Hong, Z.; Peng, J.; Chen, L. Electro-acupuncture at points of Zusanli and Quchi exerts anti-apoptotic effect through the modulation of PI3K/Akt signaling pathway. *Neurosci. Lett.* **2014**, *558*, 14–19. [CrossRef]
24. Wang, H.; Wang, L.; Liang, F.; Liu, J.; Li, J.; Lu, J.; Fu, Y.; Chen, Q.; Has, Q.; Wu, S. Effects of electroacupuncture on electrocardiogram, myocardial pathological morphology and PI3K/Akt pathway in rats with chronic myocardial ischemia. *Zhongguo Zhen Jiu* **2016**, *36*, 389–395.
25. Hwang, I.K.; Chung, J.Y.; Yoo, D.Y.; Yi, S.S.; Youn, H.Y.; Seong, J.K.; Soon, Y.S. Effects of electroacupuncture at Zusanli and Baihui on brain-derived neurotrophic factor and cyclic AMP response element-binding protein in the hippocampal dentate gyrus. *J. Vet. Med. Sci.* **2010**, *72*, 1431–1436. [CrossRef] [PubMed]
26. Zhang, H.; Qin, F.; Liu, A.; Sun, Q.; Wang, Q.; Xie, S.; Lu, S.; Zhang, D.; Lu, Z. Electro-acupuncture attenuates the mice premature ovarian failure via mediating PI3K/AKT/mTOR pathway. *Life Sci.* **2019**, *217*, 169–175. [CrossRef] [PubMed]
27. Du, J.; Wang, Q.; Hu, B.; Peng, Z.; Zhao, Y.; Ma, L.; Xiong, L.; Lu, Y.; Zhu, X.; Chen, S. Involvement of ERK 1/2 activation in electroacupuncture pretreatment via cannabinoid CB1 receptor in rats. *Brain Res.* **2010**, *1360*, 1–7. [CrossRef]
28. Xie, G.; Yang, S.; Chen, A.; Lan, L.; Lin, Z.; Gao, Y.; Huang, J.; Lin, J.; Peng, J.; Tao, J.; et al. Electroacupuncture at Quchi and Zusanli treats cerebral ischemia-reperfusion injury through activation of ERK signaling. *Exp. Ther. Med.* **2013**, *5*, 1593–1597. [CrossRef] [PubMed]
29. Wu, C.; Wang, J.; Chun, L.; Zhou, G.; Xu, X.; Zhang, X.; Lan, X. Effect of electroacupuncture on cell apoptosis and erk signal pathway in the hippocampus of adult rats with cerebral ischemia-reperfusion. *Evid. Based Complementary Altern. Med.* **2015**, 414965. [CrossRef] [PubMed]
30. Wu, C.; Li, C.; Zhou, G.; Yang, L.; Jiang, G.; Chen, J.; Li, Q.; Zhan, Z.; Xu, X.; Zhang, X. Effects of electroacupuncture on the cortical extracellular signal regulated kinase pathway in rats with cerebral ischaemia/reperfusion. *Acupunct. Med.* **2017**, *35*, 430–436. [CrossRef] [PubMed]
31. Lin, D.; Wu, Q.; Lin, X.; Boriongan, C.; He, Z.; Tan, J.; Cao, C.; Zhou, S. Brain-derived neurotrophic factor signaling pathway: Modulation by acupuncture in telomerase knockout mice. *Altern. Health Med.* **2015**, *21*, 36–46.
32. Wang, S.J.; Ma, J.; Gong, Y.X.; Wang, Y.C.; Zeng, X.L.; Liang, Y.; Sun, G.J. Effect of electroacupuncture intervention on ERK 1/2 signaling and TNF-alpha and IL-1beta protein levels in the substantia nigra in rats with Parkinson's disease. *Zhen Ci Yan Jiu* **2014**, *39*, 456–460.
33. Lan, X.; Zhang, X.; Zhou, G.P.; Wu, C.X.; Li, C.; Xu, X.H. Electroacupuncture reduces apoptotic index and inhibits p38 mitogen-activated protein kinase signaling pathway in the hippocampus of rats with cerebral ischemia/reperfusion injury. *Neural Regen. Res.* **2017**, *12*, 409–416. [CrossRef]
34. Xing, Y.; Yang, S.D.; Wang, M.M.; Dong, F.; Feng, Y.S.; Zhang, F. Electroacupuncture alleviated neuronal apoptosis following ischemic stroke in rats via midkine and ERK/JNK/p38 signaling pathway. *J. Mol. Neurosci.* **2018**, *66*, 26–36. [CrossRef]
35. Liu, W.; Wang, X.; Yang, S.; Huang, J.; Xue, X.; Zheng, Y.; Shang, G.; Tao, J.; Chen, L. Electroacupunctre improves motor impairment via inhibition of microglia-mediated neuroinflammation in the sensorimotor cortex after ischemic stroke. *Life Sci.* **2016**, *151*, 313–322. [CrossRef]
36. Xu, J.; She, Y.; Su, N.; Zhang, R.; Lao, L.; Xu, S. Effects of electroacupuncture on chronic unpredictable mild stress rats depression-like behavior and expression of p-ERK/ERK and p-P38/P38. *Evid. Based Complement Altern. Med.* **2015**, *2015*, 650729. [CrossRef] [PubMed]
37. Yang, X.; Guo, Z.; Lu, J.; Zhao, B.; Fei, Y.; Li, J.; Jiang, H.; Sun, L.; Wang, Y.; Sun, Y.; et al. The Role of MAPK and dopaminergic synapse signaling pathways in antidepressant effect of electroacupuncture pretreatment in chronic restraint stress rats. *Evid. Based Complementary Altern. Med.* **2017**, *2017*, 2357653. [CrossRef] [PubMed]
38. Duan, D.M.; Dong, X.; Tu, Y.; Liu, P. A microarray study of chronic unpredictable mild stress rat blood serum with electro-acupuncture intervention. *Neurosci. Lett.* **2016**, *627*, 160–167. [CrossRef]
39. Zhao, G.; Li, D.; Ding, X.; Li, L. Nerve growth factor pretreatment inhibits lidocaine-induced myelin damage via increasing BDNF expression and inhibiting p38 mitogen activation in the rat spinal cord. *Mol. Med. Rep.* **2017**, *16*, 4678–4684. [CrossRef] [PubMed]

40. Liao, E.T.; Lin, Y.W.; Huang, C.P.; Tang, N.Y.; Hsieh, C.L. Electric stimulation of ear reduces the effect of Toll-like receptor 4 signaling pathway on kainic acid-induced epileptic seizures in rats. *Biomed. Res. Int.* **2018**, *2018*, 5407256. [CrossRef] [PubMed]
41. Feng, X.; Yang, S.; Liu, J.; Huang, J.; Peng, J.; Lin, J.; Tao, J.; Chen, L. Electroacupuncture ameliorates cognitive impairment through inhibition of NF-κB-mediated neuronal cell apoptosis in cerebral ischemia-reperfusion injured rats. *Mol. Med. Rep.* **2013**, *7*, 1516–1522. [CrossRef]
42. Lan, L.; Tao, J.; Chen, A.; Xie, G.; Huang, J.; Lin, J.; Peng, J.; Chen, L. Electroacupuncture exerts anti-inflammatory effects in cerebral ischemia-reperfusion injured rats via suppression of the TLR4/NF-κB pathway. *Int. J. Mol. Med.* **2013**, *31*, 75–80. [CrossRef]
43. Zhu, Y.; Zeng, Y.; Wang, X.; Ye, X. Effect of electroacupuncture on the expression of mTOR and eIF4E in hippocampus of rats with vascular dementia. *Neurol. Sci.* **2013**, *34*, 1093–1097. [CrossRef]
44. Xu, T.; Li, W.; Liang, Y.; Yang, Z.; Liu, J.; Wang, Y.; Su, N. Neuroprotective effects of electro acupuncture on hypoxic-ischemic encephalopathy in newborn rats Ass. *Pak. J. Pharm. Sci.* **2014**, *27* (Suppl. 6), 1991–2000. [PubMed]
45. Oh, J.; Kim, Y.; Kim, S.; Lee, B.; Jang, J.; Kwon, S.; Park, H. Acupuncture modulates stress response by the mTOR signaling pathway in a rat post-traumatic stress disorder model. *Sci. Rep.* **2018**, *8*, 11864. [CrossRef] [PubMed]
46. Liu, W.; Zhuo, P.; Li, L.; Jin, H.; Lin, B.; Zhang, Y.; Liang, S.; Wu, J.; Huang, J.; Wang, Z.; et al. Activation of brain glucose metabolism ameliorating cognitive impairment in APP/PS1 transgenic mice by electroacupuncture. *Free. Radic. Biol. Med.* **2017**, *112*, 174–190. [CrossRef] [PubMed]
47. Kim, Y.R.; Kim, H.N.; Jang, J.Y.; Park, C.; Lee, J.H.; Shin, H.K.; Choi, Y.H.; Choi, B.T. Effects of electroacupuncture on apoptotic pathways in a rat model of focal cerebral ischemia. *Int. J. Mol. Med.* **2013**, *32*, 1303–1310. [CrossRef] [PubMed]
48. Lawan, A.; Bennett, A.M. Mitogen-activated protein kinase regulation in hepatic metabolism. *Trends Endocrinol. Metab.* **2017**, *28*, 868–878. [CrossRef] [PubMed]
49. Kim, S.N.; Kim, S.T.; Doo, A.R.; Park, J.Y.; Moon, W.; Chae, Y.; Yin, C.S.; Lee, H.; Park, H.J. Phosphatidylinositol 3-kinase/Akt signaling pathway mediates acupuncture-induced dopaminergic neuron protection and motor function improvement in a mouse model of Parkinson's disease. *Int. J. Neurosci.* **2011**, *121*, 562–569. [CrossRef]
50. Kim, S.N.; Doo, A.R.; Park, J.Y.; Bae, H.; Chae, Y.; Shim, I.; Lee, H.; Moon, W.; Lee, H.; Park, H.J. Acupuncture enhances the synaptic dopamine availability to improve motor function in a mouse model of Parkinson's disease. *PLoS ONE* **2011**, *6*, e27566. [CrossRef]
51. Li, Q.Q.; Shi, G.X.; Yang, J.W.; Li, Z.H.; Zhang, Z.H.; He, T.; Wang, J.; Liu, L.Y.; Liu, C.Z. Hippocampal cAMP/PKA/CREB is required for neuroprotective effect of acupuncture. *Physiol. Behav.* **2015**, *139*, 482–490. [CrossRef]
52. Lu, F.; Zhu, H.M.; Xie, J.J.; Zhou, H.H.; Chen, Y.L.; Hu, J.Y. Effects of electroacupuncture on behavior, plasma COR and expressions of PKA and PKC in hippocampus of the depression model rat. *Zhongguo Zhen Jiu* **2008**, *28*, 214–218.
53. Liu, J.J.; Wu, Z.F.; Sun, J.; Jiang, L.; Jiang, S.; Fu, W.B. Role of AC-cAMP-PKA cascade in antidepressant action of electroacupuncture treatment in rats. *Evid. Based Complementary Altern. Med.* **2012**, *2012*, 932414. [CrossRef]
54. Lin, R.; Lin, Y.; Tao, J.; Chen, B.; You, K.; Chen, J.; Li, X.; Chen, L.D. Electroacupuncture ameliorates learning and memory in rats with cerebral ischemia-reperfusion injury by inhibiting oxidative stress and promoting p-CREB expression in the hippocampus. *Mol. Med. Rep.* **2015**, *12*, 6807–6814. [CrossRef]
55. Ahn, S.; Kim, Y.; Kim, H.; Shin, Y.I.; Shin, H.K.; Choi, B.T. Electroacupuncture ameliorates memory impairments by enhancing oligodendrocyte regeneration in a mouse model of prolonged cerebral hypoperfusion. *Sci. Rep.* **2016**, *6*, 28646. [CrossRef] [PubMed]
56. Zhang, Y.; Lin, R.; Tao, J.; Wu, Y.; Chen, B.; You, K.; Chen, J.; Li, X.; Chen, L.D. Electroacupuncture improves cognitive ability following cerebral ischemia reperfusion injury via CaM-CaMKIV-CREB signaling in the rat hippocampus. *Exp. Ther. Med.* **2016**, *12*, 777–782. [CrossRef]
57. Yun, Y.C.; Jang, D.; Yoon, S.B.; Kim, D.; Choi, D.H.; Kwon, O.S.; Lee, Y.M.; Youn, D. Laser acupuncture exerts neuroprotective effects via regulation of Creb, Bdnf, Bcl-2, and Bax gene expressions in the hippocampus. *Evid. Based Complementary Altern. Med.* **2017**, *2017*, 7181637. [CrossRef]

58. Pak, M.E.; Jung, D.H.; Lee, H.J.; Shin, M.J.; Kim, S.Y.; Shin, Y.B.; Yun, Y.J.; Shin, H.K.; Choi, B.T. Combined therapy involving electroacupuncture and treadmill exercise attenuates demyelination in the corpus callosum by stimulating oligodendrogenesis in a rat model of neonatal hypoxia-ischemia. *Exp. Neurol.* **2018**, *300*, 222–231. [CrossRef] [PubMed]
59. Lu, J.; Liang, J.; Wang, J.R.; Hu, L.; Tu, Y.; Guo, J.Y. Acupuncture activates ERK-CREB pathway in rats exposed to chronic unpredictable mild stress. *Evid. Based Complementary Altern. Med.* **2013**, *2013*, 469765. [CrossRef]
60. Dimaras, H.; Gallie, B.L. Retinoblastoma Protein, Biological and Clinical Functions. In *Encyclopedia of Cancer*; Schwab, M., Ed.; Springer: Berlin/Heidelberg, Germany, 2011; pp. 4046–4050. [CrossRef]
61. Duval, D.; Trouillas, M.; Thibault, C.; Dembelé, D.; Diemunsch, F.; Reinhardt, B.; Mertz, A.L.; Dierich, A.; Boeuf, H. Apoptosis and differentiation commitment: Novel insights revealed by gene profiling studies in mouse embryonic stem cells. *Cell Death Differ.* **2005**, *13*, 564–575. [CrossRef]
62. Wang, Y.; Jiang, H.; Meng, H.; Li, J.; Yang, X.; Zhao, B.; Sun, Y.; Bro, T. Antidepressant mechanism research of acupuncture: Insights from a genome-wide transcriptome analysis of frontal cortex in rats with chronic restraint stress. *Evid. Based Complementary Altern. Med.* **2017**, *2017*, 1676808. [CrossRef]
63. Liu, J.; Wang, Q.; Yang, S.; Huang, J.; Feng, X.; Peng, J.; Lin, Z.; Liu, W.; Tao, W.; Chen, L. Electroacupuncture inhibits apoptosis of peri-ischemic regions via modulating p38, extracellular signal-regulated kinase (ERK1/2), and c-Jun N terminal kinases (JNK) in cerebral ischemia-reperfusion-injured rats. *Med. Sci. Monit.* **2018**, *24*, 4395–4404. [CrossRef]
64. Zhu, Y.; Deng, L.; Tang, H.; Gao, X.; Wang, Y.; Guo, K.; Kong, J.; Yang, C. Electroacupuncture improves neurobehavioral function and brain injury in rat model of intracerebral hemorrhage. *Brain Res. Bull.* **2017**, *131*, 123–132. [CrossRef]
65. Li, Z.; Zheng, X.; Li, P.; Itoua, E.S.; Moukassa, D.; Ndinga Andely, F. Effects of acupuncture on mRNA levels of apoptotic factors in perihematomal brain tissue during the acute phase of cerebral hemorrhage. *Med. Sci. Monit.* **2017**, *23*, 1522–1532. [CrossRef] [PubMed]
66. Li, X.Y.; Xu, L.; Liu, C.L.; Huang, L.S.; Zhu, X.Y. Electroacupuncture Intervention inhibits the decline of learning-memory ability and overexpression of cleaved Caspase-3 and Bax in hippocampus induced by isoflurane in APPswe/PS 1. *Zhen Ci Yan Jiu* **2016**, *41*, 24–30.
67. Wang, T.; Liu, C.Z.; Yu, J.C.; Jiang, W.; Han, J.X. Acupuncture protected cerebral multi-infarction rats from memory impairment by regulating the expression of apoptosis related genes Bcl-2 and Bax in hippocampus. *Physiol. Behav.* **2009**, *96*, 155–161. [CrossRef] [PubMed]
68. Tian, W.J.; Huang, L.N.; Wang, R.H.; An, J.M.; Zhang, M. Effects of scalp-acupuncture on astrocyte apoptosis in hippocampal CA 1 region in rats with vascular dementia. *Zhen Ci Yan Jiu* **2015**, *40*, 6–12. [PubMed]
69. Lai, H.C.; Chang, Q.Y.; Hsieh, C.L. Signal transduction pathways of acupuncture for treating some nervous system diseases. *Evid. Based Complement. Altern. Med.* **2019**, *2019*, 2909632. [CrossRef] [PubMed]
70. Fang, J.Q.; Zhu, S.X.; Zhang, Y.; Wang, F.; Zhu, Q.Y. Effects of transcutaneous electrostimulation of auricular points on behavior and hippocampal IL-1 β and TNF-α expression in temporal lobe epilepsy rats. *Acupunct. Res.* **2016**, *41*, 283–290.
71. Ding, X.; Yu, J.; Yu, T.; Fu, Y.; Han, J. Acupuncture regulates the aging-related changes in gene profile expression of the hippocampus in senescence-accelerated mouse (SAMP10). *Neurosci. Lett.* **2006**, *399*, 11–16. [CrossRef]
72. Zhang, M.; Xv, G.; Wang, W.; Meng, D.; Ji, Y. Electroacupuncture improves cognitive deficits and activates PPAR-γ in a rat model of Alzheimer's disease. *Acupunct. Med.* **2017**, *35*, 44–51. [CrossRef]
73. Jia, Y.; Zhang, X.; Yu, J.; Han, J.; Yu, T.; Shi, J.; Zhao, L.; Nie, K. Acupuncture for patients with mild to moderate Alzheimer's disease: A randomized controlled trial. *BMC Complement Altern. Med.* **2017**, *17*, 556. [CrossRef]
74. Zhou, S.; Dong, L.; He, Y.; Xiao, H. Acupuncture plus herbal medicine for Alzheimer's disease: A systematic review and meta-analysis. *Am. J. Chin. Med.* **2017**, *45*, 1327–1344. [CrossRef]
75. Zhu, W.; Wang, X.; Du, S.; Yan, C.; Yang, N.; Lin, L.; Shi, G.; Liu, C. Anti-oxidative and anti-apoptotic effects of acupuncture: Role of thioredoxin-1 in the hippocampus of vascular dementia rats. *Neuroscience* **2018**, *379*, 281–291. [CrossRef]
76. Wang, S.; Fang, J.; Ma, J.; Wang, Y.; Zeng, X.; Zhou, D.; Sun, G. Influence of electroacupuncture on p38-mitogen activated protein kinase in substantia nigra cells of rats with Parkinson disease model. *Zhongguo Zhen Jiu* **2013**, *33*, 329–333. [PubMed]

77. Krens, S.F.; Spaink, H.P.; Snaar-Jagalska, B. Functions of the MAPK family in vertebrate-development. *FEBS Lett.* **2006**, *580*, 4984–4990. [CrossRef] [PubMed]
78. Roux, P.P.; Blenis, J. ERK and p38 MAPK-activated protein kinases: A family of protein kinases with diverse biological functions. *Microbiol. Mol. Biol. Rev.* **2004**, *68*, 320–344. [CrossRef]
79. Ajibade, A.A.; Wang, Q. TAK1 negatively regulates NF-kappaB and p38 MAP kinase activation in Gr-1+CD11b+ neutrophils. *Immunity* **2012**, *36*, 43–54. [CrossRef] [PubMed]
80. Brand, S. Crohn's disease: Th1, Th17 or both? The change of a paradigm: New immunological and genetic insights implicate Th17 cells in the pathogenesis of Crohn's disease. *Gut* **2009**, *58*, 1152–1167. [CrossRef]
81. Hannigan, M.; Zhan, L. The role of p38 MAP kinase in TGF-beta1-induced signal transduction in human neutrophils. *Biochem. Biophys. Res. Commun.* **1998**, *346*, 55–58. [CrossRef]
82. Heineke, J.; Molkentin, J.D. Regulation of cardiac hypertrophy by intracellular signalling pathways. *Nat. Rev. Mol. Cell Biol.* **2006**, *77*, 589–600. [CrossRef]
83. Shiojima, I.; Walsh, K. Regulation of cardiac growth and coronary angiogenesis by the Akt/PKB signaling pathway. *Genes Dev.* **2006**, *20*, 3347–3365. [CrossRef]
84. Shioi, T.; Kang, P.M. The conserved phosphoinositide 3-kinase pathway determines heart size in mice. *EMBO J.* **2000**, *19*, 2537–2548. [CrossRef]
85. Tanike, M.; Yamaguchi, O. Apoptosis signal-regulating kinase 1/p38 signaling pathway negatively regulates physiological hypertrophy. *Circulation* **2008**, *117*, 545–552. [CrossRef] [PubMed]
86. Solinas, G.; Becattini, B. JNK at the crossroad of obesity, insulin resistance, and cell stress response. *Mol. Metab.* **2017**, *6*, 174–184. [CrossRef] [PubMed]
87. Hotamisligil, G.S.; Davis, R.J. Cell Signaling and Stress Responses. *Cold Spring Harb. Perspect. Biol.* **2016**, *8*. [CrossRef]
88. Ning, C.; Wang, X. Chicory inulin ameliorates type 2 diabetes mellitus and suppresses JNK and MAPK pathways in vivo and in vitro. *Mol. Nutr. Food Res.* **2017**, *61*. [CrossRef]
89. Koh, A.; Molinaro, A. Microbially produced imidazole propionate impairs insulin signaling through mTORC1. *Cell* **2018**, *175*, 947–961.e17. [CrossRef] [PubMed]
90. Eagleton, M.J. Inflammation in abdominal aortic aneurysms: Cellular infiltrate and cytokine profiles. *Vascular* **2012**, *20*, 278–283. [CrossRef] [PubMed]
91. Abdul-Hussien, H.; Soekhoe, R.G. Collagen degradation in the abdominal aneurysm: A conspiracy of matrixmetalloproteinase and cysteine collagenases. *Am. J. Pathol.* **2007**, *170*, 809–817. [CrossRef]
92. Saratzis, A.; Abbas, A.A. Abdominal aortic aneurysm: A review of the genetic basis. *Angiology* **2011**, *62*, 18–32. [CrossRef]
93. Saratzis, A.; Kitas, G.D. Can statins suppress the development of abdominal aortic aneurysms? A review of the current evidence. *Angiology* **2010**, *61*, 137–144. [CrossRef]
94. Papalambros, E.; Sigala, F. Immunohistochemical expression of metalloproteinases MMP-2 and MMP-9 in abdominal aortic aneurysms: Correlation with symptoms and aortic diameter. *Int. J. Mol. Med.* **2003**, *12*, 965–968. [CrossRef]
95. Petersen, E.; Gineitis, A. Activity of matrix metalloproteinase-2 and -9 in abdominal aortic aneurysms. Relation to size and rupture. *Eur. J. Vasc. Endovasc. Surg.* **2000**, *20*, 457–461. [CrossRef] [PubMed]
96. Yang, C.Q.; Li, W. MCP-1 Stimulates MMP-9 expression via ERK 1/2 and p38 MAPK signaling pathways in human aortic smooth muscle cells. *Cell Physiol. Biochem.* **2014**, *34*, 266–276. [CrossRef] [PubMed]
97. Sun, Y.; Ma, C. Metabolism: A Novel Shared Link between Diabetes Mellitus and Alzheimer's Disease. *J. Diabetes Res.* **2020**, *2020*, 4981814. [CrossRef]
98. Kyriskis, J.M.; Avruch, J. Mammalian mitogen-activated protein kinase signal transduction pathways activated by stress and inflammation. *Am. J. Physiol.* **2001**, *81*, 808–869. [CrossRef]
99. Lang, E.; Bissinger, R.; Qadri, S.M.; Lang, F. Suicidal death of erythrocytes in cancer and its chemotherapy: A potential target in the treatment of tumor-associated anemia. *Int. J. Cancer* **2017**, *141*, 1522–1528. [CrossRef]
100. Brancho, D.; Tanaka, N.; Jaeschke, A.; Ventura, J.-J.; Kelkar, N.; Tanaka, Y.; Kyuuma, M.; Takeshita, T.; Flavell, R.A.; Davis, R.J. Mechanism of p38 MAP kinase activation in vivo. *Genes Dev.* **2003**, *17*, 1969–1978. [CrossRef]
101. Krishna, M.; Narang, H. The complexity of mitogen-activated protein kinases (MAPKs) made simple. *Cell Mol. Life Sci.* **2008**, *65*, 3525–3544. [CrossRef] [PubMed]

102. Bardwell, L. Mechanisms of MAPK signalling specificity. *Biochem. Soc. Trans.* **2006**, *34*, 837–841. [CrossRef]
103. Akella, R.; Moon, T.M.; Goldsmith, E.J. Unique MAP kinase binding sites. *Biochim. Biophys. Acta* **2008**, *1784*, 48–55. [CrossRef]
104. Cuadrado, A.; Nebreda, A.R. Mechanisms and functions of p38 MAPK signalling. *Biochim. J.* **2010**, *429*, 403–417. [CrossRef]
105. Bonney, E.A. Mapping out p38MAPK. *Am. J. Reporod. Immunol.* **2017**, *77*. [CrossRef]
106. Wang, S.; Ding, L.; Ji, H.; Xu, Z.; Liu, Q.; Zheng, Y. The role of p38 MAPK in the development of diabetic cardiomyopathy. *Int. J. Mol. Sci.* **2016**, *17*, 1037. [CrossRef] [PubMed]
107. Chang, C.I.; Xu, B.E.; Cobb, M.H.; Goldsmith, E.J. Crystal structures of MAP kinase p38 complexed to the docking sites on its nuclear substrate MEF2A and activator MKK3b. *Mol. Cell* **2002**, *9*, 1241–1249. [CrossRef]
108. O'Callaghan, C.; Fanning, L.J.; Barry, O.P. p38δ MAPK: Emerging Roles of a Neglected Isoform. *Int. J. Cell Biol.* **2014**, *2014*, 272689. [CrossRef] [PubMed]
109. Sabio, G.; Arthur, J.S.C.; Kuma, Y.; Peggie, M.; Carr, J.; Murray-Tait, V.; Centeno, F.; Goedert, M.; Morrice, N.A.; Cuenda, A. p38γ regulates the localisation of SAP97 in the cytoskeleton by modulating its interaction with GKAP. *EMBO J.* **2005**, *24*, 1134–1145. [CrossRef]
110. Parker, C.G.; Hunt, J.; Diener, K.; McGinley, M.; Soriano, B.; Keesler, G.A.; Bray, J.; Yao, Z.; Wang, X.S.; Kohno, T.; et al. Identification of stathmin as a novel substrate for p38 Delta. *Biochem. Biophys. Res. Commun.* **1998**, *249*, 791–796. [CrossRef]
111. Rubin, C.I.; Atweh, G.F. The role of stathmin in the regulation of the cell cycle. *J. Cell Biochem.* **2004**, *93*, 242–250. [CrossRef]
112. Knebel, A.; Morrice, N.; Cohen, P. A novel method to identify protein kinase substrates: eEF2 kinase is phosphorylated and inhibited by SAPK4/p38δ. *EMBO J.* **2001**, *20*, 4360–4369. [CrossRef] [PubMed]
113. Goedert, M.; Hasegawa, M.; Jakes, R.; Lawler, S.; Cuenda, A.; Cohen, P. Phosphorylation of microtubule-associated protein tau by stress-activated protein kinases. *FEBS Lett.* **1997**, *409*, 57–62. [CrossRef]
114. Masuda, K.; Shima, H.; Watanabe, M.; Kikuchi, K. MKP-7, a novel mitogen-activated protein kinase phosphatase, functions as a shuttle protein. *J. Biol. Chem.* **2001**, *276*, 39002–39011. [CrossRef]
115. Kumar, G.S.; Clarkson, M.W.; Kunze, M.B.A.; Granata, D.; Wand, A.J.; Lindorff-Larsen, K.; Page, R.; Peti, W. Dynamic activation and regulation of the mitogen-activated protein kinase p38. *Proc. Natl. Acad. Sci. USA* **2018**, *115*, 4655–4660. [CrossRef]
116. Cuenda, A.; Rousseau, S. p38 MAP-Kinases pathway regulation, function and role in human disease. *Biochim. Biophys. Acta* **2007**, *1773*, 1358–1375. [CrossRef] [PubMed]
117. Wang, X.; McGowan, C.H.; He, L.; Downey, J.S.; Fearns, C.; Wang, Y.; Huang, S.; Han, J. Involvement of the MKK6-p38gamma cascade in gamma-radiation-induced cell cycle arrest. *Mol. Cell Biol.* **2000**, *20*, 4543–4552. [CrossRef]
118. Zhu, K.Q.; Zhang, S.J. Involvement of ATM/ATR-p38 MAPK cascade in MNNG induced G1-S arrest. *World J. Gastroenterol.* **2003**, *9*, 2073–2077. [CrossRef]
119. Tang, J.; Qi, X.; Mercola, D.; Han, J.; Chen, G. Essential role of p38gamma in K-Ras transformation independent of phosphorylation. *J. Biol. Chem.* **2005**, *280*, 23910–23917. [CrossRef] [PubMed]
120. Puri, P.L.; Wu, Z.; Zhang, P.; Wood, L.D.; Bhakta, K.S.; Han, J.; Feramisco, J.R.; Karin, M.; Wang, J.Y. Induction of terminal differentiation by constitutive activation of p38 MAP kinase in human rhabdomyosarcoma cells. *Genes Dev.* **2000**, *14*, 574–584. [PubMed]
121. Campbell, R.M.; Anderson, B.D.; Brooks, N.A.; Brooks, H.B.; Chan, E.M.; De Dios, A.; Gilmour, R.; Graff, J.R.; Jambrina, E.; Mader, M.; et al. Characterization of LY2228820 dimesylate, a potent and selective inhibitor of p38 MAPK with antitumor activity. *Mol. Cancer* **2014**, *13*, 364–374. [CrossRef]
122. Maimon, A.; Mogilevsky, M.; Shilo, A.; Golan-Gerstl, R.; Obiedat, A.; Ben-Hur, V.; Lebenthal-Loinger, I.; Stein, I.; Reich, R.; Beenstock, J.; et al. Mnk2 alternative splicing modulates the p38-MAPK pathway and impacts Ras-induced transformation. *Cell Rep.* **2014**, *7*, 501–513. [CrossRef] [PubMed]
123. Azijli, K.; Yuvaraj, S.; van Roosmalen, I.; Flach, K.; Giovannetti, E.; Peters, G.J.; de Jong, S.; Kruyt, F.A. MAPK p38 and JNK have opposing activities on TRAIL-induced apoptosis activation in NSCLC H460 cells that involves RIP1 and caspase-8 and is mediated by Mcl-1. *Apoptosis* **2013**, *18*, 851–860. [CrossRef] [PubMed]
124. Yuan, J.; Rozengurt, E. PKD, PKD2, and p38 MAPK mediate Hsp27 Serine-82 phosphorylation induced by neurotensin in pancreatic cancer PANC-1 cells. *J. Cell Biochem.* **2008**, *103*, 648–662. [CrossRef]

125. Cánovas, B.; Igea, A.; Sartori, A.A.; Gomis, R.R.; Paull, T.T.; Isoda, M.; Pérez-Montoyo, H.; Serra, V.; González-Suárez, E.; Stracker, T.H.; et al. Targeting p38alpha increases DNA damage, chromosome instability, and the anti-tumoral response to taxanes in breast cancer cells. *Cancer Cell* **2018**, *33*, 1094–1110.e8. [CrossRef] [PubMed]
126. Junttila, M.R.; Ala-aho, R.; Jokilehto, T.; Peltonen, J.; Kallajoki, M.; Grenman, R.; Jaakkola, P.; Westermarck, J.; Kähäri, V.-M. p38α and p38δ mitogen-activated protein kinase isoforms regulate invasion and growth of head and neck squamous carcinoma cells. *Oncogene* **2007**, *26*, 5267–5279. [CrossRef] [PubMed]
127. Ringshausen, I.; Dechow, T.; Schneller, F.; Weick, K.; Oelsner, M.; Peschel, C.; Decker, T. Constitutive activation of the MAPkinase p38 is critical for MMP-9 production and survival of B-CLL cells on bone marrow stromal cells. *Leukemia* **2004**, *18*, 1964–1970. [CrossRef] [PubMed]
128. Gao, N.; Jiang, B.H.; Leonard, S.S.; Corum, L.; Zhang, Z.; Roberts, J.R.; Antonini, J.; Zheng, J.Z.; Flynn, D.C.; Castranova, V.; et al. p38 signaling-mediated hypoxia-inducible factor 1alpha and vascular endothelial growth factor induction by Cr(VI) in DU145 human prostate carcinoma cells. *J. Biol. Chem.* **2002**, *277*, 45041–45048. [CrossRef]
129. Kim, E.S.; Sohn, Y.W.; Moon, A. TGF-beta-induced transcriptional activation of MMP-2 is mediated by activating transcription factor (ATF)2 in human breast epithelial cells. *Cancer Lett.* **2007**, *252*, 147–156. [CrossRef]
130. Hong, I.K.; Kim, Y.M.; Jeoung, D.I.; Kim, K.C.; Lee, H. Tetraspanin CD9 induces MMP-2 expression by activating p38 MAPK, JNK and c-Jun pathways in human melanoma cells. *Exp. Mol. Med.* **2005**, *37*, 230–239. [CrossRef] [PubMed]
131. Villa-Diaz, L.G.; Miyano, T. Activation of p38 MAPK during porcine oocyte maturation. *Biol. Reprod.* **2004**, *71*, 691–696. [CrossRef]
132. Lu, H.T.; Yang, D.D.; Wysk, M.; Gatti, E.; Mellman, I.; Davis, R.J.; Flavell, R.A. Defective IL-12 production in mitogen-activated protein (MAP) kinase kinase 3 (Mkk3)-deficient mice. *EMBO J.* **1999**, *18*, 1845–1857. [CrossRef]
133. Tanaka, N.; Kamanaka, M.; Enslen, H.; Dong, C.; Wysk, M.; Davis, R.J.; Flavelle, R.A. Differential involvement of p38 mitogen-activated protein kinase kinases MKK3 and MKK6 in T-cell apoptosis. *EMBO Rep.* **2002**, *3*, 785–791. [CrossRef]
134. Menon, M.B.; Gaestel, M. TPL2 meets p38MAPK: Emergence of a novel positive feedback loop in inflammation. *Biochem. J.* **2016**, *473*, 2995–2999. [CrossRef]
135. Xu, D.; Matsumoto, M.L.; MacKenzie, B.S.; Zarrin, A.A. TPL2 kinase action and control of inflammation. *Pharm. Res.* **2018**, *129*, 188–193. [CrossRef] [PubMed]
136. Liu, J.; Han, L.; Li, B.; Yang, J.; Huen, M.S.Y.; Pan, X.; Tsao, S.W.; Cheung, A.L.M. F-box only protein 31 (FBXO31) negatively regulates p38 mitogen-activated protein kinase (MAPK) signaling by mediating lysine 48-linked ubiquitination and degradation of mitogen-activated protein kinase kinase 6 (MKK6). *J. Biol. Chem.* **2014**, *289*, 21508–21518. [CrossRef] [PubMed]
137. Tanno, M.; Bassi, R. Diverse mechanisms of myocardial p38 mitogen-activated protein kinase activation: Evidence for MKK-independent activation by a TAB1-associated mechanism contributing to injury during myocardial ischemia. *Circ. Res.* **2003**, *93*, 254–261. [CrossRef] [PubMed]
138. Amantini, C.; Mosca, M.; Nabissi, M.; Lucciarini, R.; Caprodossi, S.; Arcella, A.; Giangaspero, F.; Santoni, G. Capsaicin-induced apoptosis of glioma cells is mediated by TRPV1 vanilloid receptor and requires p38 MAPK activation. *J. Neurochem.* **2007**, *102*, 977–990. [CrossRef]
139. Marrone, M.C.; Morabito, A.; Giustizieri, M.; Chiurchiù, V.; Leuti, A.; Mattioli, M.; Marinelli, S.; Riganti, L.; Lombardi, M.; Murana, E.; et al. TRPV1 channels are critical brain inflammation detectors and neuropathic pain biomarkers in mice. *Nat. Commun.* **2017**, *8*, 15292. [CrossRef]
140. Surowy, C.S.; Kym, P.R.; Reilly, R.M. Biochemical Pharmacology of TRPV1: Molecular intergrator of pain signals. In *Vanilloid Receptor TRPV1 in Drug Discovery: Targeting Pain and other Pathological Disorders*, 2nd ed.; Gomtsyan, A., Faltynek, C.R., Eds.; John Wiley & Sons, Inc.: Hoboken, NJ, USA, 2010; pp. 119–120.
141. Bianco, F.; Perrotta, C.; Novellino, L.; Francolini, M.; Riganti, L.; Menna, E.; Saglietti, L.; Schuchman, E.H.; Furlan, R.; Clementi, E.; et al. Acid sphingomyelinase activity triggers microparticle release from glial cells. *EMBO J.* **2009**, *28*, 1043–1054. [CrossRef]

142. Suter, M.R.; Berta, T.; Gao, Y.J.; Decosterd, I.; Ji, R.R. Large A-Fiber activity is required for microglial proliferation and p38 MAPK activation in the spinal cord: Different effects of resiniferatoxin and bupivacaine on spinal microglial changes after spared nerve injury. *Mol. Pain* **2009**, *5*, 53. [CrossRef]
143. Liao, H.Y.; Hsieh, C.L.; Huang, C.P. Electroacupuncture Attenuates CFA-induced Inflammatory Pain by suppressing Nav1.8 through S100B, TRPV1, Opioid, and Adenosine Pathways in Mice. *Sci. Rep.* **2017**, *13*, 42531. [CrossRef]
144. Zhou, T.T.; Wu, J.R.; Chen, Z.Y.; Liu, Z.X.; Miao, B. Effects of dexmedetomidine on P2X4Rs, p38-MAPK and BDNF in spinal microglia in rats with spared nerve injury. *Brain Res.* **2014**, *1568*, 21–30. [CrossRef]
145. Keller, A.F.; Beggs, S.; Salter, M.W.; De Koninck, Y. Transformation of the output of spinal lamina I neurons after nerve injury and microglia stimulation underlying neuropathic pain. *Mol. Pain.* **2007**, *3*, 27. [CrossRef] [PubMed]
146. Liang, J.; Deng, G.; Huang, H. The activation of BDNF reduced inflammation in a spinal cord injury model by TrkB/p38 MAPK signaling. *Exp. Med.* **2019**, *17*, 1688–1696. [CrossRef] [PubMed]
147. Cheng, C.Y.; Lin, J.G.; Su, S.Y.; Tang, N.Y.; Kao, S.T.; Hsieh, C.L. Electroacupuncture-like stimulation at Baihui and Dazhui acupoints exerts neuroprotective effects through activation of the brain-derived neurotrophic factor-mediated MEK1/2/ERK1/2/p90RSK/bad signaling pathway in mild transient focal cerebral ischemia in rats. *BMC Complement Altern. Med.* **2014**, *14*, 92. [CrossRef]
148. Schmidt, C.E.; Shastri, V.R.; Vacanti, J.P.; Langer, R. Stimulation of neurite outgrowth using an electrically conducting polymer. *Proc. Natl. Acad. Sci. USA* **1997**, *94*, 8948–8953. [CrossRef] [PubMed]
149. Jaffe, L.F.; Poo, M.M. Neurites grow faster towards the cathode than the anode in a steady field. *J. Exp. Zool.* **1979**, *209*, 115–128. [CrossRef] [PubMed]
150. Patel, N.; Poo, M.M. Orientation of neurite growth by extracellular electric fields. *J. Neurosci.* **1982**, *2*, 483–496. [CrossRef]
151. Kerns, J.M.; Fakhouri, A.J.; Weinrib, H.P.; Freeman, J.A. Electrical stimulation of nerve regeneration in the rat: The early effects evaluated by a vibrating probe and electron microscopy. *Neuroscience* **1991**, *40*, 93–107. [CrossRef]
152. Kerns, J.M.; Lucchinetti, C. Electrical field effects on crushed nerve regeneration. *Exp. Neurol.* **1991**, *117*, 71–80. [CrossRef]
153. Todorov, A.T.; Yogev, D.; Qi, P.; Fendler, J.H.; Rodziewicz, G.S. Electric-field-induced reconnection of severed axons. *Brain. Res.* **1992**, *582*, 329–334. [CrossRef]
154. Pomeranz, B.; Campbell, J.J. Weak electric current accelerates motoneuron regeneration in the sciatic nerve of ten-month-old rats. *Brain. Res.* **1993**, *603*, 271–278. [CrossRef]
155. Chen, Y.S.; Hu, C.L.; Hsieh, C.L.; Lin, J.G.; Tsai, C.C.; Chen, T.H.; Yao, C.H. Effects of percutaneous electrical stimulation on peripheral nerve regeneration using silicone rubber chambers. *J. Biomed. Mater. Res.* **2001**, *57*, 541–549. [CrossRef]
156. Chen, Y.S.; Hsieh, C.L.; Tsai, C.C.; Chen, T.H.; Cheng, W.C.; Hu, C.L.; Yao, C.H. Increased success of peripheral nerve regeneration using silicone rubber chambers filled with an extracellular gel containing collagen, laminin and fibronectin. *Biomaterials* **2000**, *21*, 1541–1547. [CrossRef]
157. Greer, R.; Daniel, J.; Uemura, E.; Kudej, R.; Chen, Y.S.; Chung, C.H. Use of a multiple lumen cuff for nerve regeneration. *Mat. Res. Soc. Symp. Proc.* **1994**, *331*, 3–11. [CrossRef]
158. Chen, Y.S.; Miller, C.; Greer, M.H.; Quinones, M.; Greer, R.T. Development of a multiple-lumen nerve cuff utilizing growth stimulant patterns for controlled regeneration. *Mat. Res. Soc. Symp. Proc.* **1999**, *550*, 303–312. [CrossRef]
159. Zhang, R.; Lao, L.; Ren, K.; Berman, B.M. Mechanisms of acupuncture-electroacupuncture on persistent pain. *Anesthesiology* **2014**, *120*, 482–503. [CrossRef] [PubMed]
160. Silva, J.R.T.; Silva, M.L.; Prado, W.A. Analgesia induced by 2- or 100-Hz electroacupuncture in the rat tail-flick test depends on the activation of different descending pain inhibitory mechanisms. *J. Pain* **2011**, *12*, 51–60. [CrossRef] [PubMed]
161. Wang, Q.; Wang, F.; Li, X.; Yang, Q.; Li, X.; Xu, N.; Huang, Y.; Zhang, Q.; Gou, X.; Chen, S.; et al. Electroacupuncture pretreatment attenuates cerebral ischemic injury through α7 nicotinic acetylcholine receptor-mediated inhibition of high-mobility group box 1 release in rats. *J. Neuroinflammation* **2012**, *9*, 24. [CrossRef]

162. Cheng, C.Y.; Lin, J.G.; Tang, N.Y.; Kao, S.T.; Hsieh, C.L. Electroacupuncture-like stimulation at the Baihui (GV20) and Dazhui (GV14) acupoints protects rats against subacute-phase cerebral ischemia-reperfusion injuries by reducing S100B-mediated neurotoxicity. *PLoS ONE* **2014**, *9*, e91426. [CrossRef]
163. Chen, H.C.; Chen, M.Y.; Hsieh, C.L.; Wu, S.Y.; Hsu, H.C.; Lin, Y.W. TRPV1 is a responding channel for acupuncture manipulation in mice peripheral and central nerve system. *Cell. Physiol. Biochem.* **2018**, *49*, 1813–1824. [CrossRef]
164. Ashwell, J. The many paths to p38 mitogen-activated protein kinase activation in the immune system. *Nat. Rev. Immunol.* **2006**, *6*, 532–540. [CrossRef]
165. Zhang, C.N.; Rahimnejad, S. Molecular characterization of p38 MAPK from blunt snout bream (*Megalobrama amblycephala*) and its expression after ammonia stress, and lipoplysaccaride and bacterial challenge. *Fish Shellfish Immunol.* **2019**, *84*, 848–856. [CrossRef]
166. Sreekanth, G.P.; Chuncharunee, A. SB203580 modulates p38 MAPK signaling and Dengue virus-induced liver injury by reducing MAPKAPK2, HSP27, and ATF2 phosporylation. *PLoS ONE* **2016**, *11*, e0149486. [CrossRef] [PubMed]
167. Beardmore, V.A.; Hinton, H.J. Generation and characterization of p38beta (MAPK11) gene-targeted mice. *Mol. Cell Biol.* **2005**, *25*, 10454–10464. [CrossRef] [PubMed]
168. Cheng, J.; Ji, R. Intracellular Signaling in Primary Sensory Neurons and Persistent Pain. *Neurochem. Res.* **2008**, *33*, 1970–1978. [CrossRef] [PubMed]
169. Mizukoshi, K.; Sasakia, M.; Izumia, Y.; Miuraa, M.; Watanabe, M.; Amaya, F. Activation of p38 mitogen-activated protein kinase in the dorsal root ganglion contributes to pain hypersensitivity after plantar incision. *Neuroscience* **2013**, *234*, 77–87. [CrossRef]
170. Tsuda, M. Microglia in the spinal cord and neuropathic pain. *J. Diabetes Investig.* **2016**, *7*, 17–26. [CrossRef]
171. Suzuki, N.; Hasegawa-Moriyama, M. Lidocaine attenuates the development of diabetic-induced tactile allodynia by inhibiting microglial activation. *Anesth. Analg.* **2011**, *113*, 941–946. [CrossRef]
172. Cheng, K.I.; Wang, H.C. Persistent mechanical allodynia positively correlates with an increase in activated microglia and increased P-p38 mitogen-activated protein kinase activation in streptozotocin-induced diabetic rats. *Eur. J. Pain* **2014**, *18*, 162–173. [CrossRef]
173. Hsu, H.C.; Yang, N.Y.; Lin, Y.W.; Ki, T.C.; Liu, H.J.; Hsieh, C.L. Effect of electroacupuncture on rats with chronic constriction injury-Induced neuropathic pain. *Sci. World J.* **2014**, *2014*, 129875. [CrossRef]
174. Jiang, S.W.; Lin, Y.W.; Hsieh, C.L. Electroacupuncture at Hua Tuo Jia Ji acupoints reduced neuropathic pain and increased $GABA_A$ receptors in rat spinal cord. *Evid. Based Complement Altern. Med.* **2018**, *2018*, 8041820. [CrossRef]
175. Huang, C.P.; Lin, Y.W.; Lee, D.Y.; Hsieh, C.L. Electroacupuncture relieves CCI-induced neuropathic pain involving excitatory and inhibitory neurotransmitters. *Evid. Based Complement Altern. Med.* **2019**, *2019*, 6784735. [CrossRef]
176. Lin, J.G.; Lo, M.W.; Wen, Y.R.; Hsieh, C.L.; Tsai, S.K.; Sun, W.Z. The effect of high and low frequency electroacupuncture in pain after lower abdominal surgery. *Pain* **2002**, *99*, 509–514. [CrossRef]
177. Wang, B.; Tang, J.; White, P.F.; Naruse, R.; Sloninsky, A.; Kariger, R.; Gold, J.; Wender, R.H. Effect of the intensity of transcutaneous acupoint electrical stimulation on the postoperative analgesic requirement. *Anesth. Analg.* **1997**, *85*, 406–413. [PubMed]
178. Chen, W.H.; Hsieh, C.L.; Huang, C.P.; Lin, T.J.; Tzen, J.T.C.; Ho, T.Y.; Lin, Y.W. Acid-sensing ion channel 3 mediates peripheral anti-hyperalgesia effects of acupuncture in mice inflammatory pain. *J. Biomed. Sci.* **2011**, *18*, 82. [CrossRef] [PubMed]
179. Chen, W.H.; Tzen, J.T.C.; Hsieh, C.L.; Chen, Y.H.; Lin, T.J.; Chen, S.Y.; Lin, Y.W. Attenuation of TRPV1 and TRPV4 expression and function in mouse inflammatory pain models using electroacupuncture. *J. Biomed. Sci.* **2012**, *2012*. [CrossRef]
180. Huang, C.P.; Chen, H.N.; Su, H.L.; Hsieh, C.L.; Chen, W.H.; Lai, Z.R.; Lin, Y.W. Electroacupuncture reduces carrageenan- and CFA-induced inflammatory pain accompanied by changing the expression of Nav1.7 and Nav1.8, rather than Nav1.9, in mice dorsal root ganglia. *Evid. Based Complement Altern. Med.* **2013**, *2013*, 312184. [CrossRef]
181. Wu, S.Y.; Chen, W.H.; Hsueh, C.H.; Lin, Y.W. Abundant expression and functional participation of TRPV1 at Zusanli acupoint (ST36) in mice: Mechanosensitive TRPV1 as an acupuncture-responding channel. *BMC Complement Altern. Med.* **2014**, *14*, 96. [CrossRef]

182. Lu, K.W.; Hsu, C.K.; Hsieh, C.L.; Yang, J.; Lin, Y.W. Probing the effects and mechanisms of electroacupuncture at ipsilateral or contralateral ST36-ST37 acupoints on CFA-induced inflammatory pain. *Sci. Rep.* **2016**, *24*, 22123. [CrossRef]
183. Liao, H.Y.; Hsieh, C.L.; Huang, C.P.; Lin, Y.W. Electroacupuncture attenuates induction of inflammatory pain by regulating opioid and adenosine pathways in mice. *Sci. Rep.* **2017**, *7*, 15679. [CrossRef]
184. Yang, J.; Hsieh, C.L.; Lin, Y.W. Role of transient receptor potential vanilloid 1 in electroacupuncture analgesia on chronic inflammatory pain in mice. *Biomed Res. Int.* **2017**, *2017*, 5068347. [CrossRef]
185. Yen, C.M.; Wu, T.C.; Hsieh, C.L.; Huang, Y.W.; Lin, Y.W. Distal electroacupuncture at the LI4 acupoint reduces CFA-induced inflammatory pain via the brain TRPV1 signaling pathway. *Int. J. Mol. Sci.* **2019**, *20*, 4471. [CrossRef]
186. Hsu, H.C.; Hsieh, C.L.; Wu, S.Y.; Lin, Y.W. Toll-like receptor 2 plays an essential role in electroacupuncture analgesia in a mouse model of inflammatory pain. *Acupunct. Med.* **2019**, *37*, 356–364. [CrossRef] [PubMed]
187. Yang, C.P.; Hsieh, C.L.; Wang, N.H.; Li, T.C.; Hwang, K.L.; Yu, S.C.; Chang, M.H. Acupuncture in patients with carpal tunnel syndrome: A randomized controlled trial. *Clin. J. Pain.* **2009**, *25*, 327–333. [CrossRef] [PubMed]
188. Yang, C.P.; Wang, N.H.; Li, T.C.; Hsieh, C.L.; Chang, H.H.; Hwang, K.L.; Ko, W.S.; Chang, M.H. A randomized clinical trial of acupuncture versus oral steroids for carpal tunnel syndrome: A long-term follow-up. *J. Pain* **2011**, *12*, 272–279. [CrossRef] [PubMed]
189. Yang, C.P.; Chang, M.H.; Liu, P.E.; Li, T.C.; Hsieh, C.L.; Hwang, K.L.; Chang, H.H. Acupuncture versus topiramate in chronic migraine prophylaxis: A randomized clinical trial. *Cephalalgia* **2011**, *31*, 1510–1521. [CrossRef]
190. Walder, R.Y.; Rasmussen, L.A.; Rainier, J.D.; Light, A.R.; Wemmie, J.A.; Sluka, K.A. ASIC1 and ASIC3 play different roles in the development of hyperalgesia after inflammatory muscle injury. *J. Pain* **2010**, *11*, 210–218. [CrossRef]
191. Black, J.A.; Liu, S.; Tanaka, M.; Cummins, T.R.; Waxman, S.G. Changes in the expression of tetrodotoxin-sensitive sodium channels within dorsal root ganglia neurons in inflammatory pain. *Pain* **2004**, *108*, 237–247. [CrossRef]
192. Yu, L.; Yang, F.; Luo, H.; Liu, F.Y.; Han, J.S.; Xing, G.G.; Wan, Y. The role of TRPV1 in different subtypes of dorsal root ganglion neurons in rat chronic inflammatory nociception induced by complete Freund's adjuvant. *Mol. Pain* **2008**, *4*, 61. [CrossRef]
193. Goldman, N.; Chen, M.; Fujita, T.; Xu, Q.; Peng, W.; Liu, W.; Jensen, T.; Pei, Y.; Wang, F.; Han, X.; et al. Adenosine A1 receptors mediate local anti-nociceptive effects of acupuncture. *Nat. Neurosci.* **2010**, *13*, 883–888. [CrossRef]
194. Silberstein, S.D. Migraine pathophysiology and its clinical implications. *Cephalalgia* **2004**, *24* (Suppl. 2), 2–7. [CrossRef]
195. Burstein, R.; Noseda, R.; Borsook, D. Migraine: Multiple processes, complex pathophysiology. *J. Neurosci.* **2015**, *35*, 6619–6629. [CrossRef]
196. Sabino, G.S.; Santos, C.M.; Francischi, J.N.; de Resende, M.A. Release of endogenous opioids following transcutaneous electric nerve stimulation in an experimental model of acute inflammatory pain. *J. Pain* **2008**, *9*, 157–163. [CrossRef] [PubMed]
197. King, E.W.; Audette, K.; Athman, G.A.; Nguyen, H.O.; Sluka, K.A.; Fairbanks, C.A. Transcutaneous electrical nerve stimulation activates peripherally located alpha-2A adrenergic receptors. *Pain* **2005**, *115*, 364–373. [CrossRef] [PubMed]
198. Ainsworth, L.; Budelier, K.; Clinesmith, M.; Fiedler, A.; Landstrom, R.; Leeper, B.J.; Moeller, L.; Mutch, S.; O'Dell., K.; Ross, J.; et al. Transcutaneous electrical nerve stimulation (TENS) reduces chronic hyperalgesia induced by muscle inflammation. *Pain* **2006**, *120*, 182–187. [CrossRef]
199. Sekido, R.; Ishimaru, K.; Sakita, M. Differences of electroacupuncture-induced analgesic effect in normal and inflammatory conditions in rats. *Am. J. Chin. Med.* **2003**, *31*, 955–965. [CrossRef] [PubMed]
200. Zhao, W.; Liu, M.; Kirkwood, K.L. p38alpha stabilizes interleukin-6 mRNA via multiple AU-rich elements. *J. Biol. Chem.* **2008**, *283*, 1778–1785. [CrossRef] [PubMed]
201. Tudor, C.; Marchese, F.P. p38 mitogen-activated protein kinase inhibits tristetraprolin-directed decay of the mRNA of the anti-inflammatory cytokine interleukin-10. *FEBS Lett.* **2009**, *583*, 1933–1938. [CrossRef]

202. Berger, C.; von Kummer, R. Does NO regulate the cerebral blood flow response in hypoxia? *Acta Neurol. Scand.* **2009**, *97*, 118–125. [CrossRef]
203. Cheng, C.Y.; Lin, J.G.; Tang, N.Y.; Kao, S.T.; Hsieh, C.L. Electroacupuncture at different frequencies (5Hz and 25Hz) ameliorates cerebral ischemia-reperfusion injury in rats: Possible involvement of p38 MAPK-mediated anti-apoptotic signaling pathways. *BMC Complement Altern. Med.* **2015**, *15*, 241. [CrossRef]
204. Armstrong, S.C.; Delacey, M.; Ganote, C.E. Phosphorylation state of hsp27 and p38 MAPK during preconditioning and protein phosphatase inhibitor protection of rabbit cardiomyocytes. *J. Mol. Cell Cardiol.* **1999**, *31*, 555–567. [CrossRef]
205. Marais, E.; Genade, S.; Salie, R.; Huisamen, B.; Maritz, S.; Moolman, J.A.; Lochner, A. The temporal relationship between p38 MAPK and HSP 27 activation in ischaemic and pharmacological preconditioning. *Basic Res. Cardiol.* **2005**, *100*, 35–47. [CrossRef]
206. Fan, W.; Gao, X.K. Hsp70 interacts with mitogen-activated protein kinase (MAPK)-activated protein kinase 2 to regulate p38MAPK stability and myoblast differentiation during skeletal muscle regeneration. *Mol. Cell Biol.* **2018**, *38*. [CrossRef] [PubMed]
207. Chang, Q.Y.; Lin, Y.W.; Hsieh, C.L. Acupuncture and neuroregeneration in ischemic stroke. *Neural Regen. Res.* **2018**, *13*, 573–583. [CrossRef] [PubMed]
208. Xu, H.; Sun, H.; Chen, S.H.; Zhang, Y.M.; Piao, Y.L.; Gao, Y. Effects of acupuncture at Baihui (DU20) and Zusanli (ST36) on the expression of heat shock protein 70 and tumor necrosis factor α in the peripheral serum of cerebral ischemia-reperfusion-injured rats. *Chin. J. Integr. Med.* **2014**, *20*, 369–374. [CrossRef]
209. Dayalan Naidu, S.; Sutherland, C.; Zhang, Y.; Risco, A.; de la Vega, L.; Caunt, C.J.; Hastie, C.J.; Lamont, D.J.; Torrente, L.; Chowdhry, S.; et al. Heat Shock Factor 1 is a substrate for p38 mitogen-activated protein kinase. *J. Mol. Cell Biol.* **2016**, *36*, 2403–2417. [CrossRef] [PubMed]
210. Jin, X.; Qiao, A.; Moskophidis, D.; Mivechi, N.F. Modulation of Heat Shock Factor 1 Activity through Silencing of Ser303/Ser307 Phosphorylation Supports a Metabolic Program Leading to Age-Related Obesity and Insulin Resistance. *Mol. Cell Biol.* **2018**, *38*, e00095-18. [CrossRef] [PubMed]
211. Ni, H.; Wang, X.S. MAPKAPK5, a novel mitogen-activated protein kinase (MAPK)-activated protein kinase, is a substrate of the extracellular-regulated kinase (ERK) and p38 kinase. *Biochem. Biophys. Res. Comm.* **1998**, *243*, 492–496. [CrossRef]
212. Sahadevan, P.; Allen, B.G. MK5: A novel regulator of cardiac fibroblast function? *Iubmb Life* **2017**, *69*, 785–794. [CrossRef]
213. Shiryaev, A.; Moens, U. Mitogen-activated protein kinase p38 and MK2, MK3 and MK5: Ménage à trois or ménage à quatre. *Cell Signal.* **2010**, *22*, 1185–1192. [CrossRef]
214. Liu, C.H.; Lin, Y.W.; Tang, N.Y.; Liu, H.J.; Hsieh, C.L. Neuroprotective Effect of Uncaria rhynchophylla in kainic acid-induced epileptic seizures by modulating hippocampal mossy fiber sprouting, neuron survival, astrocyte proliferation, and S100B expression. *Evid. Based Complement Altern. Med.* **2012**, *2012*, 194790. [CrossRef]
215. Kim, S.T.; Jeon, S.; Park, H.J.; Hong, M.S.; Jeong, W.B.; Kim, J.H.; Kim, Y.; Lee, H.J.; Park, H.J.; Chung, J.H. Acupuncture inhibits kainic acid-induced hippocampal cell death in mice. *J. Physiol. Sci.* **2008**, *58*, 31–38. [CrossRef]
216. Kim, S.T.; Doo, A.R.; Kim, S.N.; Kim, S.Y.; Kim, Y.Y.; Kim, J.H.; Lee, H.; Yin, C.S.; Park, H.J. Acupuncture suppresses kainic acid-induced neuronal death and inflammatory events in mouse hippocampus. *J. Physiol. Sci.* **2012**, *62*, 377–383. [CrossRef] [PubMed]
217. Bae, C.H.; Kim, D.S.; Jun, Y.L.; Kwon, S.; Park, H.J.; Hahm, D.H.; Lee, H.; Kim, S.T. Proteomic analysis of the effect of acupuncture on the suppression of kainic acid-induced neuronal destruction in mouse hippocampus. *Evid. Based Complement Altern. Med.* **2013**, *2013*, 436315. [CrossRef] [PubMed]
218. Liu, C.H.; Lin, Y.W.; Hsu, H.C.; Liu, H.J.; Lin, W.J.; Hsieh, C.L. Electroacupuncture at ST36-ST37 and at ear ameliorates hippocampal mossy fiber sprouting in kainic acid-induced epileptic seizure rats. *Biomed Res. Int.* **2014**, *2014*, 756019. [CrossRef] [PubMed]
219. Hsu, H.C.; Tang, N.Y.; Liu, C.H.; Hsieh, C.L. Antiepileptic Effect of Uncaria rhynchophylla and Rhynchophylline involved in the initiation of c-Jun N-terminal kinase phosphorylation of MAPK signal pathways in acute seizures of kainic acid-treated rats. *Evid. Based Complement Altern. Med.* **2013**, *2013*, 961289. [CrossRef] [PubMed]

220. Lin, Y.W.; Hsieh, C.L. Auricular electroacupuncture reduced inflammation-related epilepsy accompanied by altered TRPA1, pPKCα, pPKCε, and pERk1/2 signaling pathways in kainic acid-treated rats. *Mediat. Inflamm.* **2014**, *2014*, 493480. [CrossRef]
221. Liao, E.T.; Tang, N.Y.; Lin, Y.W.; Hsieh, C.L. Long-term electrical stimulation at ear and electro-acupuncture at ST36-ST37 attenuated COX-2 in the CA1 of hippocampus in kainic acid-induced epileptic seizure rats. *Sci. Rep.* **2017**, *7*, 472. [CrossRef]
222. Inprasit, C.; Lin, Y.W.; Huang, C.P.; Wu, S.Y.; Hsieh, C.L. Targeting TRPV1 to relieve motion sickness symptoms in mice by electroacupuncture and gene deletion. *Sci. Rep.* **2018**, *8*, 10365. [CrossRef] [PubMed]
223. Maione, S.; Cristino, L.; Migliozzi, A.; Georgiou, A.; Starowicz, K.; Salt, T.; Marzo, V. TRPV1 channels control synaptic plasticity in the developing superior colliculus. *J. Physiol.* **2009**, *587*, 2521–2535. [CrossRef]
224. Puig, B.; Gomez-Isla, T. Expression of stress-activated kinases c-Jun N-terminal kinase (SAPK/JNK-P) and p38 kinase (p38-P), and tau hyperphosphorylation in neurites surrounding betaA plaques in APP Tg2576 mice. *Neuropathol. Appl. Neurobiol.* **2004**, *30*, 491–502. [CrossRef]
225. Risco, A.; Cuenda, A. New Insights into the p38γ and p38δ MAPK Pathways. *J. Signal Transduct.* **2012**, *2012*, 520289. [CrossRef]
226. Escós, A.; Risco, A. p38γ and p38δ Mitogen Activated Protein Kinases (MAPKs), New Stars in the MAPK Galaxy. *Front. Cell Dev. Biol.* **2016**, *4*, 31. [CrossRef]
227. Maphis, N.; Jiang, S. Selective suppression of the alpha isoform of p38 MAPK rescues late-stage tau pathology. *Alzheimers Res.* **2016**, *8*, 54. [CrossRef] [PubMed]
228. Lin, Y.W.; Hsieh, C.L. Electroacupuncture at Baihui acupoint (GV20) reverses behavior deficit and long-term potentiation through N-methyl-d-aspartate and transient receptor potential vanilloid subtype 1 receptors in middle cerebral artery occlusion rats. *J. Integr. Neurosci.* **2010**, *9*, 269–282. [CrossRef]
229. Dong, W.; Guo, W.; Zheng, X.; Wang, F.; Chen, Y.; Zhang, W.; Shi, H. Electroacupuncture improves cognitive deficits associated with AMPK activation in SAMP8 mice. *Metab. Brain Dis.* **2015**, *30*, 777–784. [CrossRef] [PubMed]
230. Song, J.J.; Lee, Y.J. Role of the ASK1-SEK1-JNK1- HIPK1 signal in Daxx trafficking and ASK1 oligomerization. *J. Biol. Chem.* **2003**, *278*, 47245–47252. [CrossRef] [PubMed]
231. Chang, H.Y.; Nishitoh, H.; Yang, X.; Ichijo, H.; Baltimore, D. Activation of apoptosis signal-regulating kinase 1 (ASK1) by the adapter protein Daxx. *Science* **1988**, *281*, 1860–1863. [CrossRef] [PubMed]
232. Akterin, S.; Cowburn, R.F.; Miranda-Vizuete, A.; Jimenez, A.; Bogdanovic, N.; Winblad, B.; Cedazo-Minguez, A. Involvement of glutaredoxin-1 and thioredoxin-1 in amyloid toxicity and Alzheimer's disease. *Cell Death Differ.* **2006**, *13*, 1454–1465. [CrossRef]
233. Takahashi-Niki, K.; Niki, T.; Taira, T.; Iguchi-Ariga, S.M.M.; Ariga, H. Reduced anti-oxidative stress activities of DJ-1 mutants found in Parkinson's disease patients. *Biochem. Biophys. Res. Commun.* **2004**, *320*, 389–397. [CrossRef]
234. Junn, E.; Taniguchi, H.; Jeong, B.S.; Zhao, X.; Ichijo, H.; Mouradian, M.M. Interaction of DJ-1 with Daxx inhibits apoptosis signal-regulating kinase 1 activity and cell death. *Proc. Natl. Acad. Sci. USA* **2005**, *102*, 9691–9696. [CrossRef]
235. Tang, J.; Liu, J.; Li, X.; Zhong, Y.; Zhong, T.; Liu, Y.; Wang, J.H.; Jiang, Y. PRAK Interacts with DJ-1 and prevents oxidative stress-induced cell death. *Oxid. Med. Cell. Longev.* **2014**, 735618. [CrossRef]
236. Karunakaran, S.; Diwakar, L. Activation of apoptosis signal regulating kinase 1 (ASK1) and translocation of death-associated protein, Daxx, in substantia nigra pars compacta in a mouse model of Parkinson's disease: Protection by alpha-lipoic acid. *FASEB J.* **2007**, *21*, 2226–2236. [CrossRef] [PubMed]
237. Lu, K.W.; Yang, J.; Hsieh, C.L.; Hsu, Y.C.; Lin, Y.W. Electroacupuncture restores spatial learning and downregulates phosphorylated N-methyl-D-aspartate receptors in a mouse model of Parkinson's disease. *Acupunct. Med.* **2017**, *35*, 133–141. [CrossRef] [PubMed]
238. Lin, J.G.; Hsieh, C.L.; Lin, Y.W. Analgesic effect of electroacupuncture in a mouse fibromyalgia model: Roles of TRPV1, TRPV4, and pERK. *PLoS ONE* **2015**, *10*, e0128037. [CrossRef] [PubMed]
239. Lu, K.W.; Hsieh, C.L.; Yang, J.; Lin, Y.W. Effects of electroacupuncture in a mouse model of fibromyalgia: Role of N-methyl-D-aspartate receptors and related mechanisms. *Acupunct. Med.* **2017**, *35*, 59–68. [CrossRef]

4

Use of Acupuncture for the Treatment of Sports-Related Injuries in Athletes

Ji-Won Lee [1], Jun-Hwan Lee [2,3,*] and Song-Yi Kim [1,*]

1 College of Korean Medicine, Gachon University, Seongnam 13120, Korea; behelia11@gmail.com
2 Clinical Medicine Division, Korea Institute of Oriental Medicine, Daejeon 34054, Korea
3 Korean Medicine Life Science, University of Science & Technology (UST), Campus of Korea Institute of Oriental Medicine, Daejeon 34054, Korea
* Correspondence: omdjun@kiom.re.kr (J.-H.L.); songyi@gachon.ac.kr (S.-Y.K.)

Abstract: Acupuncture is one of the representative complementary and alternative medicine treatments used for various types of pain. This systematic review summarized and analyzed clinical case reports/series utilizing acupuncture for treating sports injuries in athletes, thereby providing the basis for further research to establish clinical evidence on acupuncture treatment in sports medicine. A comprehensive literature search was conducted in Embase including MEDLINE up to 21 August 2019 without language and publication date restrictions. Due to the heterogeneity of each study, explanatory and descriptive analyses were performed. As a result, in each case report/series, it was confirmed that acupuncture was applied for treating various types of sports injuries experienced by athletes. Acupuncture can help relieve short-term pain and recover from dysfunction and has been used as a useful, noninvasive, and conservative modality for managing sports injuries such as lateral meniscus rupture, femoral acetabular impingement, ganglion cysts, and sports hernia. In addition, acupuncture has been suggested as a treatment worth trying for diseases such as yips and delayed onset muscle soreness. The included cases showed some potential of acupuncture in the treatment of various types of sports injuries, beyond pain control in musculoskeletal disorders. However, considering that this review was based on case reports/series, a limited understanding of the clinical value of acupuncture in athletes is required. In the future, more specific research questions and hypotheses should be addressed to generate evidence based on experimental research.

Keywords: sports injury; athlete; acupuncture; case report; case series; review

---

1. Introduction

In recent years, exercise has served a multitude of functions, in addition to promoting health [1]. Regular exercise not only improves an individual's health, but is also considered as a "therapy" for people from all walks of life, such as the pediatric and elderly population, those with chronic diseases, or those with obesity [2,3]. Exercise generally has obvious benefits, but it also requires proper techniques, strength, and frequency [1]. At present, as the population of sports enthusiasts increases, sports injuries have become a prevalent affliction [4]. Musculoskeletal disorders account for most sports injuries and tend to recur frequently [5,6]. Although rare compared to musculoskeletal diseases, sports medicine encompasses various kinds of diseases that preclude sports activities, including psychological issues [7].

In comparison to recreational athletes or non-athletes, elite athletes are deemed to possess more specific goals and are more motivated for improving performance [8]. It is natural that sports injuries are very crucial to elite athletes because they directly affect their careers and economic profit. Therefore, an athlete-centered, long-term, return-to-play (RTP) strategy for those with sports injuries is deemed to be of utmost priority [9]. The objective of an athlete's treatment and rehabilitation is to return to their respective sports with minimal performance loss, whereas that of non-athletes is to return to normal daily activities [9]. Accordingly, athletes' sports injuries often lead to complicated considerations in the doctors' decision-making process [10].

Regarding therapeutic approach for sports injuries, it is important to consider the patient background, including the type of sport and nature of the injury (acute or overuse), or their usual training or match schedules, as well as whether they belong to professional or recreational sports [11]. Thus, practitioners need to know the wealth of clinical evidence about sports-specific profiles and various treatment options [12]. Experimental studies, including randomized controlled trials (RCTs) or controlled clinical trials (CCTs), commonly provide valuable evidence [13] but may have limitations, especially in athletes. Although little has been studied about the motivations of elite athletes to participate in clinical studies, the benefits, generally considered being patients' motivations in clinical study, including access to health care and personal benefit, altruism, and monetary incentives [14], may not be attractive to elite athletes. This could be the reason why experiments conducted on athletes were mainly uncontrolled trials involving the participation of an entire team or experiments conducted with young nonprofessional athletes or in a heterogeneous group of athletes. Another limitation is that the research inclusion criteria required by RCTs are often too restrictive for a wide range of sports injuries, and the statistical results of RCTs can often be regarded as ignoring or equalizing the participants' background characteristics [13]. A case report is a detailed report of an individual patient's diagnosis, treatment, response to treatment, and follow-up, while a case series aggregates individual cases who received similar treatments into one report [15]. Essentially, clinical case reports or series (case reports/series) not only belong at the bottom of the hierarchy of evidence-based medicine (EBM), but also provide a lower causal relationship compared to RCTs [16]. However, they can provide important and beneficial clues about potential treatments for athletes. In addition, case reports/series are the primary sources of information on new treatment options, responses to treatment, details of management, long-term follow-up, and unexpected adverse events (AEs) of treatment [17].

Acupuncture is a nonpharmaceutical therapy known to induce pain control, especially in the musculoskeletal system [18]. Various therapeutic effects of acupuncture are associated with central and systemic mechanisms involving the brain or autonomic nervous system as well as local effects at the acupuncture site [19]. Previous studies have shown that acupuncture changes the levels of neurotransmitters or hormones such as beta-endorphin, dopamine, serotonin, and cortisol [20–22] and has a specific effect on the limbic system or emotional area of the brain [19,23]. Also, other studies have further elucidated that acupuncture may be beneficial in treating chronic pain with depression [24], drug addiction [25], and degenerative disorders such as Alzheimer disease [26].

At present, with regard to potential advantages of acupuncture, case reports/series on acupuncture in athletes have been published steadily [27–30]. However, limited reviews with a comprehensive perspective on the use of acupuncture in athletes have been reported. Therefore, this systematic review aimed to summarize and analyze clinical case reports/series utilizing acupuncture for treating sports injuries of athletes, thereby providing the basis for further research to establish clinical evidence and expand the scope of acupuncture treatment in sports medicine. Furthermore, this study sought to provide useful insights for practitioners willing to utilize acupuncture in the clinical practice.

2. Materials and Methods

2.1. Search Strategy

To establish the search strategy that could comprehensively include clinical studies of athletes receiving acupuncture treatment for sports injuries, taking into account the search term sensitivity and specificity, a preliminary search was conducted in PubMed (https://pubmed.ncbi.nlm.nih.gov/)

and domestic databases (Research Information Sharing Service (RISS, http://www.riss.kr/), National Digital Science Library (NDSL, http://www.ndsl.kr/), and Oriental Medicine Advanced Searching Integrate System (OASIS, https://oasis.kiom.re.kr/)). Based on these results, the following search terms were selected. The search terms used consisted of a combination of traditional Korean medicine treatment ("traditional Korean medicine", "traditional Chinese medicine", "acupuncture", "herb*", "moxibustion", "cupping", or "pharmacopuncture" ("aqua acupuncture", "herb* acupuncture", or "acupoint injection")) and sports injury ((("wound", "medicine", or "injury") and ("athletic" or "sport")), "athletic injury", "sports injury", or "sports medicine"). Finally, a literature search was conducted in Embase (www.embase.com) including MEDLINE up to 21 August 2019 without language and publication date restrictions. Furthermore, the reference lists of related reviews were screened to ensure that there were no missing studies. We also manually identified additional records through other sources, including Google Scholar. All searched studies were listed and organized using Microsoft Excel (Microsoft, Redmond, WA, USA).

2.2. *Study Selection, Data Extraction, and Data Analysis*

The inclusion criteria were clinical case reports or series that studied the effects of treatment, including acupuncture, on sports injuries of athletes. To clarify this inclusion criterion, we reviewed and established several definitions among the authors. Firstly, we included manual acupuncture (MA), electroacupuncture (EA), auricular acupuncture, laser acupuncture (LA), acupressure, catgut embedding, dry needling, and transcutaneous electrical nerve stimulation (TENS) in the category of "acupuncture". It is controversial whether TENS can be classified as a type of acupuncture; hence, we only included it in the analysis when the TENS was applied to the acupuncture points. Secondly, we defined case reports/series as a descriptive study based on uncontrolled observations containing detailed information on the diagnosis, treatment, response to treatment, and follow-up of individual patients. Several steps were taken based on the following exclusion criteria to select a study whose study design was a case report or a case series, regardless of the number of cases in an individual patient. The exclusion criteria were as follows: (1) Studies not targeted for humans (i.e., in vitro studies or animal studies), (2) research that did not collect original primary data (review, protocol, editorial, letter, etc.), (3) cross-sectional study or prevalence research, (4) experimental study with control (i.e., randomized controlled trials, controlled clinical trials), (5) no acupuncture-related treatment interventions (defined in advance) were used, (6) not targeted for athletes, (7) full text of the research results were not provided (i.e., conference poster abstract), and (8) studies not written in English, Chinese, or Korean. Since case reports/series are mostly retrospective observational studies, in many cases, different combination treatments are commonly used together, and it is ambiguous to distinguish which treatment was employed as the primary or adjuvant treatment. Therefore, we included all studies where the use of acupuncture as the main treatment was uncertain, but conducted a rigorous evaluation in the screening process to ensure that acupuncture was used for treatment in each individual study.

The records were screened accordingly and independently by two authors (J.-W.L. and S.-Y.K.) based on the title, abstract, or full text. First, all duplicate records belonging to the same title and author were removed. Grounded on the above inclusion/exclusion criteria, studies that were unrelated to sports medicine or studies that focused on doping, which fall into the category of sports medicine but failed to satisfy the inclusion criteria for this study, were first excluded for convenience. Next, the studies that corresponded to the exclusion criteria were removed to finally screen appropriate studies for our review analysis.

2.3. *Data Extraction and Data Analysis*

Data extraction was performed by one author (J.-W.L.) using predefined data extraction forms and then reviewed by another author (S.-Y.K.). If there was a discrepancy or further discussion was needed, it was resolved by another investigator (J.-H.L.), who was not involved in the extraction and review process. The data were extracted by classifying the following categories. These categories were modified based on some of the topic and checklist items in the CAse REport (CARE) guideline [31]: patient information, therapeutic intervention, follow-up, and outcomes were extracted. In the "patient information," main concerns and symptoms of the patient including duration of the disorder, relevant past interventions, and patients' demographic data such as type of sports, age, and gender were collected. For "therapeutic intervention", types of acupuncture and acupuncture points, types of co-intervention, administration of intervention (such as treatment duration and number of treatment sessions), and changes in intervention with rationale were extracted. In relation to "follow-up and outcomes", the outcome measures used in each study, their results, and AEs were collected, and information on RTP, recurrence, and conclusions from the authors of each study were summarized and analyzed.

The included sports were analyzed based on static components during competition according to the sports classification by Mitchell et al. [32]. If such sports did not quite match up to Mitchell et al.'s classification, we classified the sports in a consensus discussion between the authors.

Our study was not homogeneous enough to quantitatively synthesize the results of each individual study as not limited to a specific disease and did not include a control group. Therefore, it was not possible to evaluate the effectiveness by estimating the size of the effect or by statistically pooling and calculating the results between studies, and only descriptive and narrative results of qualitative analysis on the role of "acupuncture" described in each individual study were provided.

3. Results

Our screening process is illustrated in Figure 1. Initially, 1954 potentially relevant articles were searched through the database, and 36 additional records were identified by manual searching. After removing duplicates (n = 31) from a total of 1990 records identified using the search strategy, 1959 studies were screened in view of the title, abstract, or full text, and 1937 were discarded (1558 studies were unrelated to sports medicine; 142 studies were not primary studies; 100 studies were experimental studies; 30 studies were not related to intervention using acupuncture points, etc.).

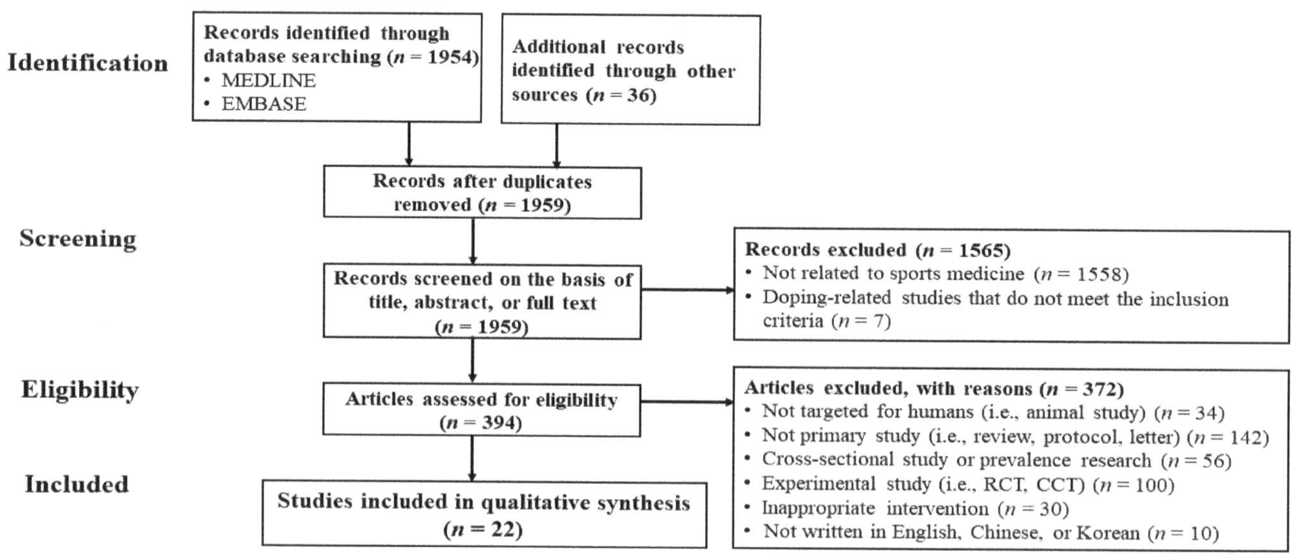

Figure 1. Flow diagram. CCT, controlled clinical trial; RCT, randomized controlled trial.

Finally, 22 case reports/series were included in our review [27–30,33–50]. The summary of the characteristics of the inclusion studies based on the items in the CARE checklist is shown in Table 1.

Table 1. Summary of included case reports/series.

Study		Demographic Information				Main Concerns and Symptoms of the Patient		Medical History	Administration of Intervention	Follow-up and Outcomes				
No	Study ID	Coun. (Lang)	Sports type	Age (yr)	No. of Cases	Disorders	Duration	Previous Interventions	① Interventions ② Duration ③ No. of sessions	Outcome measures	Results	Adverse events	① Return to play ② Recurrence (f/u)	Authors' comments for acupuncture treatments
Diseases of the musculoskeletal system and connective tissue														
1	Dlin, 1980 [33]	Israel (Eng.)	ND	12–44 (mean = 2(5)	22	Musculotendinous syndromes of the chronic exertion type (shoulder, knee, anterior tibia, back pain)	Few wks-several mon	At least a 2 to 3 wk period: [all patients] heat application, rest; [as needed] oral anti-inflammatory medication (indomethacin), physiotherapy (ultrasound, or local steroid injections)	① TENS ② ND ③ 2–6	(1) Pain questionnaire (2) Pain grade	(1) Complete pain relief (n = 1(5), good (>50% reduction) (n = (4), fair (30–50% reduction) (n = (1), poor (<30% reduction) (n = (2) (2) Grade 0 (n = 17), 2 grades reduction (good result) (n = (2), 1 grade reduction (fair result) (n = (1), No changes (n = (2)	None	① 18 of 22 subjects returned to full sports activity ② 10-day-2-mon after return to full sports activity (n = 6)	*TENS stimulation of acupuncture points may be effective in the therapy of painful sports injuries of the athletic exertion type.*
2	Sternfeld, 1992 [34]	Israel (Eng.)	Long-distance running	16	1	Runner's stitch syndrome	Several mon	Analgesics and NSAIDs	① MA ② 31-day [1/day (3-day)+1/wk (4-wk)] ③ 7	Symptoms	Complete and permanent recovery	ND	① Resuming all activities and achievements in competitive sports ② None (several wks)	*We suggest acupuncture as a preferred therapy for cases involving runner's stitch syndrome.*
3	Seplow, 1996 [35]	USA (Eng.)	Basketball	17	1	Lateral meniscus injury (a tear of the posterior horn of the lateral meniscus)	3-day	Ice, rest, NSAIDs (2-day)	① EA + others ② Initial 2-wk ③ ND	Symptoms	Walk without limp or pain and range of knee flexion returned to 130°	ND	① Return to training in 5-wks, full participation in 8-wks ② ND	*When tears are diagnosed, conservative methods may be effective in treating these athletes and may in fact be more effective in many cases.*

Table 1. *Cont.*

	Study	Demographic Information				Main Concerns and Symptoms of the Patient		Medical History	Administration of Intervention	Follow-up and Outcomes				
4	Hoven, 2000 [36]	USA (Eng.)	Ski	19	1	Peroneal nerve entrapment and ankle sprain	ND	Pelvic/lower extremity chiropractic manipulation, interferential current, cryotherapy (3-day)	① MA + others ② 5-day ③ 5	Symptoms	Pain and weakness alleviated after 3-day of care	ND	①, ② ND	*It appears that chiropractic manipulation of the lumbar, pelvis and lower extremity, combined with interferential current, cryotherapy, acupuncture and trigger point therapy played a significant role in alleviating the peroneal neuropathy experienced by this elite junior national skier.*
5	Young, 2005 [38]	UK (Eng.)	Rugby	#1: 19; #2: 32	2	#1: Calf strain/mild chronic compartment syndrome; #2: Tennis elbow/muscle tightness	#1: 6-mon; #2: ND	ND	① EA + MA + others ② #1: 6-wk #2: 4-wk (2/wk) ③ #1: 12; #2: 8	Symptoms	#1: Completion of the full training without pain #2: Training at ease	ND	① #1: Playing games without pain; #2: Playing at ease ② ND	*Even though using acupuncture is very effective in treatment, there comes a time in the treatment of an injury when you will need to open the channels physically to allow qi and blood to flow smoothly and to return the shortened muscle back to its normal length.*
6	Martínez-Silvestrini, 2006 [39]	Puerto Rico (Eng.)	ND	11	1 *	CRPS after lower extremity trauma and clinical depression	Few wks	(For CRPS treatment) Hydrotherapy, electrical stimulation, ultrasound to the Achilles tendon, stretching, active assisted range of motion, weight bearing, opioid analgesics, corticosteroids	① MA + others ② 3-mon ③ ND	Symptoms	The clinics discharge without any deficits	ND	①, ② ND	*ND*

Table 1. *Cont.*

	Study	Demographic Information				Main Concerns and Symptoms of the Patient		Medical History	Administration of Intervention	Follow-up and Outcomes				
7	Yan, 2008 [41]	China (Chin.)	Football	Mean = 21	19 **	Sports injury in knee joint medial collateral ligament	ND	ND	① EA + others ② ND (one course comprised 7-day) ③ ND	(1) Recovery time (2) Therapeutic effect (3) The overall efficiency	(1) Rapid (23%); moderate (50%) (2) Recovered (40%); partly recovered (53%) (3) 93%	ND	①, ② ND	*ND*
8	Osborne, 2010 [42]	UK (Eng.)	Volleyball	23–27 (mean = 2(5)	4	Anterior/ anterolateral shoulder pain (1)	#1: 2 mon.; #2: 6 yr.; #3: 18 mon.; #4: 6-mon	Conservative treatment (#1: Thera band, stretching; #2, #3: ND; #4: exercises, stretching)	① MA + others ② 1-mon-long intense competitive phase ③ #1, #3, #4: 1; #2: 2	(1) Functional assessment (MPQ) (2) ROM (3) Verbal pain scores (4) Muscle strength	(1)-(4) All scores improved	ND	① Continuing overhead activities ② ND	*These cases support the use of dry needling in elite athletes during a competitive phase with short-term pain relief and improved function in shoulder injuries.*
9	Pearcey, 2013 [46]	Canada (Eng.)	ND	31	1	Exertional rhabdomyolysis	Few days	Intravenous hydration with sodium bicarbonate and blood work [3 days]	① MA + others ② 2 day ③ ND	CK levels	Declined by 45%	ND	① 1 mon. after the diagnosis, the subject slowly returned to high-intensity resistance training (>2/wk.) without any complications ② ND	*ND*
10	Woitzik, 2013 [47]	Canada (Eng.)	Cycle	45	1	Ganglion cyst of the foot	10-day	ND	① EA ② 4-wk (1/wk) ③ 4	Symptoms	Resolution of the cyst (11 day after final treatment)	ND	①, ② ND	*EA may be a novel and non-invasive conservative approach for the treatment of ganglion cysts.*
11	Morimoto, 2013 [45]	Japan (Eng.)	Various sports (2)	17–77 (mean = 39)	41	Jumper's knee, lateral/medial epicondylitis, Achilles tendinitis, adductor muscle injury, rotator cuff injuries, etc. (3)	ND	ND	① LA + others ② ND ③ 2–10 (mean = 4.(1)	Pain Relief Score	5 or less (n = 27,66%)	ND	①, ② ND	*Low-level LA is an effective treatment for sports injuries, particularly jumper's knee, tennis elbow and Achilles tendinitis.*

Table 1. *Cont.*

	Study		Demographic Information			Main Concerns and Symptoms of the Patient		Medical History	Administration of Intervention	Follow-up and Outcomes				
12	Gliedt, 2014 [49]	USA (Eng.)	Basketball	41	1	Sub-acute left elbow tendinopathy	5 wk	Self-massage, OTC NSAIDs	① MA + others ② ND (1/wk) ③ 2	Symptoms	Reduced left elbow swelling and left wrist extensor muscle hypertonicity, and no pain	ND	① A return to normal recreational athletic activities including basketball ② None (6-wk)	*The patient's outcomes indicated a quick resolution of subjective complaints and objective findings with the chosen treatment.*
13	Jayaseelan, 2014 [50]	USA (Eng.)	Running	#1: 70; #2: 69	2	Proximal hamstring tendinopathy	#1: 7 mon; #2: 5 mon	Eccentric training of hamstrings, lumbopelvic stabilization exercises, patient education (2-wk: "Phase 1" treatment)	① MA + others ② #1: 3 wk; #2: 4 wk ("Phase 2" treatment) (1/wk) ③ 3	(1) Pain (NRS) (2) Global rating of change (3) Lower Extremity Functional Scale (4) Tenderness (5) Strength	(1)–(5) All score improvement, significant function improvement	ND	① Each patient returned to running and sitting without symptoms ② None (6 mon)	*In these 2 runners, eccentric loading of the hamstrings, lumbopelvic stabilization exercises, and trigger point dry needling provided short- and long-term pain reduction and functional benefits.*
14	MacIntyre, 2015 [27]	Canada (Eng.)	Ice hockey	22	1	FAI	4 yr	None	① EA + others ② 6-wk (1–2/wk) ③ 8	Symptoms	No pain [at rest, daily activities (including exercise), all stress tests used for initial physical examination]; despite having less pain, the hip scour and FADIR tests still provided a hard end-feel and palpable click at extreme ROM	ND	① At 8 wk ② None (6 mon)	*Conservative management utilizing a multimodal approach, as described in the case, should be first line treatment.*
Exercise-induced fatigue														

Table 1. *Cont.*

Study		Demographic Information				Main Concerns and Symptoms of the Patient		Medical History	Administration of Intervention	Follow-up and Outcomes				
15	Chen, 2008 [40]	China (Chin.)	Rowing, track and field, swimming, table tennis (4)	15–26 (mean = 20)	41	Exercise-induced fatigue	N/A	N/A	① Catgut embedding ② 90–120 day ③ 6	(1) Training-related condition (2) Changes level of blood testosterone and hemoglobin	(1) Significantly improved (2) Significantly increased	ND	①, ② N/A	*Catgut implantation at acupoints can significantly improve exercise fatigue in the player and the mechanism is possibly related with increase of testosterone and hemoglobin levels.*
16	Garlanger, 2017 [29]	USA (Eng.)	Nordic ski	14–17	15	Exercise-related DOMS and sense of well-being	N/A	N/A	① MA + others ② 2 wk ③ 1–5	(1) Time required by research staff on treatment days (2) Cost (3) AEs (4) Participant/ provider ratio (5) Effect on DOMS 6) Effect on sense of well-being	(1) 90 min (2) 1500 USD (3) (See next column) (4) 7:1 (5) significantly improved ($p <$ 0.05) 6) NS	No severe AEs; Minor AEs (73%, site pain, etc.)	①, ② N/A	*Providing acupuncture to adolescent Nordic ski athletes in the practice field under extreme temperature is feasible with the appropriate resources.*
17	Luetmer, 2019 [30]	USA (Eng.)	Football	13–18 (mean = 16)	42	Exercise-related DOMS and sense of well-being	N/A	N/A	① MA + others ② 5-day ③ 5 (n = 1(1); 4 (n = 1(3); 3 (n = 8); 2 (n = 6); 1 (n = (4)	Same as above	(1) 75 min (2) 700 USD (3) (See next column) (4) 7–10:1 (5) significantly improved ($p <$ 0.001) (6) NS	No severe AEs; Minor AEs (55%, mild focal numbness or tingling)	①, ② N/A	*Effectively providing acupuncture to multiple adolescent football players in their training environment is feasible with appropriate staff and resources.*
Others														

Table 1. *Cont.*

	Study	Demographic Information				Main Concerns and Symptoms of the Patient		Medical History	Administration of Intervention	Follow-up and Outcomes				
18	Abe, 2014 [48]	Brazil (Eng.)	Various sports (Paralympic athletes) (5)	Mean = 35	7	Persistent pain (shoulder, elbow, spine, or knee) (6)	#1: 4-wk; #2-#4, #6: chronic, intermittent; #5: 2-wk; #7: 8-wk	Oral/topical NSAIDs, muscle relaxant, physiotherapy, immobilization (7)	① MA + others ② 6 wk (2/wk) ③ 12	(1) Pain (VAS) (2) Pain (MPQ)	(1), (2) Significant pain reduction	No severe AEs; Minor AEs (episodic local bleeding); One athlete died of liver cancer after this study	①, ② ND	*Pain symptoms were reduced with acupuncture. The mean duration required for improvement was eight acupuncture sessions.*
19	Lin, 2016 [28]	USA (Eng.)	#1: Ice hockey #2: Field hockey and lacrosse #3: Soccer	#1: 8; #2: 15; #3: 18	3	Sport-related postconcussive symptoms	#1,#2: 1 mon; #3: 1.5 mon	Physical therapy, medications (8)	① MA + EA + others ② #1, #2, 6-wk; #3, 14-wk (1/wk) ③ #1, #2, 6; #3, 14	(1) Pain (VAS) (2) Pain (BPI) (3) Postconcussive symptoms questionnaire	(1)-(3) Satisfactory symptomatic reduction in all patients	None	① #1, #2: ND; #3: Return to all sports activities (All patients returned to their physical, social, and school activities) ② ND	*Acupuncture with conventional medication appeared to reduce the postconcussive symptoms in the 3 patients.*
20	Yuill, 2012 [44]	Canada (Eng.)	#1: Soccer #2, #3: Soccer and hockey	#1: 23; #2: 18; #3: 29	3	Sports hernia (chronic groin pain)	#1: 5 wk; #2: 3-mon; #3: 5-wk	#1: None; #2: Ice, interferential current, ultrasound (2 mon); #3: Physiotherapy, adductor stretching/ strengthening, interferential current, ultrasound	① MA + EA + others ② 6–8-wk (1–2/wk) ③ 6–16	(1) Pain (VAS) (2) Resisted muscle testing	(1) 0/10 in all cases at the time of patient discharge (2) All positive tests changed to negative	ND	① Within 3–4 days of last therapy ② None (2 yr)	*Three soccer players, of varying levels of ability, presenting with a suspected sports hernia were relieved of their pain after 8 weeks of conservative care.*
21	Donoyama, 2011 [43]	Japan (Eng.)	Middle- and long-distance running	26	1	Amenorrhoea	Several mon	A norgestrel-ethinyl estradiol combination (2-wk]	① MA + others ② 13 mon ③ 46	(1) Menstrual blood flow (2) Basal Body Temperature (3) Body Weight (4) Body Fat Rate (5) BMI	(1) Amount and duration of menstrual flow increased at regular intervals (2) Moved close to the biphasic pattern (3)-(5) NS	ND	①, ② ND	*Acupuncture treatment may be a feasible treatment option in the field of sports medicine to help competitive athletes with amenorrhoea.*

Table 1. *Cont.*

Study		Demographic Information				Main Concerns and Symptoms of the Patient		Medical History	Administration of Intervention	Follow-up and Outcomes				
22	Rosted, 2005 [37]	UK (Eng.)	Golf	65	1	Yips	2 yr	None	① MA ② Few weeks (1/wk+1/2-wk) ③ 8	Symptoms	Symptoms disappeared after 1 treatment	ND	① Playing golf using his right hand without symptoms ② None (2 yr)	*Acupuncture may be worth trying in patients with the yips since this condition is otherwise difficult to treat.*

AE, adverse event; BMI, body mass index; BPI, brief pain inventory; Coun, country; Chin., Chinese; CRPS, complex regional pain syndrome; DOMS, delayed onset muscle soreness; EA, electroacupuncture; Eng., English; FADIR test, flexion-adduction-internal rotation test; FAI, Femoroacetabular impingement; f/u, follow-up; L, left; LA, laser acupuncture; lang, language; MA, manual acupuncture; min, minutes; mon, month; MPQ, McGill pain questionnaire; N/A, not applicable; ND, not described; NRS, numeric rating scale; NSAID, nonsteroidal anti-inflammatory drug; OTC, over-the-counter; R, right; ROM, range of motion; SLAP, superior labrum tear from anterior to posterior; TENS, transcutaneous electrical nerve stimulation; VAS, visual analogue scale; wk, week; yr, year. *Of all three cases, one was treated with acupuncture. ** Of all 30 cases, 19 were treated with acupuncture. (1) #1: Intermittent discomfort. #2: Partial nonrepaired SLAP lesion but with no functional impact. #3: Right arthroscopic capsular tightening, intermittent pain. #4: Intermittent pain in right shoulder. (2) Golf (n = 6), martial arts (n = 4), basketball (n = 4), marathon (n = 3), aerobics (n = 2), ski (n = 2), softball (n = 2), dance (n = 2), tennis (n = 2), triathlon (n = 2), volleyball (n = 2), etc. (n = 10). (3) Jumper's knee (n = 8), lateral epicondylitis of humerus (n = 3), Achilles tendinitis (n = 3), adductor muscle injury (n = 2), medial epicondylitis of humerus (n = 2), rotator cuff injuries (n = 2), etc. (n = 21). (4) Rowing (n = 7), track and field (n = 20), Swimming (n = 12), table tennis (n = 2); (5) #1, #4-#6: Basketball #2: Swimming and volleyball. #3: Swimming. #7: Track and field (paralympic athletes). (6) #1: Right shoulder and Right elbow. #2: Spine. #3: Left knee, shoulders, and spine. #4: Left shoulder. #5: Shoulders and spine. #6: Shoulders. #7: Left shoulder. (7) #1: Oral and topical NSAIDs (three days after onset). #2, #3: NSAIDs and physiotherapy (immediately after onset). #4, #6: NSAIDs (immediately after onset); #5: muscle relaxant and NSAIDs, physiotherapy (cryotherapy), immobilization (immediately after onset). #7: NSAIDs (four weeks; intermittent); (8) #1: Physical therapy and medications (acetaminophen, ibuprofen, or amitriptyline) (20 mg/day). #2: Acetaminophen (every day), ibuprofen (only for severe headaches), amitriptyline (20 mg/day), physical therapy, vestibular therapy; #3: Ibuprofen (as needed, ~2/wk), physical therapy (2/wk).

From 1980 to 2019, the number of relevant studies increased steadily with one study in the 1980s, two in the 1990s, six in the 2000s, and 13 in the 2010s. (Figure 2a). The studies were conducted in eight countries, with the largest number of studies in the United States (n = 7, 31.8%); followed by Canada (n = 4); the UK (n = 3); China, Israel, and Japan (n = 2, respectively); and Brazil and Puerto Rico (n = 1, respectively) (Figure 2b). Two studies conducted in China [40,41] were written in Chinese and the rest were written in English.

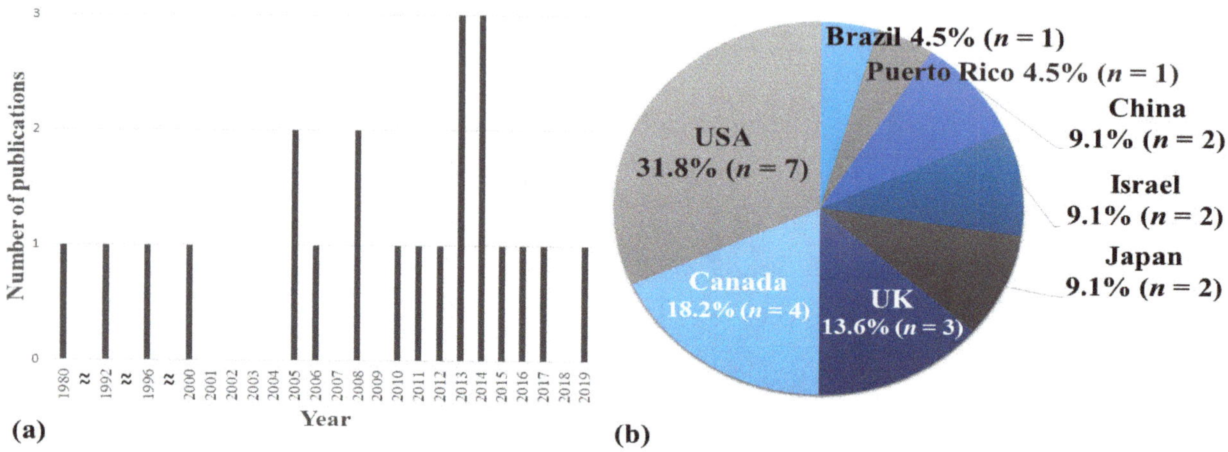

Figure 2. Characteristics of the included studies. (**a**) Number of published case reports/series by year; (**b**) frequency by country in which case reports/series were performed.

3.1. Demographic Information, Main Concerns, and Symptoms of the Patient

All subjects included in this review were athletes, and sports injuries were reported in various sports such as basketball (n = 4, 9 cases); running, skiing, or volleyball (n = 3, respectively); and field hockey, golf, soccer, football, ice hockey, swimming, or track and field (n = 2, respectively). The details of each sport are shown in Figure 3. Most studies (n = 14) reported cases for one-sport type of athlete, but five studies included athletes of various types of sports, and three studies did not report any specific sport types.

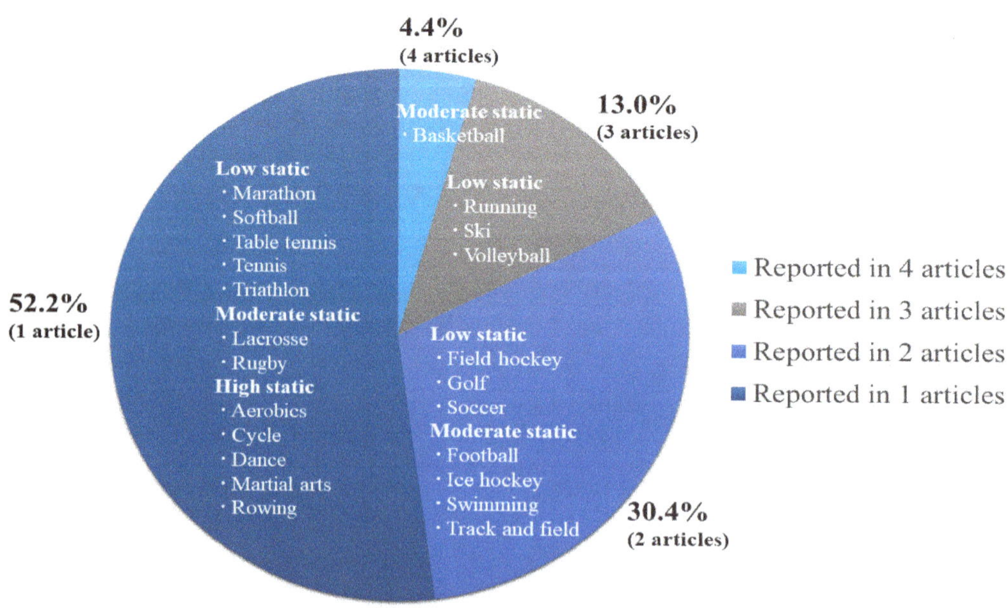

Figure 3. Type of sports. This figure shows how many case reports/series were performed according to the type of sports. For example, there were four case reports/series for basketball players, and three case reports/series for runners, skiers, and volleyball players, respectively. Each type of sports was classified and described according to the static components during competition.

The total number of athletes included in our review was 211, of which 119 (56.4%) were men. The athletes' ages ranged from 8 to 77 years old (mean = 24.8).

Figure 4 shows the main concerns and symptoms of athletes in the included studies. Of the 211 cases of sports injuries, musculoskeletal system and connective tissue diseases accounted for the highest proportion of primary symptoms reported in each case report/series (98 cases, $n = 14$ (46.4 %)). The most injured body regions were the knees (medial collateral ligament injury (19 cases), jumper's knee (8 cases), lateral meniscus injury (1 case)), followed by the elbows (lateral epicondylitis (4 cases), medial epicondylitis (2 cases), tendinopathy (1 case)), and shoulders (pain (4 cases), rotator cuff injury (2 cases)). In addition, studies of diverse musculoskeletal disorders were reported, including musculotendinous syndrome with chronic pain in multiple body regions (22 cases), complex regional pain syndrome, exertional rhabdomyolysis, and ganglion cysts of the foot (1 case, respectively) (Figure 5). On the other hand, sports injuries other than the musculoskeletal system were as follows. There were two studies [29,30] on exercise-related delayed onset muscle soreness (DOMS, 57 cases) and one study [40] on exercise-induced fatigue (41 cases) in athletes. Two studies reported mental and behavioral disorders such as yips for golfers (1 case) [37] and postconcussive symptoms (3 cases) [28]. Other studies included persistent pain in para-athletes (7 cases) [48], sports hernias (3 cases) [44], and amenorrhea (1 case) [43].

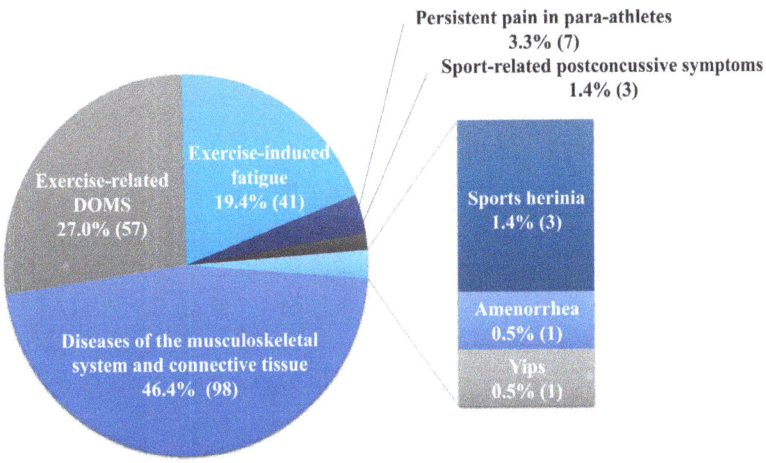

Figure 4. Main concerns and symptoms of the patients.

The duration of the athletes' disorder or symptoms varied from the day of onset to four years. According to relevant past interventions in each case report/series, among the patients of the included cases, except for seven studies, three cases had no past intervention, and all the other patients received conservative treatment such as physical therapy or medications for the symptoms. Of the seven studies excluded above, three studies conducted simply to observe the changes during the training periods did not require records for past intervention. The remaining four studies did not report relevant past interventions. The details are described in Table 1.

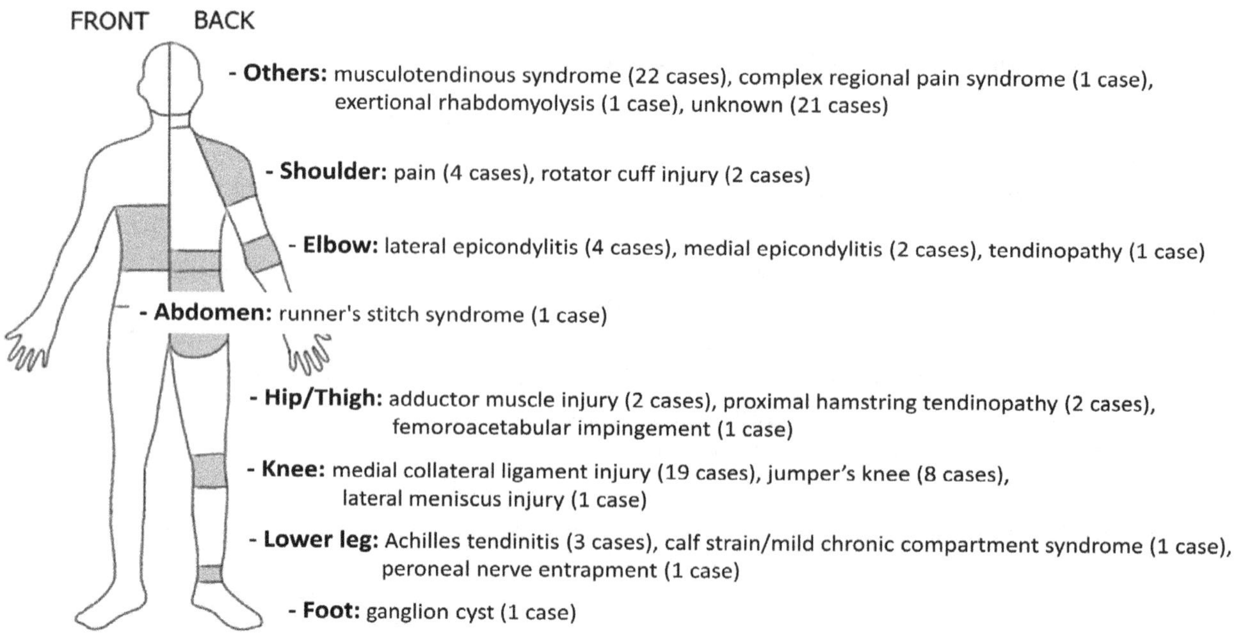

Figure 5. Injured body regions of musculoskeletal disease.

3.2. Therapeutic Intervention

3.2.1. Acupuncture

Twelve of the 22 studies included in our review reported the use of MA at acupoints or myofascial trigger points (MTrPs). For EA, four studies used EA alone, while three studies used MA with EA. Other studies demonstrated catgut embedding, TENS at acupoints or MTrPs, or low-level LA at acupoints or ashi points (acupuncture site, not given a specific name or definite location, determined by tenderness or other pathological reactions).

Some trends were observed between the types of acupuncture and the category of diseases utilized. For example, MA with acupoints was used in various symptoms in our review, such as yips, amenorrhea, or sports hernia, in addition to musculoskeletal disorders. On the other hand, studies in which MA was applied only to MTrP, study that used EA alone without MA, TENS study, and LA study were mainly used for athletes with diseases of the musculoskeletal system and connective tissue.

The treatment sites were reported in detail as specific acupoints in 15 studies (Table 2 remaining seven studies, six described treatment sites, not as particular acupoints, but as muscles or ranges. In addition, one study did not describe any treatment sites.

Table 2. Details of acupuncture and co-intervention.

No.	Study ID	Sports Type	Disorders	Details of Acupuncture (Acupuncture Sites)	Co-Intervention
Diseases of the musculoskeletal system and connective tissue					
1	Dlin, 1980 [33]	ND	Musculotendinous syndromes of the chronic exertion type (shoulder, knee, anterior tibia, and back pain)	TENS (MTrPs or acupoints)	None
2	Sternfeld, 1992 [34]	Long-distance running	Runner's stitch syndrome	MA (PC3, LR14, ST36, SP9, LR2, SP3)	None
3	Seplow, 1996 [35]	Basketball	Lateral meniscus injury (a tear of the posterior horn of the lateral meniscus)	EA (ST41, GB43, BL54, BL60)	Ice, kinesiology, resistance bands
4	Hoven, 2000 [36]	Ski	Peroneal nerve entrapment and ankle sprain	MA (ST40, GB34, GB35, GB36)	Chiropractic manipulation (lumbar spine, pelvis, lower extremity), interferential current, cryotherapy, soft tissue mobilization
5	Young, 2005 [38]	Rugby	#1: Calf strain and mild chronic compartment syndrome #2: Tennis elbow and muscle tightness	#1: - EA (BL55-BL57, BL57-GB35) - MA (BL40, BL57, BL58, BL60, BL65, GB34, GB41, LI4) #2: - EA (ashi points, EX-B2 from C3 to L5) - MA (ashi points, GB21, LI15, TE14, TE5, LI10, LI11, LI12, LI5, LI4, LI3, TE3)	#1: Tuina (gun-fa, rolling technique; rou-fa, kneading; plucking (frictions)), stretching, patient education #2: Tuina (gun-fa), cupping (epicondyle)
6	Martínez-Silvestrini, 2006 [39]	ND	CRPS after lower extremity trauma and clinical depression	(for clinical depression and pain disorder treatment) MA (ND)	(for clinical depression and pain disorder treatment) Fluoxetine (SSRIs)

Table 2. *Cont.*

No.	Study ID	Sports Type	Disorders	Details of Acupuncture (Acupuncture Sites)	Co-Intervention
7	Yan, 2008 [41]	Football	Sports injury in knee joint medial collateral ligament	EA (EX-LE2, EX-LE5, GB34)	Massage, physiotherapy, cold pack, electric stimulation, external preparation, surgery, splint, rehabilitation training (as needed)
8	Osborne, 2010 [42]	Volleyball	Anterior/anterolateral shoulder pain	MA (MTrPs: scapulohumeral muscles)	Soft tissue therapy around the shoulder, post-training icing strategies, exercises and stretching
9	Pearcey, 2013 [46]	ND	Exertional rhabdomyolysis	MA (from shoulder to hand)	Intravenous hydration with sodium bicarbonate and blood work
10	Woitzik, 2013 [47]	Cycle	Ganglion cyst of the foot	EA (ST36, LR3, 2 needles inserted into the cyst on opposite sides stimulated at 5 Hz)	None
11	Morimoto, 2013 [45]	Various sports	Jumper's knee, lateral epicondylitis of humerus, Achilles tendinitis, adductor muscle injury, medial epicondylitis of humerus, rotator cuff injuries, etc	LA (low level laser therapy at points of pain/or acupuncture points)	Medication (NSAIDs) or a poultice (as needed)
12	Gliedt, 2014 [49]	Basketball	Sub-acute left elbow tendinopathy	MA (palpated areas of tenderness, just distal to the insertion site of the common wrist extensor muscles)	HVLA spinal manipulation (thoracic spine), ART (elbow), home exercise program (Brugger's exercises for postural dysfunction)
13	Jayaseelan, 2014 [50]	Running	Proximal hamstring tendinopathy	MA (MTrPs: medial/lateral hamstrings, adductor magnus muscle)	Eccentric training of hamstrings, lumbopelvic stabilization exercises, patient education

Table 2. *Cont.*

No.	Study ID	Sports Type	Disorders	Details of Acupuncture (Acupuncture Sites)	Co-Intervention
14	MacIntyre, 2015 [27]	Ice hockey	FAI	EA (2 Hz, L2-L5 bilaterally, and hip muscles and nerves, SP12, LR10, GB29, BL53, BL54)	Soft tissue therapy, spinal manipulative therapy, MWM and rehabilitation exercises
Exercise-induced fatigue					
15	Chen, 2008 [40]	Rowing, track and field, swimming, table tennis	Exercise-induced fatigue	Catgut embedding (CV4, BL23, GV4, ST36, SP6 and etc.)	None
16	Garlanger, 2017 [29]	Nordic ski	Exercise-related DOMS and sense of well-being	MA (when underlying muscle soreness occurred: SP10, ST34, SP9, ST36, GB34, BL56; if no specific muscle soreness: ST36, GB34, ST34)	NSAIDs (24–48 h prior to the study, $n = 6$; between treatment days 2 and 3, $n = 3$; between treatment days 4 and 5, $n = 1$)
17	Luetmer, 2019 [30]	Football	Exercise-related DOMS and sense of well-being	MA (when underlying muscle soreness occurred: SP10, ST34, SP9, ST36, GB34, BL56; if no specific muscle soreness: ST36, GB34, ST34)	NSAIDs or acetaminophen (before day 1, $n = 7$; between day 1 and 2, $n = 7$; between days 2 and 3, $n = 10$; between days 3 and 4, $n = 8$; between days 4 and 5, $n = 9$)
Others					
18	Abe, 2014 [48]	Various sports (Paralympic athletes)	Persistent pain (shoulder, elbow, spine, or knee)	MA (CV12, CV3, LI4, LU7, HT7, SP10, ST36, LR2, KI3)	The training schedule and the usual treatment regimens maintained
19	Lin, 2016 [28]	Ice hockey, field hockey, lacrosse, soccer	Sport-related postconcussive symptoms	- MA (#1: LI4, ST36, LR3, TE5, Ashi points; #2: LI4, ST36, LR3, TE5, SP6, Yin-Tang, Ashi points; #3: LI4, ST36, SP6, LR3, TE23, GV20, Yin-Tang, TE5, LI11, ST7, BL4, BL6, TE9, GB21, GB20, Ashi points) - EA(2-Hz, ST 36)	Cupping (Back Shu points), Gua sha (Back Shu points, treatment involving repeated pressured strokes over body surface with a smooth edged tool), conventional medical therapies maintained

Table 2. *Cont.*

No.	Study ID	Sports Type	Disorders	Details of Acupuncture (Acupuncture Sites)	Co-Intervention
20	Yuill, 2012 [44]	Soccer, hockey	Sports hernia (chronic groin pain)	- EA (2 Hz, L2-L4, T10-T12 bilaterally) - MA (#1: SP 13, ST 29, ST30, KI11, GB28 #2: ST29, ST30, LR9, LR10 #3: ST30, LR10)	Soft tissue therapy, laser therapy and microcurrent (site of the chief complaint), stretching, Wobenzyme (2400mg tabs, 2/day, 2 weeks), rehabilitation therapy, plyometric training (3/week, 8 weeks)
21	Donoyama, 2011 [43]	Middle- and long-distance running	Amenorrhoea	MA (CV6, CV12, LR3, LR14, BL17, BL18, BL23, SP6, SP10)	A norgestrel-ethinyl estradiol combination (as needed)
22	Rosted, 2005 [37]	Golf	Yips	MA (GV20, EX-HN-1, TE5)	None

ART, active release techniques; BL, bladder meridian; CRPS, Complex regional pain syndrome; CV, conception vessel meridian; DOMS, Delayed onset muscle soreness; EA, electroacupuncture; EX-B, extra point (back); EX-HN, extra point (head and neck); EX-LE, extra point (lower extremity); FAI, Femoroacetabular impingement; GB, gallbladder meridian; GV, governor vessel meridian; HT, heart meridian; HVLA, high-velocity low-amplitude; KI, kidney meridian; LA, laser acupuncture; LI, large intestine meridian; LR, liver meridian; LU, lung meridian; MA, manual acupuncture; MTrPs, myofascial trigger points; MWM, Mulligan Mobilizations with Movement; ND, not described; NSAID, nonsteroidal anti-inflammatory drug; PC, pericardium meridian; SP, spleen meridian; SSRIs, selective serotonin reuptake inhibitors; ST, stomach meridian; TE, triple energizer meridian; TENS, transcutaneous electrical nerve stimulation.

3.2.2. Other Intervention (Co-Intervention)

In 12 studies that applied MA, only two studies that described golfer's yips and runner's stitch syndrome used MA alone, and all other studies used a variety of co-interventions with acupuncture. Moreover, excluding three studies applying TENS for musculotendinous syndromes, catgut embedding for exercise-induced fatigue, or EA for ganglion cysts of the foot, the other 10 studies used a combination of co-interventions with acupuncture. The types of co-intervention differed depending on the disease; most commonly used were medication, Tuina, and various physical therapies (Table 2).

3.2.3. Treatment Duration and Session

The duration of treatment and follow-up periods for patients in each study varied from a few days to 13 months. With the exception of four studies that did not report the number of treatments, the study that provided the largest number of acupuncture treatments was the amenorrhea study in female runners (46 acupuncture treatment sessions over 13 months). Most of the others showed fewer than 10 treatment sessions.

Of the 11 studies reporting treatment frequency, the most common was a once- or twice-a-week regimen. Administration of treatment once a day or once every two weeks was reported in only one study, respectively.

Two studies showed that acupuncture was used only for some of the treatment periods: one study [50] used acupuncture in the second phase of the total three-phase treatment course, and the other study [35] used acupuncture only during the first two weeks.

3.3. *Follow-Up and Outcomes*

3.3.1. Outcome Measures

The outcome measures used in the studies can be categorized as follows: (1) Subjective outcome measures, (2) objective outcome measures, (3) AEs, (4) information on RTP, and (5) recurrence rates, including follow-up results.

Many studies described narratively regarding the alteration or improvement of patients' symptoms ($n = 9$). Different types of pain scales were used for an array of diseases that involve pain, including those of the musculoskeletal system, as follows ($n = 7$): Numerical rating scale (NRS), brief pain inventory (BPI), visual analog scale (VAS), pain relief score (PRS), McGill Pain Questionnaire (MPQ). There were also some objective outcome measures, such as blood test results, blood flow changes, body temperature, or numerical motor function evaluation outcome measures, including range of motion (ROM) ($n = 6$). Additionally, in some cases, results were comprehensively described on treatment days and cost for treatment, AEs, participants/providers ratio, effects on training, and recovery time, for the purpose of validity and feasibility evaluation of treatment intervention [29,30].

3.3.2. Results

Most of the main outcomes focused on positive changes in patients. This can also be confirmed by the authors' comments within each study on acupuncture treatment (Table 1). Of the 13 studies on the diseases of the musculoskeletal system and connective tissue, three studies used acupuncture only as an adjunctive treatment and acupuncture was not mentioned in the authors' conclusions [39,41,46]. Several studies reported that MA played a significant role in the treatment of shoulder pain, elbow tendinopathy, proximal hamstring tendinopathy, or peroneal nerve entrapment. EA was highly recommended as a conservative intervention for the treatment of femoroacetabular impingement [27], lateral meniscus injury [35], and ganglion cysts of the foot [47]. According to Young [38], EA plus MA is very effective in the treatment of calf strain and tennis elbow. LA and TENS are effective in musculoskeletal disorders involving several regions.

In mental and behavioral disorders, MA for golfer's yips and MA plus EA for sports-related postconcussive symptoms appeared to significantly reduce the symptoms. MA is beneficial and feasible for treating exercise-related DOMS in adolescent athletes and persistent pain in para-athletes. Catgut implantation at acupoints for sports fatigue or MA plus EA on soccer players with sports hernias appeared to significantly alleviate symptoms. As a result of Donoyama's study [43], acupuncture or hormone replacement therapy for amenorrhea was not effective as a single intervention, but only when used in combination.

3.3.3. Adverse Events

AEs were reported in five studies (22.7%), of which two reported no AEs, and the remaining three reported only minor AEs such as bleeding, pain, or numbness at the acupuncture site.

3.3.4. Return to Play and Recurrence

Results of the patients' RTP were reported in 12 studies (54.5%). In contrast, relatively less follow-up data related to relapse were collected, with only seven studies (31.8%) recording follow-up results to estimate recurrence rates (2-year follow-up period, $n = 2$; less than 6 months follow-up period, $n = 5$). As a result, only one study [33] reported that there was recurrence within the follow-up period; it was reported that six of 22 athletes treated for musculotendinous syndrome recurred between 10 days and two months after return to play.

4. Discussion

This systematic review summarized and analyzed case reports/series and series using acupuncture for sports injuries in athletes. Although the causal relationship of the effectiveness of acupuncture treatment was unclear due to the nature of the case report/series, it was confirmed that acupuncture was applied to a variety of sports injuries for athletes, ranging from yips of golf players to sports hernias of soccer players. The types of acupuncture also varied, including MA, EA, TENS, LA, and catgut embedding. The authors who performed each case report/series reported on the value of acupuncture as follows: (1) Short-term pain relief and recovery from dysfunction in each injured body region observed after acupuncture treatment could be beneficial in competitive elite athletes; (2) acupuncture has also been recognized for its clinical value as a useful noninvasive, conservative management for sports injuries such as lateral meniscus rupture, femoroacetabular impingement, ganglion cysts, and sports hernias; (3) acupuncture is worth trying for psychoneuromuscular impediments such as yips, which are poorly treated, and for exercise-related DOMS in athletes, and it has been suggested as an accessible treatment with appropriate resource (including cost and time).

Several previous RCTs have shown that acupuncture is effective in controlling pain in sports injuries in athletes, and it has been reported that the symptoms of rotator cuff tendinitis [51], shoulder impingement syndrome [52], shin splints [53], and plantar fasciitis [54] were improved by acupuncture. As of late, research on the effects and mechanisms of acupuncture tended to focus on pain control, but, clinically, it has been applied to various diseases and symptoms other than pain. Many studies related to pain control in acupuncture, which have been reported so far, have elucidated well the systemic and local mechanisms of acupuncture through mediators such as the central or autonomic nervous systems [19]. Nevertheless, research and discussion on the very complex elements involved in performing "acupuncture" are still in progress, and research on the specific mechanisms of the different diseases is still required.

As with the complexity of acupuncture, the scope of sports injuries is difficult and extensive to establish clearly. [55,56]. There are many different terms for sports injury, such as "sports impairment", "sports trauma", "sports incapacity", "sports disease", and "sports illness". If it can be recognized that each of these terms may have subtle differences in meaning, it can be seen that the need for a very complex perspective and a multidisciplinary approach in the field of sports medicine is inevitable. In fact, sports injury is known to require a systematic and multidisciplinary approach to treatment due to its complex etiology and various symptoms [7]. For example, overuse injuries in athletes are difficult to treat because symptoms are often extensive and uncharacteristic [57]. Another factor to consider in the treatment of sports injury in athletes is that they need not only recovery of the injured body part, but also recovery of their function to perform the sport again [15]. For athletes to return to play, systematic rehabilitation is necessary following successful treatment [58]. Physical and muscle strength, muscular endurance, flexibility, and agility need to be improved again as well as management of anxiety and depression caused by injury, if necessary [17]. Therefore, for sports injuries of elite athletes, an "RTP strategy" is required, and, for this, it has been discussed that the conservative method using a multimodal approach should be considered first [27]. However, apart from the lack of evidence of recommendations for various conservative treatment options [59], there are still limitations in the application of drug therapy, one of the most used conservative managements, to all cases of the RTP strategy [60]. The case studies included in this review suggest that acupuncture is one of the conservative approaches that would merit consideration in the field of sports and may be worth trying even for unexpected disorders that are not easy to treat [27–30,33–50].

Interestingly, case reports/series included in this review were mainly performed in the Americas and Europe, but not in the East Asian countries where acupuncture is primarily used in clinical practice. However, this does not denote that acupuncture treatments are not applied to sports injuries in East Asian countries. In Korea, acupuncture has been used formally or informally in sporting events since the early 1990s. In international sports competitions held in Korea that encompass a variety of sports, team doctors treated Korean athletes (sometimes including foreign athletes) with acupuncture and expressed satisfaction [61–63]. This positive experience has led to an opportunity for acupuncture to be introduced into the official medical treatment of the Olympic Village polyclinic in the 2018 PyeongChang Winter Olympics [64].

For a critical interpretation of this review, we suggest that careful consideration of the following limitations is essential. Firstly, the distinctive advantage of this review, but also an intricate disadvantage, was that we analyzed "sports injury" research on "athletes". Defining the terms "sports injury" and "athlete" involves a multitude of controversial concepts. [65] Thus, future research suggesting an accurate terminology will provide a clearer perspective. Second, it should be taken into account that the data we analyzed were derived from case reports/series. For our research to provide useful insights for clinical acupuncture for sports medicine practitioners, it is necessary to establish specific recommendations for which acupuncture is an effective treatment for the different types of sports injuries. This cannot be presented based only on case reports/series. The third limitation is linked to the second limitation. It should be noted that acupuncture treatment may not be a "study only to verify the effectiveness of acupuncture" in each case study. Since a number of studies included in this review used acupuncture as a co-intervention, or an adjunctive treatment, and not a stand-alone intervention, the effect of acupuncture can be a response to a multimodal conservative treatment. Fourth, our research showed that acupuncture can be applied to a variety of diseases within the sports injury category in athletes, but should not be misleading in the sense that acupuncture is effective for all variety of diseases. Experimental research such as RCTs for athletes, or systematic review based on it, can give a clear answer to the effectiveness of acupuncture. A recent systematic review of the effects of acupuncture treatment on DOMS reported that acupuncture had small-to-moderate effects compared to the no-treatment group and presented insufficient data for meta-analysis [66]. Further well-designed studies assessing acupuncture's efficacy in sports medicine are warranted to establish a strong evidence and to support clinical practice.

This study provided minor clues about the possibility of applying acupuncture to various types of sports injuries in athletes. In the future, we need to clarify which types of injuries are more effective in acupuncture through a detailed classification of sports injuries. As previously stated, it is very difficult to clearly identify the causes or symptoms of sports injuries. Nevertheless, in order to propose a more practical application of acupuncture, research that can generate evidence through more specific research questions and hypotheses should be conducted.

5. Conclusions

In this review, we endeavored to identify the potential of acupuncture for managing discomfort in athletes and their return to exercise through case reports/series on sports injuries in athletes. The included cases showed some potential of acupuncture in the treatment of various types of sports injuries, beyond pain control in musculoskeletal disorders. In addition, this review will assist practitioners who wish to use acupuncture to treat sports injuries and enable practical clinical applications of acupuncture, thereby allowing the use of novel therapeutic options for patients. This is the first review, to our knowledge, to systematically search, summarize, and analyze clinical case reports/series on the potential application of acupuncture in the treatment of sports injuries of athletes.

Author Contributions: Conceptualization, S.-Y.K. and J.-H.L.; methodology, validation, formal analysis, investigation, and data curation, J.-W.L. and S.-Y.K.; resources, J.-H.L.; writing—original draft preparation, J.-W.L.; writing—review and editing, S.-Y.K. and J.-H.L.; visualization, J.-W.L. and S.-Y.K.; supervision, S.-Y.K.; project administration, S.-Y.K.; funding acquisition, J.-H.L. All authors have read and agreed to the published version of the manuscript.

Acknowledgments: A special thanks to Gyeong Hwan Hyeon (Gachon University) for helping in preparing the figures.

References

1. Warburton, D.E.R.; Bredin, S.S.D. Health benefits of physical activity: A systematic review of current systematic reviews. *Curr. Opin. Cardiol.* **2017**, *32*, 541–556. [CrossRef] [PubMed]
2. Pedersen, B.K.; Saltin, B. Exercise as medicine—Evidence for prescribing exercise as therapy in 26 different chronic diseases. *Scand. J. Med. Sci. Sports* **2015**, *25*, 1–72. [CrossRef] [PubMed]
3. Petridou, A.; Siopi, A.; Mougios, V. Exercise in the management of obesity. *Metabolism* **2019**, *92*, 163–169. [CrossRef] [PubMed]
4. Parkkari, J.; Kujala, U.M.; Kannus, P. Is it possible to prevent sports injuries? Review of controlled clinical trials and recommendations for future work. *Sports Med.* **2001**, *31*, 985–995. [CrossRef] [PubMed]
5. Patel, D.R.; Baker, R.J. Musculoskeletal injuries in sports. *Prim. Care Clin. Off Pract.* **2006**, *33*, 545–579. [CrossRef] [PubMed]
6. Alessandrino, F.; Balconi, G. Complications of muscle injuries. *J. Ultrasound* **2013**, *16*, 215–222. [CrossRef] [PubMed]
7. Khan, K.; Brukner, P. *Brukner & Khan's Clinical Sports Medicine*; McGraw-Hill Education: New York, NY, USA, 2011.
8. Šmela, P.; Pačesová, P.; Kraček, S.; Hájovský, D. Performance Motivation of Elite Athletes, Recreational Athletes and Non-Athletes. *Acta Fac. Educ. Phys. Univ. Comen.* **2017**, *57*, 125–133. [CrossRef]
9. Zippelius, K.; Schwarzinger, A. Sports injuries-improved healing processes due to integrative TCM therapy. *Eur. J. Orient. Med.* **2017**, *8*, 28–33.
10. Herring, S.A.; Kibler, W.B.; Putukian, M. The team physician and the return-to-play decision: A consensus statement-2012 update. *Med. Sci. Sports Exerc.* **2012**, *44*, 2446–2448. [CrossRef]
11. Ting, J.H.; Wallis, D.H. Medical management of the athlete: Evaluation and treatment of important issues in sports medicine. *Clin. Podiatr. Med. Surg.* **2007**, *24*, 127–158. [CrossRef]
12. Doyscher, R.; Kraus, K.; Finke, B.; Scheibel, M. Acute and overuse injuries of the shoulder in sports. *Orthopade* **2014**, *43*, 202–208. [CrossRef]
13. Krauss, A. Why all randomised controlled trials produce biased results. *Ann. Med.* **2018**, *50*, 312–322. [CrossRef]
14. Dainesi, S.M.; Goldbaum, M. Reasons behind the participation in biomedical research: A brief review. *Rev. Bras. Epidemiol.* **2014**, *17*, 842–851. [CrossRef]
15. Grimes, D.A.; Schulz, K.F. Descriptive studies: What they can and cannot do. *Lancet* **2002**, *359*, 145–149. [CrossRef]
16. Kuchar, E. The importance of case reports in current pediatric endocrinology and metabolism literature—The

analysis of publications indexed in Medline in the years 2004–2009. *Pediatr. Endocrinol. Diabetes Metab.* **2010**, *16*, 119–122.

17. Gopikrishna, V. A report on case reports. *J. Conserv. Dent.* **2010**, *13*, 265–271. [CrossRef]
18. Yuan, Q.-L.; Wang, P.; Liu, L.; Sun, F.; Cai, Y.-S.; Wu, W.-T.; Ye, M.-L.; Ma, J.-T.; Xu, B.-B.; Zhang, Y.-G. Acupuncture for musculoskeletal pain: A meta-analysis and meta-regression of sham-controlled randomized clinical trials. *Sci. Rep.* **2016**, *6*, 30675. [CrossRef]
19. Filshie, J.; White, A.; Cummings, M. *Medical Acupuncture: A Western Scientific Approach*, 2nd ed.; Elsevier: Amsterdam, The Netherlands, 2016.
20. Han, J.-S. Acupuncture and endorphins. *Neurosci. Lett.* **2004**, *361*, 258–261. [CrossRef]
21. Cheng, K.J. Neurobiological Mechanisms of Acupuncture for Some Common Illnesses: A Clinician's Perspective. *J. Acupunct. Meridian Stud.* **2014**, *7*, 105–114. [CrossRef]
22. Pirnia, B.; Bazargan, N.M.; Hamdieh, M.; Pirnia, K.; Malekanmehr, P.; Maleki, F.; Zahiroddin, A. The Effectiveness of Auricular Acupuncture on the Levels of Cortisol in a Depressed Patient. *Iran. J. Public Health* **2019**, *48*, 1748–1750. [PubMed]
23. Hui, K.K.; Marina, O.; Liu, J.; Rosen, B.R.; Kwong, K.K. Acupuncture, the limbic system, and the anticorrelated networks of the brain. *Auton. Neurosci.* **2010**, *157*, 81–90. [CrossRef] [PubMed]
24. MacPherson, H.; Vickers, A.; Bland, M.; Torgerson, D.; Corbett, M.S.; Spackman, E.; Saramago, P.; Woods, B.; Weatherly, H.; Sculpher, M.; et al. Acupuncture for chronic pain and depression in primary care: A programme of research. *Program. Grants Appl. Res.* **2017**, *5*, 1–316. [CrossRef]
25. Cui, C.-L.; Wu, L.-Z.; Luo, F. Acupuncture for the Treatment of Drug Addiction. *Neurochem. Res.* **2008**, *33*, 2013–2022. [CrossRef]
26. Huang, Q.; Luo, D.; Chen, L.; Liang, F.X.; Chen, R. Effectiveness of Acupuncture for Alzheimer's Disease: An Updated Systematic Review and Meta-analysis. *Curr. Med Sci.* **2019**, *39*, 500–511. [CrossRef] [PubMed]
27. MacIntyre, K.; Gomes, B.; MacKenzie, S.; D'Angelo, K. Conservative management of an elite ice hockey goaltender with femoroacetabular impingement (FAI): A case report. *J. Can. Chiropr. Assoc.* **2015**, *59*, 398–409.
28. Lin, K.; Tung, C. Acupuncture for Recovery from Pediatric Sport-Related Concussion. *Med Acupunct.* **2016**, *28*, 217–222. [CrossRef]
29. Garlanger, K.L.; Fredericks, W.H.; Do, A.; Bauer, B.A.; Laskowski, E.R. The Feasibility and Effects of Acupuncture in an Adolescent Nordic Ski Population. *PM R* **2017**, *9*, 795–803. [CrossRef]
30. Luetmer, M.T.; Do, A.; Canzanello, N.C.; Bauer, B.A.; Laskowski, E.R. The Feasibility and Effects of Acupuncture on Muscle Soreness and Sense of Well-being in an Adolescent Football Population. *Am. J. Phys. Med. Rehabil.* **2019**, *98*, 964–970. [CrossRef]
31. Riley, D.S.; Barber, M.S.; Kienle, G.S.; Aronson, J.K.; von Schoen-Angerer, T.; Tugwell, P.; Kiene, H.; Helfand, M.; Altman, D.G.; Sox, H.; et al. CARE guidelines for case reports: Explanation and elaboration document. *J. Clin. Epidemiol.* **2017**, *89*, 218–235. [CrossRef]
32. Mitchell, J.H.; Haskell, W.L.; Raven, P.B. Classification of sports. *J.Am. Coll. Cardiol.* **1994**, *24*, 864–866. [CrossRef]
33. Dlin, R.A.; Benmair, J.; Hanne, N. Pain Relief in Sports Injuries—Application of TENS to Acupuncture Points. *Int. J. Sports Med.* **1980**, *1*, 203–206. [CrossRef]
34. Sternfeld, M.; Finkelstein, Y.; Eliraz, A.; Hod, I. Runner's stitch syndrome successfully treated by acupuncture. *Am. J. Acupunct.* **1992**, *20*, 213–215.
35. Seplow, W. Management of Lateral Meniscus Injury. *Sports Chiropr. Rehabil.* **1996**, *10*, 86–88.
36. Hoven, J.; Snyder, R.; Andrew, T. Management of peroneal nerve entrapment in an elite skier: A case report. *J. Sports Chiropr. Rehabil.* **2000**, *14*, 70–74.
37. Rosted, P. Acupuncture for treatment of the yips?—A case report. *Acupunct. Med.* **2005**, *23*, 188–189. [CrossRef]
38. Young, K. Sports Injuries and TCM. *J. Chin. Med.* **2005**, *78*, 1–10.
39. Martinez-Silvestrini, J.A.; Micheo, W.F. Complex regional pain syndrome in pediatric sports: A case series of three young athletes. *Boletín la Asoc Médica Puerto Rico* **2006**, *98*, 31–37.
40. Chen, Y.Z.; Xu, Y.; Yang, W.B.; Lu, Y.H.; Fang, H.B. Observation on therapeutic effect of catgut implantation at acupoints on exercise fatigue and study on the mechanism. *Zhongguo Zhen Jiu* **2008**, *28*, 656–658.

41. Yan, X.N.; Ren, C.X. Cause and treatment of sports injury in knee joint medial collateral ligament. *Zhongguo Zuzhi Gongcheng Yanjiuyu Linchuang Kangfu* **2008**, *12*, 5567–5570.
42. Osborne, N.J.; Gatt, I.T. Management of Shoulder Injuries Using Dry Needling in Elite Volleyball Players. *Acupunct. Med.* **2010**, *28*, 42–45. [CrossRef]
43. Donoyama, N.; Hotoge, S.; Ohkoshi, N. Acupuncture Might Have Contributed to Improving Amenorrhoea in a Top Athlete. *Acupunct. Med.* **2011**, *29*, 304–306. [CrossRef] [PubMed]
44. Yuill, E.A.; Pajaczkowski, J.A.; Howitt, S.D. Conservative care of sports hernias within soccer players: A case series. *J. Bodyw. Mov. Ther.* **2012**, *16*, 540–548. [CrossRef]
45. Morimoto, Y.; Saito, A.; Tokuhashi, Y. Low level laser therapy for sports injuries. *Laser Ther.* **2013**, *22*, 17–20. [CrossRef] [PubMed]
46. Pearcey, G.E.P.; Bradbury-Squires, D.J.; Power, K.E.; Behm, D.G.; Button, D.C. Exertional Rhabdomyolysis in an Acutely Detrained Athlete/Exercise Physiology Professor. *Clin. J. Sport Med.* **2013**, *23*, 496–498. [CrossRef]
47. Woitzik, E.; Kissel, J. Ganglion cyst of the foot treated with electroacupuncture: A case report. *J. Can. Chiropr. Assoc.* **2013**, *57*, 310–315.
48. Abe, G.C.; Yonamine, B.T.S.; Mello, C.A.D.S.; Ramos, P.E.; Conde, M.S.; Oliveira, A.S.B. Acupuncture for Treating Persistent Pain in Brazilian Para-Athletes. *Med Acupunct.* **2014**, *26*, 50–56. [CrossRef]
49. Gliedt, J.A.; Daniels, C.J. Chiropractic management of elbow tendinopathy following a sports related trauma. *J. Can. Chiropr. Assoc.* **2014**, *58*, 52–57.
50. Jayaseelan, D.J.; Moats, N.; Ricardo, C.R. Rehabilitation of Proximal Hamstring Tendinopathy Utilizing Eccentric Training, Lumbopelvic Stabilization, and Trigger Point Dry Needling: 2 Case Reports. *J. Orthop. Sports Phys. Ther.* **2014**, *44*, 198–205. [CrossRef] [PubMed]
51. Kleinhenz, J.; Streitberger, K.; Windeler, J.; Güssbacher, A.; Mavridis, G.; Martin, E. Randomised clinical trial comparing the effects of acupuncture and a newly designed placebo needle in rotator cuff tendinitis. *Pain* **1999**, *83*, 235–241. [CrossRef]
52. Kamali, F.; Sinaei, E.; Morovati, M. Comparison of Upper Trapezius and Infraspinatus Myofascial Trigger Point Therapy by Dry Needling in Overhead Athletes With Unilateral Shoulder Impingement Syndrome. *J. Sport Rehabil.* **2019**, *28*, 243–249. [CrossRef]
53. Callison, M. Clinical study: Acupuncture & tibial stress syndrome (Shin splints). *J. Chin. Med.* **2002**, *70*, 24–28.
54. Karagounis, P.; Tsironi, M.; Prionas, G.; Tsiganos, G.; Baltopoulos, P. Treatment of plantar fasciitis in recreational athletes: Two different therapeutic protocols. *Foot Ankle Spec.* **2011**, *4*, 226–234. [CrossRef]
55. Timpka, T.; Jacobsson, J.; Bickenbach, J.; Finch, C.F.; Ekberg, J.; Nordenfelt, L. What is a sports injury? *Sports Med.* **2014**, *44*, 423–428. [CrossRef]
56. Joseph, C.W.; Finch, C.F. *Sports Injuries. International Encyclopedia of Public Health*, 2nd ed.; Quah, S.R., Cockerham, W.C., Eds.; Academic Press: Cambridge, MA, USA, 2017; pp. 79–86.
57. Renström, P.; Johnson, R.J. Overuse injuries in sports. A review. *Sports Med.* **1985**, *2*, 316–333. [CrossRef]
58. Crockett, B. Rehabilitation of the athlete. *Mo. Med.* **2011**, *108*, 173–175.
59. Babatunde, O.O.; Jordan, J.L.; Van der Windt, D.A.; Hill, J.C.; Foster, N.E.; Protheroe, J. Effective treatment options for musculoskeletal pain in primary care: A systematic overview of current evidence. *PLoS ONE* **2017**, *12*, e0178621. [CrossRef]
60. Mehallo, C.J.; Drezner, J.A.; Bytomski, J.R. Practical management: Nonsteroidal antiinflammatory drug (NSAID) use in athletic injuries. *Clin. J. Sport Med.* **2006**, *16*, 170–174. [CrossRef]
61. Jeon, M.S.; Bae, S.Y. The Study of Athlete Patients Visited Korean Medical Clinic in CheongJu-Gym at the 2016 CheongJu World Martial Arts. *J. Sports Korean Med.* **2016**, *16*, 51–56.
62. Oh, M.J.; Son, I.M.; Shin, J.M.; Cho, J.H. The Study of Patients Visited Korean Medical Clinic in Athletes' Village Hospital at The 28th Univesiade Gwanju Korea. *J. Sports Korean Med.* **2016**, *16*, 1–7.
63. Yang, C.; Lee, E.; Hwang, E.H.; Kwon, O.; Lee, J.H. Management of Sport Injuries with Korean Medicine: A Survey of Korean National Volleyball Team. *Evid. Based Complement. Alternat. Med.* **2016**, *2016*, 1–7. [CrossRef]
64. Kim, D.S.; Lee, Y.H.; Bae, K.S.; Baek, G.H.; Lee, S.Y.; Shim, H.; On, M.G.; Rhie, S.J.Y. PyeongChang 2018 Winter Olympic Games and athletes' usage of 'polyclinic' medical services. *BMJ Open Sport Exerc. Med.* **2019**, *5*, e000548. [CrossRef]

65. Araujo, C.G.; Scharhag, J. Athlete: A working definition for medical and health sciences research. *Scand. J. Med. Sci. Sports* **2016**, *26*, 4–7. [CrossRef]
66. Chang, W.D.; Chang, N.J.; Lin, H.Y.; Wu, J.H. Effects of Acupuncture on Delayed-Onset Muscle Soreness: A Systematic Review and Meta-Analysis. *Evid. Based Complement. Alternat. Med.* **2020**, *2020*, 5864057. [CrossRef]

5

Association of Acupuncture Treatment with Mortality of Type 2 Diabetes in China: Evidence of a Real-World Study

Mengyun Sui, Long Xue and Xiaohua Ying *

NHC Key Laboratory of Health Technology Assessment, School of Public Health, Fudan University, Dongan Road 130, Shanghai 200032, China; 18111020027@fudan.edu.cn (M.S.); 18111020030@fudan.edu.cn (L.X.)

* Correspondence: xhying@fudan.edu.cn

Abstract: The prevalence and mortality rates of diabetes are increasing globally, posing severe challenges to health systems. Acupuncture is used worldwide as a non-drug treatment for diabetes. However, empirical evidence of the effect of combined acupuncture and drug treatments on diabetic-associated mortality is limited. This study aimed to examine this association of acupuncture treatment with mortality of type 2 diabetes based on real-world data. A four-year cohort study was conducted in Shanghai between 2015 and 2018, The database consisted of 37,718 patients (acupuncture group: 6865 type 2 diabetes mellitus (T2DM) patients, non-acupuncture (control) group: 30,853 T2DM patients) in 2016. The objective was to analyze the impact of receiving acupuncture prescriptions for diabetes in 2016 on all-cause mortality in 2018 based on real-world data. An Inverse Probability Weighted Regression Adjustment (IPWRA) and Propensity Score Matching (PSM) were used to minimize the bias due to potential confounding variables to increase the reliability of differences in comparisons between the two groups. Our inverse probability weighted regression results suggest that the coefficient of the key dependent variable of accepted acupuncture in 2016 was negative (coefficient: −0.0002; 95% CI: −0.0024–0.0019, $p = 0.857$), but it is not statistically significant. In robustness check, PSM with the nearest-neighbor method with replacement at a 1:4 ratio and 1:3 ratio and kernel matching showed that the average treatment effect was negative. Therefore, there was a negative correlation between acupuncture combined with other drugs and the mortality of diabetic patients, but it was not statistically significant.

Keywords: diabetes mellitus; acupuncture; mortality; traditional Chinese medicine

1. Introduction

1.1. *Prevalence of Diabetes*

Diabetes mellitus has shown an alarming increase, becoming a global epidemic [1]. According to the most recent International Diabetes Federation (IDF) Diabetes Atlas 2019, the prevalence of diabetes worldwide tripled from 151 million in 2000 to 463 million in 2019 and is projected to reach 700 million by 2045. Diabetes is expected to be present in 10.9% of the global population by 2045 [2]. Patients with diabetes are prone to microvascular complications (nephropathy, retinopathy, and neuropathy) and macrovascular complications (concomitant atherosclerosis and coronary artery disease) [3]. The number of deaths resulting from diabetes and its complications was estimated to be 4.2 million in 2019. The ultimate value of diabetes prevention lies in reduced blood sugar, incidence of complications, and mortality [4].

1.2. Introduction of Acupuncture

Acupuncture therapy is a significant part of traditional Chinese medicine (TCM). There are various types of acupuncture, including manual acupuncture, electroacupuncture, ear acupuncture, moxibustion, and acupoint injection [5]. It involves the treatment of disease by inserting needles along specific pathways or meridians, according to the disease being treated. Acupuncture is widely practiced globally, including in countries such as Japan, Taiwan, China, and the United States [6–8]. Many patients use a combination of conventional medicine and acupuncture to treat diabetes [9]. Acupuncture has unique advantages. For example, its approach is holistic in that it hinges on the belief that the human body is an organic whole, which is mainly connected by the meridian system [10].

1.3. Strengthening Acupuncture in China

The World Health Organization (WHO) recommends that countries take effective measures to prevent and treat diabetes [11]. Accordingly, the WHO and the National Institutes of Health reported that acupuncture could be an effective means to treat diabetes [12]. As acupuncture is indigenous to China, the Chinese government is paying more attention to its development and promotion. In the Chinese Guidelines for the Prevention and Treatment of type 2 diabetes mellitus (T2DM) (2017 edition), TCM treatment has been included. China is increasing the coverage of acupuncture in community health service centers and family doctor teams. Meanwhile, with the internationalization of TCM, it is necessary to prove the effectiveness of this practice.

To meet the demand for acupuncture in diabetes treatment, top-down policies from the Chinese government have been promulgated [13]. For example, in 2009, the State Administration of TCM issued an implementation plan for appropriate TCM technology [14]. In 2016, the State Administration of TCM announced a project that promotes the integration of acupuncture into the regular diabetic care provided by the family physician [15]. Since then, an increasing number of patients with diabetes have been using acupuncture as an alternative medical therapy.

Shanghai is a pioneer city for the family doctor system and TCM services. The family doctor team usually has one or two core general practitioners and is equipped with a TCM physician, public health physician, nurse, and physician assistant [16]. The government is committed to providing acupuncture knowledge and skills training to family doctors, thereby increasing the number of TCM doctors and expanding the integration of acupuncture into family doctor teams. The family doctor provides Western medicine, TCM, acupuncture and moxibustion and other related services. In 2018, a total of 6.66 million family doctors in Shanghai had signed contracts with 30% of permanent residents; moreover, more than 84% of patients with diabetes had signed contracts [17]. Acupuncture is frequently applied in conjunction with Western medicine to relieve symptoms in patients with diabetes.

1.4. The Purpose of the Study

Previous studies have reported the relationship between acupuncture and blood glucose levels and complications in patients with diabetes [18,19]. However, there is insufficient evidence to support these results because of the small sample size, uncertain outcomes, and a lack of real-world situations. Although many people enjoy using acupuncture, the mainstream scientific approach based on evidence and outcome reproduction cannot fully demonstrate the value of acupuncture, and the evidence of the contribution of acupuncture to health is limited.

To bridge the gap between acupuncture therapy and its effect on type 2 diabetes mellitus (T2DM), the participants of this study were categorized into two groups—control and acupuncture groups. Only one goal has been considered in this study. The objective was to analyze the impact of received acupuncture for diabetes in 2016 on all-cause mortality in 2018 based on real-world data. We used baseline characteristics of patients in 2016 to estimate diabetes death in 2018. We explored the long-term health effects of receiving acupuncture prescriptions. The hypothesis of this study was compared with that of the control group; the acupuncture group had a lower mortality rate. The mortality rate was the primary outcome of the research.

2. Materials and Methods

2.1. Study Design

In this study, we utilized a three-stage sampling design to select T2DM patients (stratified by the community health center, family physician team, and T2DM patients). First, out of the 240 community health service centers in the 16 administrative regions of Shanghai, one-third were included in the study. These 80 centers were selected through stratified sampling of the administrative divisions. Then, three family physician teams were drawn from each center, and a total of 240 teams were included. Finally, 150 patients with T2DM who received TCM were chosen from the family physician team by simple random sampling. We defined the treatment group as those who received acupuncture therapy. The study population selection is shown in Figure 1.

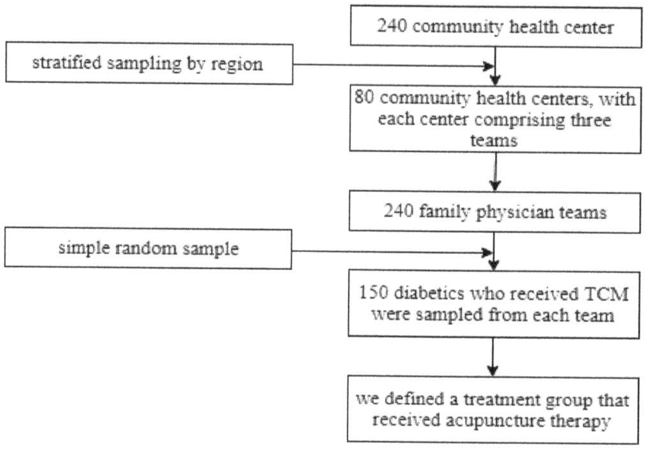

Figure 1. The sampling protocol of this study. TCM: traditional Chinese medicine.

2.2. Data Source and Population Selection

This study used panel data deposited in the Health Information Center Database of Shanghai, from patients who received TCM from 1 January 2015 to 31 December 2018. Quarterly records of patients over these four years were collected, but we ended up using the year data as the unit of analysis. The datasets consisted of demographic characteristics, outpatient and inpatient health service utilization of different hospital types (primary, secondary, tertiary hospital), number of acupuncture prescriptions, cost of different hospital types, death, and information on complications. We defined disease according to the International Classification of Diseases, 10th Revision (ICD-10). The database consisted of 37,718 patients (acupuncture group: 6865 T2DM patients, non-acupuncture (control) group: 30,853 T2DM patients) in 2016.

2.3. Research Variables

2.3.1. Dependent Variable

We included one critical outcome—i.e., occurrence of mortality, as a dependent variable. Mortality is a binary variable, and it was recognized when the patient died in 2018.

2.3.2. Independent Variable

The key variable was the choice of which group should receive acupuncture—defined as "1" for acupuncture and "0" for the control group. Categorial variables consisted of patients' gender, age, other chronic diseases, treatment cost, and residential location. Gender was categorized as male and female; four age ranges were stratified (<60, 60–69, 70–79, and ≥80 years); four levels of other chronic diseases were categorized (0, 1, 2 and ≥3 chronic diseases); two classes for the residential location were categorized (urban and outskirts); the cost per year was divided into four groups (≤2000, 2001–7000, 7001–15,000 and ≥15,001 yuan). We collected information on other chronic diseases, such as hypertension, coronary heart disease, stroke, arrhythmia, and angina. The complication variable was binary, with "yes" and "no" as options.

The regression formula is as follows:

$$Y_i = \beta_0 + \beta_1 Treat + \beta X_i + \varepsilon_i$$

where Y_i refers to diabetic i who died or not; treat denotes whether they received acupuncture treatment; X_i indicates covariate variables, including gender, cost, age, residential location and other chronic disease. ε_i is the error term.

2.4. Statistical Analysis

Descriptive statistics were used to demonstrate the baseline characteristics of the patients with T2DM. Percentages were used to analyze categorical data, and means were adopted to analyze continuous data.

In this study, we used baseline data for diabetes in 2016 and death data for 2018 to estimate the effect. Due to the retrospective cohort design of our study and the possibility of selection bias, we considered that the demographic characteristics and disease status of the patients could affect the results. Therefore, an Inverse Probability Weighted Regression Adjustment (IPWRA) and Propensity Score Matching (PSM) were used to minimize the bias due to potential confounding variables to increase the reliability of differences in comparisons between the two groups [16,17]. We used IPWRA to estimate the relationship of whether received outpatient visits of traditional Chinese Medicine for diabetes in 2016 with all-cause mortality in 2018. IPWRA is one approach to estimate unbiased treatment effects when we have confounding factors. Firstly, the IPWRA method generated IP (Inverse Probability) weights according to individual's values of treatment and covariate and assigns the inverse of probability of treatment for treated individuals and the inverse probability of not being treated for control individuals [20,21]. Then, it re-estimates the outcome model using these new weights. In this study, we use gender, age, residential location, cost and other chronic disease to estimate IP weights, then new weights and a logistic regression model were used to estimate outcomes.

In a robustness check, we used three methods to estimate the Average Treatment Effect (ATE)—PSM of a 1:4 ratio, 1:3 ratio and kernel matching, respectively. We used baseline data from patients with diabetes in 2016 for matching. Patients'gender, age, other chronic, cost, residential location are matching variables. Propensity score, logistic regression on patients' demographics information for each eligible subject was matched according to the score by using the nearest-neighbor method at a 1:4 ratio with 0.02 in the caliper [22]. The 50 times bootstrap method was employed to obtain the robust standard error.

For all data sets, differences were considered statistically significant when the p value < 0.05. All analyses were performed using STATA software (version 16.0).

3. Results

3.1. Baseline T2DM Patient Characteristics

Table 1 describes the baseline patient characteristics of the treatment and control groups. Both the acupuncture and control groups had a higher proportion of females. The average age of the acupuncture group was two years older than that of the control group. A higher proportion of patients in the acupuncture group had other chronic diseases. The results indicated that people with T2DM and other chronic conditions are more likely to seek non-drug treatment. Overall, acupuncture group patients were more likely to be older, female, have other chronic disease. The outpatient and inpatient visits in the treatment group were higher than those in the control group. In the treatment group, mean prescriptions of acupuncture were 3.26 ± 4.74 per year, and medical expenses in the same period were approximately 1.6 times that of the control group.

Table 1. Baseline characteristics of type 2 diabetes mellitus (T2DM) patients in 2016.

Characteristics	Acupuncture Group (N = 6865)			Non-Acupuncture Group (N = 30,853)		
	Mean	SE	95%CI	Mean	SE	95% CI
Gender (%)						
Male	34.64	0.006	33.43–35.87	40.98	0.002	40.44–41.53
Female	65.35	0.006	64.13–66.57	59.01	0.002	58.46–59.56
Age (years)						
Mean	70.04	0.125	69.79–70.28	67.91	0.057	67.79–68.02
<60	9.96	0.003	9.27–10.69	19.29	0.002	18.85–19.73
60–69	33.38	0.006	32.28–34.51	38.79	0.003	38.25–39.34
70–79	25.53	0.005	24.51–26.58	27.09	0.003	26.60–27.59
≥80	31.11	0.006	30.03–32.22	14.81	0.002	14.42–15.21
Residential location (%)						
Urban	44.22	0.006	42.95–45.49	34.93	0.002	34.39–35.46
Suburban	55.77	0.006	54.50–57.04	65.07	0.002	64.53–65.60
Chronic (%)						
0	9.77	0.003	9.09–10.49	20.18	0.002	19.73–20.63
1	19.16	0.004	18.25–20.11	29.91	0.002	29.40–30.42
2	23.10	0.005	22.12–24.11	23.92	0.002	23.44–24.40
≥3	47.95	0.006	46.77–49.13	25.99	0.002	25.50–26.48
Total cost (yuan)						
Mean	16,571.99	177.64	16,223.74–16,920.24	10,098.17	61.94	9976.74–10,219.60
≤2000	5.07	0.002	4.57–5.61	20.32	0.002	19.87–20.77
2001–7000	16.35	0.004	15.50–17.25	31.53	0.003	31.01–32.05
7001–15,000	29.30	0.005	28.24–30.39	27.76	0.003	27.26–28.26
≥15,001	49.26	0.006	48.08–50.44	20.39	0.002	19.94–20.84
Outpatient visits						
Number of primary-level hospitals	39.51	0.355	38.81–40.21	26.63	0.135	26.36–26.90
Number of secondary-level hospitals	7.43	0.138	7.16–7.71	5.35	0.052	5.25–5.45
Number of tertiary-level hospitals	8.82	0.144	8.53–9.10	6.50	0.056	6.39–6.61
Inpatient visits						
Number of primary-level hospitals	0.012	0.002	0.01–0.02	0.012	0.000	0.01–0.01
Number of secondary-level hospitals	0.278	0.012	0.25–0.30	0.145	0.003	0.13–0.15
Number of tertiary-level hospitals	0.271	0.010	0.25–0.29	0.149	0.003	0.14–1.56
Total prescriptions of acupuncture	3.26	0.062	3.14–3.38	0.00	0.000	0.00

3.2. *Inverse Probability Weighted Regression Results*

In 2018, there was 45 diabetes patients in the acupuncture group who died—a mortality of 0.67%; in the control group there were 186 diabetes patients who died—a mortality of 0.61%. After controlling for confounders, the results were collected and are shown in Table 2. Our inverse probability weighted regression results suggest that the coefficient of the key dependent variable of accepted acupuncture in 2016 was negative (coefficient: −0.0002; 95% CI: −0.0024–0.0019, $p = 0.857$), but it is not statistically significant. Compared with women, being a man is a risk factor for death in diabetes. Age is also a dangerous factor for diabetes, and the older the person with diabetes, the greater the probability of death. An age over 70 years old increases the threat to diabetic patients significantly (coefficient: 0.0056; 95% CI: 0.0030–0.0082, $p < 0.001$).

Table 2. Inverse probability weighted regression results.

Death in 2018	Coefficient	95%CI	SE	*p*-Value
Treat 2016	−0.0002	−0.0024–0.0019	0.0011	0.857
Gender (%)				
Male	0.0040 ***	0.0016–0.0064	0.0012	0.001
Age (%)				
60–69	0.0016	−0.0005–0.0038	0.0011	0.140
70–79	0.0056 ***	0.0030–0.0082	0.0013	0.000
≥80	0.0192 ***	0.0144–0.0239	0.0024	0.000

Table 2. *Cont.*

Death in 2018	Coefficient	95%CI	SE	*p*-Value
Chronic (%)				
1	0.0004	0.0032–0.0024	0.0014	0.774
2	0.0003	0.0042–0.0035	0.0019	0.850
≥3	0.0025	0.0061–0.0008	0.0017	0.145
Residential location (%)				
Urban	−0.0024 ***	−0.0046–−0.0003	0.0011	0.027
Cost (%)				
2001–7000	0.0050 ***	0.0022–0.0007	0.0014	0.000
7001–15,000	0.0049 ***	0.0019–0.0079	0.0015	0.001
≥15,001	0.0063 ***	0.0029–0.0095	0.0016	0.000
Constant	−0.0026	−0.0055–0.0002	0.0014	0.075

*** $p < 0.01$, CI: Confidence Interval, SE: Standard Error.

3.3. Robust Test Results

After using the PSM method at 1:4 ratio, 970 patients were assigned to the acupuncture group and successfully matched with 5823 patients in the control group. After matching, the mortality rate in the acupuncture group was 0.74% and that in the control group was 1.02%. While many differences were statistically significant before the PSM procedure ($p < 0.05$, Table 3), there were few substantively important differences between the acupuncture group and the control group after adjustment ($p > 0.05$). As shown in Table 4, the average treatment effect in the PSM of 1:4 method was negative but not statistically significant (coefficient: −0.0014, 95% CI: −0.0072, 0.0042, $p = 0.611$). Using the PSM method at 1:3 ratio, the coefficient is also negative (coefficient: −0.0034, 95% CI: −0.0105, 0.0036, $p = 0.344$). In the Kernel Matching, the coefficient is −0.0002.

Table 3. Comparable characteristics between the two groups before and after matching.

Characteristics	Before Matching			After Matching		
	Acupuncture Group	Non-Acupuncture Group	*p* Value	Acupuncture Group	Non-Acupuncture Group	*p* Value
Gender (%)						
Male	34.57	40.97	<0.001	34.57	34.57	1.000
Age (%)						
60–69	39.15	38.84	0.647	39.15	39.15	1.000
70–79	29.95	27.11	<0.001	29.95	29.95	1.000
≥80	19.25	14.78	<0.001	19.25	19.25	1.000
Chronic (%)						
1	22.49	29.92	<0.001	22.49	22.49	1.000
2	27.07	24.01	<0.001	27.07	27.07	0.979
≥3	39.12	26.10	<0.001	39.12	39.12	0.981
Cost (%)						
2001–7000	19.13	31.61	<0.001	19.13	19.13	1.000
7001–15,000	34.39	27.88	<0.001	34.39	34.39	1.000
≥15,001	40.62	20.48	<0.001	0.62	0.62	1.000
Residential location (%)						
Urban	44.22	34.88	<0.001	44.22	44.22	1.000

Table 4. The average treatment effect of the three methods.

Method	Coefficient	95%CI	Standard Error	Z	*p*
1:4 PSM (bootstrap 50 times)	−0.0014	−0.0072, 0.0042	0.0029	−0.51	0.611
1:3 PSM (bootstrap 50 times)	−0.0034	−0.0105, 0.0036	0.0036	−0.95	0.344
Kernel Matching	−0.0002	−0.0022, −0.0016	0.0009	−0.30	0.766

PSM: Propensity Score Matching.

4. Discussion

This nationwide study analyzed the impact of receiving acupuncture for diabetes in 2016 on all-cause mortality in 2018 based on real-world data from mainland China. The results suggest a negative correlation between acupuncture combined with other drugs and the mortality of diabetes, but it was not statistically significant. The mortality rate was lower in the acupuncture combined with other drug groups than in the control group, but the difference was not significant. To the authors' knowledge, this study is one of the few to suggest that acupuncture reduces T2DM mortality using real-world data. There are reasons why there is a negative relationship between acupuncture treatment and mortality among patients with T2DM. First, acupuncture can improve insulin function, glucose metabolism, and glucose-related hormone levels by stimulating acupoints, thus achieving the goal of lowering blood glucose. At the same time, acupuncture can stimulate the biological activity of mitochondrial respiratory chain-related enzymes, improve mitochondrial function, and thus enhance the sensitivity of islet cells. These related mechanisms provide theoretical support for the acupuncture treatment of diabetes [5,23]. Western medicine can reduce the blood sugar levels of patients with diabetes and the incidence of complications, but it is not possible to achieve a complete cure. Acupuncture, in combination with Western medicine, has better efficacy and fewer side effects than single medicine alone, consequently reducing damage to the body caused by drugs administered to diabetic patients.

Our conclusion is that a negative correlation between acupuncture combined with other drugs and the mortality of diabetic, to some extent, can support the previous literature, comprising studies based on diabetic model rats, clinical trials, and meta-analyses. For example, some studies have clarified the mechanism and potential advantages of acupuncture in improving diabetic patients' blood sugar and its complications through animal experiments [24]. The compound laser acupuncture–moxibustion had positive effects on the regulation of hyperglycemia and insulin resistance in T2DM rats [25,26]. In terms of clinical indicators, a study involving 1943 people with diabetes showed that acupuncture baseline treatments reduced fasting blood sugar (FBS), 2-h blood glucose, and glycated hemoglobin levels [18]. Participants in the acupuncture group of another study were needled at CV-12 and showed a significant drop in random blood glucose levels [19]. Yet another study showed that a combination of metformin and acupuncture improves the body mass index; body weight; fasting insulin, FBS, triglyceride, low-density lipoprotein cholesterol, and high-density lipoprotein cholesterol levels [27]. In terms of treating complications, the findings of the acupuncture trial may establish the value of acupuncture therapy for the improvement of peripheral nerve function and subjective perception relative to diabetic peripheral neuropathy [28–31]. Acupuncture treatment is also a cost-effective option. Acupuncture therapy improves vascular circulation and wound healing as an alternative therapy for the treatment of diabetic foot [32].

Our study has three advantages. First, based on the perspective of evidence-based medicine, combined with real-world data, we answered one key question. We chose mortality as the outcome indicator that could reflect the relationship between real-world acupuncture treatment and the mortality rate in patients with T2DM. At present, most articles have utilized process indicators. Second, our study sample came from a credible source (Shanghai Health Information Statistics Center) and was sufficiently large, had good representativeness, and less missing data. Third, confounding factors were eliminated by the IPWRA and PSM. IPWRA and PSM are popular econometric methods at present. Nonetheless, our study has a few limitations. First, although we used IPWRA and PSM to eliminate the differences between the two groups, we might not have eliminated potential confounding factors entirely, including patients' lifestyle habits such as smoking, drinking, and exercise. Second, the conclusion drawn by IPWRA and PSM is not a causal relationship, and thus further research is required. Third, our data represent a retrospective cohort, and the study has not yet been prospectively designed.

5. Conclusions

We have demonstrated that the association of acupuncture combined with other-drug groups with mortality is negative but statistical insignificance. Further studies with a larger sample of patients with T2DM and using econometric methods combined with the current popular big data machine learning methods would validate the impact of acupuncture on the mortality rate in patients with T2DM and provide objective evidence for acupuncture treatment of diabetes.

Author Contributions: M.S. and X.Y. contributed to the conceptualization and study design. M.S. performed the literature review. M.S. analyzed the data and wrote the draft. L.X. contributed to software development. All authors have read and agreed to the published version of the manuscript.

Acknowledgments: Thanks to all the authors who contributed to this paper.

References

1. Standl, E.; Khunti, K.; Hansen, T.B.; Schnell, O. The global epidemics of diabetes in the 21st century: Current situation and perspectives. *Eur J. Prev Cardiol* **2019**, *26* (Suppl. 2), 7–14. [CrossRef] [PubMed]
2. Federation, I.D. IDF Diabetes Atlas, 9th edn. 2019. Available online: http://www.diabetesatlas.org (accessed on 25 July 2020).
3. Stolar, M. Glycemic control and complications in type 2 diabetes mellitus. *Am. J. Med.* **2010**, *123* (Suppl. 3), S3–S11. [CrossRef]
4. Diabetes Prevention Program Research Group. Long-term effects of lifestyle intervention or metformin on diabetes development and microvascular complications over 15-year follow-up: The Diabetes Prevention Program Outcomes Study. *Lancet Diabet Endocrinol* **2015**, *3*, 866–875. [CrossRef]
5. Feng, Y.; Fang, Y.; Wang, Y.; Hao, Y. Acupoint Therapy on Diabetes Mellitus and Its Common Chronic Complications: A Review of Its Mechanisms. *BioMed Res. Int.* **2018**, *2018*, 3128378. [CrossRef] [PubMed]
6. Upchurch, D.M.; Rainisch, B.W. A sociobehavioral wellness model of acupuncture use in the United States, 2007. *J. Alternat Complement. Med. (New York, N.Y.)* **2014**, *20*, 32–39. [CrossRef] [PubMed]
7. Ishizaki, N.; Yano, T.; Kawakita, K. Public status and prevalence of acupuncture in Japan. *Evid Based Complement. Alternat Med.* **2010**, *7*, 493–500. [CrossRef] [PubMed]
8. Wu, M.Y.; Lee, Y.C.; Lin, C.L.; Huang, M.C.; Sun, M.F.; Yen, H.R. Trends in use of acupuncture among adults in Taiwan from 2002 to 2011: A nationwide population-based study. *PLoS ONE* **2018**, *13*, e0195490. [CrossRef]
9. Poon, T.Y.; Ong, K.L.; Cheung, B.M. Review of the effects of the traditional Chinese medicine Rehmannia Six Formula on diabetes mellitus and its complications. *J. Diabet* **2011**, *3*, 184–200. [CrossRef]
10. Shi, L.; Feng, L.; Yang, Y.; Li, X.; Zhang, M.; Zhang, Y.; Ni, Q. Prevention of type 2 diabetes mellitus with acupuncture: Protocol for a systematic review and meta-analysis. *Medicine* **2018**, *97*, e13355. [CrossRef]
11. Shu, Z.; Wang, L.; Sun, X. An evaluation of the effects of general practitioner-supported patient noncommunicable diseases control model in Shanghai, China. *Int J. Health Plann. Manage.* **2019**, *34*, 947–959. [CrossRef]
12. Meyer-Hamme, G.; Friedemann, T.; Greten, H.J.; Plaetke, R.; Gerloff, C.; Schroeder, S. ACUDIN—ACUpuncture and laser acupuncture for treatment of DIabetic peripheral Neuropathy: A randomized, placebo-controlled, partially double-blinded trial. *BMC Neurol.* **2018**, *18*, 40. [CrossRef] [PubMed]
13. Chung, V.C.; Ma, P.H.; Wang, H.H.; Wang, J.J.; Hong, L.C.; Wei, X.; Wong, S.Y.; Tang, J.L.; Griffiths, S.M. Integrating traditional Chinese medicine services in community health centers: Insights into utilization patterns in the pearl river region of China. *Evid. Based Complement. Alternat Med.* **2013**, *2013*, 426360. [CrossRef] [PubMed]

14. National Administration of Traditional Chinese Medicine. Implementation Plan for Popularizing Appropriate Technology of Traditional Chinese Medicine for Common and Frequently-Occurring Diseases at Grassroots Level (2009–2010). 2009. Available online: http://yzs.satcm.gov.cn/gongzuodongtai/2018-03-25/6558.html (accessed on 27 July 2020).
15. National Administration of Traditional Chinese Medicine. 13th Five-year plan for the development of traditional Chinese medicine. In Medicine, S.A. o. T. C. Ed. 2016. Available online: http://www.gov.cn/xinwen/2016-08/11/content_5098934.htm (accessed on 27 July 2020).
16. Fang, Y. *Study of the Family-Doctor System in Shanghai*; Shanghai University of Engineering Science: Shanghai, China, 2016.
17. Network, C.B. The Signing Rate of Family Doctors in Shanghai is 30%. 2019. Available online: https://www.yicai.com/news/100095345.html (accessed on 5 August 2020).
18. Chen, C.; Liu, J.; Sun, M.; Liu, W.; Han, J.; Wang, H. Acupuncture for type 2 diabetes mellitus: A systematic review and meta-analysis of randomized controlled trials. *Complement. Ther. Clin. Pract.* **2019**, *36*, 100–112. [CrossRef]
19. Kumar, R.; Mooventhan, A.; Manjunath, N.K. Immediate effect of needling at CV-12 (Zhongwan) acupuncture point on blood glucose level in patients with type 2 diabetes mellitus: A pilot randomized placebo-controlled trial. *J. Acupunct. Meridian Stud.* **2017**, *10*, 240–244. [CrossRef] [PubMed]
20. Mansournia, M.A.; Altman, D.G. Inverse probability weighting. *BMJ* **2016**, *352*, i189. [CrossRef]
21. Strumpf, E.; Ammi, M.; Diop, M.; Fiset-Laniel, J.; Tousignant, P. The impact of team-based primary care on health care services utilization and costs: Quebec's family medicine groups. *J. Health Econ.* **2017**, *55*, 76–94. [CrossRef]
22. Xian, W.; Xu, X.; Li, J.; Sun, J.; Fu, H.; Wu, S.; Liu, H. Health care inequality under different medical insurance schemes in a socioeconomically underdeveloped region of China: A propensity score matching analysis. *BMC Public Health* **2019**, *19*, 1373. [CrossRef] [PubMed]
23. Zhang, R. *The Clinical Study of Laser Acupuncture and Moxibustion in Treating Type 2 Diabetes with Deficiency of Qi and Yin*; Nanjing University of Traditional Chinese Medicine: Nanjing, China, 2020. [CrossRef]
24. Pan, H.; Huang, H.; Zhang, L.; Ma, S.; Yang, H.; Wang, H. "Adjusting internal organs and dredging channel" electroacupuncture treatment prevents the development of diabetic peripheral neuropathy by downregulating glucose-related protein 78 (GRP78) and caspase-12 in streptozotocin-diabetic rats. *J. Diabetes* **2019**, *11*, 928–937. [CrossRef]
25. Li, Y.; Qian, Z.Y.; Cheng, K.; Zhao, L.; Shen, X.Y.; Deng, H.P. Effect of Compound Laser Acupuncture-Moxibustion on Blood Glucose, Fasting Insulin and Blood Lipids Levels in Type 2 Diabetic Rats. *Chin. J. Integrat. Med.* **2020**, *26*, 33–38. [CrossRef]
26. Cornejo-Garrido, J.; Becerril-Chávez, F.; Carlín-Vargas, G.; Ordoñez-Rodríguez, J.M.; Abrajan-González Mdel, C.; de la Cruz-Ramírez, R.; Ordaz-Pichardo, C. Antihyperglycaemic effect of laser acupuncture treatment at BL20 in diabetic rats. *Acupunct Med. J. Brit. Med. Acupunct Soc.* **2014**, *32*, 486–494. [CrossRef]
27. Firouzjaei, A.; Li, G.C.; Wang, N.; Liu, W.X.; Zhu, B.M. Comparative evaluation of the therapeutic effect of metformin monotherapy with metformin and acupuncture combined therapy on weight loss and insulin sensitivity in diabetic patients. *Nutr. Diabet.* **2016**, *6*, e209. [CrossRef]
28. Wang, L.Q.; Chen, Z.; Zhang, K.; Liang, N.; Yang, G.Y.; Lai, L.; Liu, J.P. Zusanli (ST36) Acupoint Injection for Diabetic Peripheral Neuropathy: A Systematic Review of Randomized Controlled Trials. *J. Alternat. Complement. Med.* **2018**, *24*, 1138–1149. [CrossRef]
29. Zhang, C.; Ma, Y.X.; Yan, Y. Clinical effects of acupuncture for diabetic peripheral neuropathy. *J. Tradit. Chin. Med.* **2010**, *30*, 13–14. [CrossRef]
30. Nash, J.; Armour, M.; Penkala, S. Acupuncture for the treatment of lower limb diabetic peripheral neuropathy: A systematic review. *Acupunct Med. J. Brit. Med. Acupunct Soc.* **2019**, *37*, 3–15. [CrossRef]
31. Lee, S.; Kim, J.H.; Shin, K.M.; Kim, J.E.; Kim, T.H.; Kang, K.W.; Lee, M.; Jung, S.Y.; Shin, M.S.; Kim, A.R.; et al. Electroacupuncture to treat painful diabetic neuropathy: Study protocol for a three-armed, randomized, controlled pilot trial. *Trials* **2013**, *14*, 225. [CrossRef]
32. Lee, M.; Li, H.; Liu, D. Acupuncture as adjuvant therapy for diabetic foot: A protocol for systematic review. *Medicine* **2020**, *99*, e19502. [CrossRef] [PubMed]

6

Nonspecific Feelings Expected and Experienced during or Immediately after Electroacupuncture: A Pilot Study in a Teaching Situation

David F. Mayor [1,*], Lara S. McClure [2] and J. Helgi Clayton McClure [2]

1 Department of Allied Health Professions and Midwifery, School of Health and Social Work, University of Hertfordshire, Hatfield AL10 9AB, UK

2 Northern College of Acupuncture, York YO1 6LJ, UK; LaraMcClure@chinese-medicine.co.uk (L.S.M.); helgi.claytonmcclure@oxon.org (J.H.C.M.)

* Correspondence: davidmayor@welwynacupuncture.co.uk

Academic Editors: Gerhard Litscher and William Chi-shing Cho

Abstract: Background: Some feelings elicited by acupuncture-type interventions are "nonspecific", interpretable as resulting from the placebo effect, our own self-healing capacities—or, indeed, the flow of *qi*. Expectation is thought to contribute to these nonspecific effects. Here we describe the use of two innovative 20-item questionnaires ($EXPre_{20}$ and $EXPost_{20}$) in a teaching situation. **Methods:** Respondents were acupuncture students or practitioners on electroacupuncture (EA) training courses (N = 68). $EXPre_{20}$ and $EXPost_{20}$ questionnaires were completed before and after receiving individualised treatment administered by colleagues. Respondents were also asked about their prior experience of EA or transcutaneous electroacupuncture stimulation (TEAS). **Results:** Respondents *expected* significantly more items to change than not to change, but significantly fewer were *experienced* as changing. Increases in given questionnaire items were both expected and experienced significantly more often than decreases. "Tingling", "Relaxation", and "Relief" or "Warmth" were most often expected to increase or were experienced as such, and "Pain" and "Tension" to decrease or experienced as decreasing. Expectations of change or no change were confirmed more often than not, particularly for "Tingling" and "Tension". This was not the result of the personal respondent style. Cluster analysis suggested the existence of two primary feeling clusters, "Relaxation" and "Alertness". **Conclusions:** Feelings experienced during or immediately after acupuncture-type interventions may depend both on prior experience and expectation.

Keywords: electroacupuncture; nonspecific feelings; expectation; placebo; *qi*; cluster analysis

---

1. Introduction

Writings about acupuncture often mention its "nonspecific" effects, although even those familiar with the literature on these effects vary in their interpretation of the term [1]. The placebo effect is sometimes considered as evidence for an activation of what some consider as our "nonspecific" self-healing capacities [2–4]. There are also accounts of how, in response to placebo (more accurately, sham) acupuncture, bodily sensations of warmth, tingling, pulsing, flow (spreading, radiating), and electricity have been elicited—warmth and tingling being particularly associated with treatment efficacy [5,6]. Such sensations are also reported in other complementary and alternative medicine (CAM) modalities such as "biofield energy healing" [7], and have been interpreted by many CAM practitioners as resulting from the flow of *qi*, the immanent life force of the body and the world (part agency, part image or form, part metaphor), of key importance in acupuncture and Chinese culture as a whole, as well as being central to Western traditions of vitalism, where it has many other names [8,9].

The expectation of a positive outcome is thought to be a major contributor to nonspecific effects of treatment [10], partly because it alters how bodily sensations are identified [11]. However, no independently developed pre-existing questionnaires were found that could be used to assess expectation or experience of the nonspecific feelings that may arise in response to acupuncture-type interventions, although scales have been developed to evaluate the common specific sensations elicited by acupuncture [12–21]. Our objectives in this study were therefore to use two previously developed 20-item questionnaires, $EXPre_{20}$ and $EXPost_{20}$, to investigate differences in response patterns between respondent subgroups and identify any patterns of change (both expected and experienced) for particular nonspecific feelings. For further explanation on these "EXP_{20}" questionnaires and their precursors, $EXPre_{32}$ and $EPost_{32}$, see Section 2, Materials and Methods, below, and for the questionnaires themselves, see Appendixs A and B).

Research questions and hypotheses

1. Firstly, the study aims to address the question of fulfillment of expectation. Our central hypothesis is that there will be strong, generally positive correlations between the expected and experienced feelings—in other words, that expectation in this context is generally fulfilled [10,11]. (This should not be conflated with the association between expectation of treatment *effectiveness* and its outcome, or benefit [22–24]).

2. We aim to establish whether there are trends across responses to different questionnaire items. For instance, there might be significant overall differences between the numbers of "Yes" and "No" responses, or between the numbers of "increase" and "decrease" responses, given to the various nonspecific feelings assessed by the questionnaires. For example, feelings of "Relaxation" have been reported in response to acupuncture treatment [25], and feelings of "Aliveness" might be associated on theoretical grounds with an improvement in the flow of *qi* [8]. Would both these be found to increase in this context?

3. We also aim to address the question of prior experience effects. Those with prior experience of electroacupuncture (EA) or transcutaneous electrical nerve stimulation (TENS) might report generally different expectations or experiences of feelings elicited by EA/TEAS (transcutaneous electroacupuncture stimulation) than are reported by those without. Related to this, students might report different expectations or experiences than those reported by practitioners. Our use of Continuing Professional Development (CPD) practitioner versus Student respondent groups, as well as recording the presence versus absence of prior experience of EA/TENS, will allow us to explore the effects of the treatment experience in two different ways (general and specific).

Of course, differences by respondent group or by prior experience might be detected *between* questionnaire items also.

4. A final key aim of the present study is to identify any significant associations among the different feelings assessed by the questionnaires. A cluster analysis will enable us to better understand these associations, through an exploration of the relationships between them. For example, using the language of Chinese medicine, some feelings could be considered more "*yang*" (masculine, positive, expansive) and others more "*yin*" (feminine, negative, withdrawing) [26]. Are these ideational associations reflected in the clusters found?

2. Materials and Methods

2.1. Recruitment, Questionnaires, and Treatments

Respondents were recruited during pre-arranged electroacupuncture (EA) teaching sessions in the UK, three of these being university-affiliated undergraduate acupuncture training courses and two independently organised CPD courses for acupuncture practitioners (in Nottingham and Brighton). The basic structure of the sessions was similar on all courses, although one of the undergraduate courses (CICM) was only a half-day rather than a full-day session. The same lecturer—an acupuncturist with over 30 years of experience—presented and supervised all the courses.

Respondents were asked to complete two 20-item questionnaires: an initial expectation questionnaire ($EXPre_{20}$) at the beginning of the teaching session, and a follow-up experience questionnaire ($EXPost_{20}$) after receiving a short treatment from a fellow attendee (a flow chart of this sequence is shown in Figure 1).

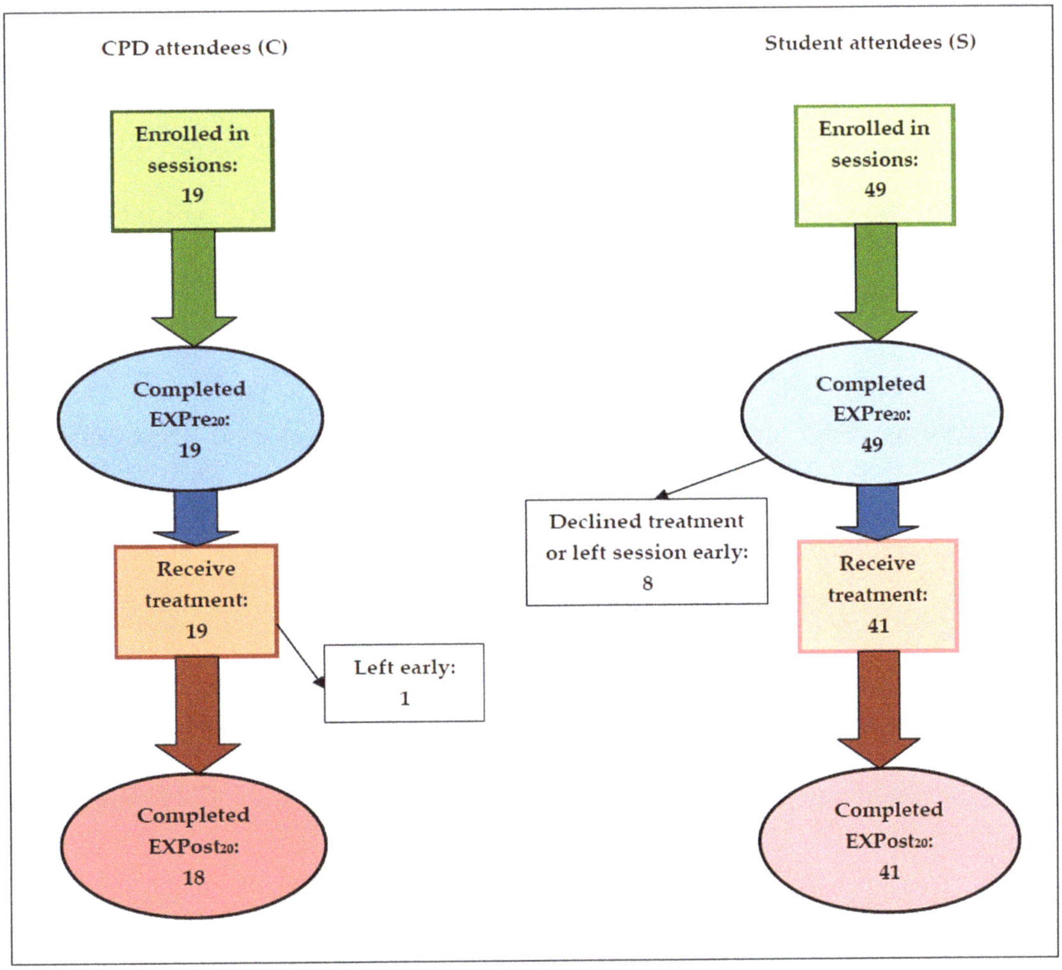

Figure 1. Study flow chart for CPD (C) and Student (S) attendees. Key: $EXPre_{20}$ = initial expectation questionnaire; $EXPost_{20}$ = follow-up experience questionnaire.

Pilot Studies: development of the EXP_{20} questionnaires from earlier 32-item versions

In earlier research, two longer 32-item questionnaires had been piloted in three cohorts of acupuncture and other complementary health practitioners and students familiar with acupuncture, who received EA or TEAS (transcutaneous electroacupuncture stimulation as against the usual "nerve stimulation", TENS) in experimental studies or a classroom situation ($N = 204$). They were designed to assess expectation ($EXPre_{32}$) and experience ($EXPost_{32}$) of the relatively nonspecific feelings (bodily, emotional, or mental) that may arise in response to acupuncture-type interventions, in particular the established methods of EA and TEAS [27]. Findings on their content validity and reliability, together with a cluster analysis, have been presented elsewhere [28]. The salient results were that significant numbers of feelings experienced by respondents were those they expected, and that significant numbers of feelings not experienced were those not expected. It should be noted that many of the participants in this earlier study had no prior experience of EA/TEAS, although nearly all were familiar with acupuncture.

Following this, 20 experienced acupuncture practitioners and researchers rated items in the original 32-item questionnaires as either "essential", "useful but not essential", or "not necessary". These ratings, together with the analysis of actual questionnaire usage, were used to reduce the original questionnaires from 32 to 20 items [29]. More information on the development of the EXP_{20} questionnaires can be found in the publications cited [28–30].

Treatment was supervised but participants were free in this teaching situation to use their own choice of acupuncture points and stimulation parameters (frequency, amplitude, mode, pulse, and overall stimulation duration). They were also encouraged to use several different EA/TEAS stimulators, of which 11 were provided for their use. Treatments were carried out in small groups of 3–4 participants. Information on the treatments received is provided in the Supplementary Material Table S1.

2.2. Ethics Approval

Ethics approval was granted under an application for a related study by the Health and Human Sciences Ethics Committee of the University of Hertfordshire, UK (Protocol HEPEC/07/11/93), approved 5 July 2011, 24 Aug 2012 . Permission was also received from course organisers and respondents.

2.3. Questionnaire Administration

The present paper describes and analyses the use of the shorter 20-item questionnaires in a teaching situation ($N = 68$).

The questionnaires (Appendix B) were printed with items in randomised order, so it was unlikely that they would appear in the same order in both $EXPre_{20}$ and $EXPost_{20}$ for a particular respondent. These two were also distributed and collected separately, so that they could not be seen at the same time, reducing the likelihood of respondents basing their replies to $EXPost_{20}$ on their earlier replies to $EXPre_{20}$.

In $EXPre_{20}$, respondents were asked "Relative to how you feel NOW, during or immediately following EA/TEAS do you expect to experience any change AT ALL in the feeling of . . . " (a particular feeling). Possible responses were "Yes", "No", or "don't know/can't say" ("DK", i.e., no particular expectation). If they answered "Yes", they were then asked if they expected the feeling to increase or decrease. Similarly, in $EXPost_{20}$, respondents were asked "Relative to how you felt when you completed the earlier questionnaire, during or immediately following EA/TEAS did you experience a change in the feeling of . . . ".

Questionnaires were collated using pre-printed ID codes double-checked against respondents' signatures/initials and writing styles.

2.4. Statistical Analysis

Anonymised scores for each questionnaire item were analysed using Excel and SPSS v20. Binomial and χ^2 (chi-square) tests were used to assess significance of differences; to assess the degree of association, Cramer's V and Pearson's r were used (both with a range of 0 to 1). Three methods of hierarchical cluster analysis appropriate for binary data were used: Jaccard's index (or "similarity ratio"), Sokal and Sneath's index 5 (range 0 to 1) [31,32], and Ward's method. For the first two methods, distances were calculated using average linkage (both between and within groups), nearest neighbour (single linkage), and furthest neighbour (complete linkage). Squared Euclidean distances were used for Ward's method. Appropriate numbers of clusters were estimated visually from the dendrograms for each method, particularly where there was apparent agreement among them for the largest reasonable (readily interpretable) number of clusters [32].

3. Results

3.1. Respondents

The present study sample consisted of acupuncture practitioners undertaking continuous professional development courses (hereafter CPD or practitioners) and students of acupuncture (Students). The two groups were composed of respondents from five training centres (CPD: Brighton, Nottingham; Students: the College of Integrated Chinese Medicine, Reading (CICM), London South bank University (LSBU), and the Northern College of Acupuncture, York (NCA)).

Student respondents were obliged to attend EA sessions as part of their acupuncture training, whereas practitioner respondents signed up for EA courses voluntarily (all respondents were informed that they did not need to complete the questionnaires if they did not wish to). Training centre, age, gender (where known), prior experience of EA and/or TENS, and numbers completing the two questionnaires are shown in Table 1. All attendees completed the initial questionnaire. A few attendees declined treatment because of known contraindications (e.g., pregnancy or a heart condition), an aversion to "non-traditional" EA/TEAS, or to electricity itself. Some students left the sessions early, and thus were not present to complete $EXPost_{20}$ questionnaires. The flow chart in Figure 1 shows the numbers at the start of the EA sessions and those at the end.

Table 1. Respondent cohorts, showing age (mean, SD), gender, whether practitioner/CPD (C) or student (S), prior experience of electroacupuncture (EA) and/or transcutaneous electrical nerve stimulation (TENS), and numbers completing each of the two questionnaires, $EXPre_{20}$ and $EXPost_{20}$, as well as both EXP questionnaires.

Training Centre	Total *N*	Age	Gender	C/S	Prior	No Prior	$EXPre_{20}$	$EXPost_{20}$
LSBU (19.10.13)	14	37.8, 8.3	11 F, 2 M	S	8	6	14	11
Nottingham (23.11.13)	8	52.1, 5.7	n/a [a]	C	6	2	8	7
Brighton (06.04.14)	11	45.9, 7.9	9 F, 2 M	C	6 [b]	4 [b]	11	11
CICM (07.04.14)	24	39.7, 9.5	19 F, 5 M	S	10	14	24	19
NCA (12.04.14)	11	39.8, 9.8	9 F, 2 M	S	6	5	11	11
CPD N	*19*	*48.3, 7.6*	*9–17 F, 2–10 M* [a]	*C*	*12*	*6*	*19*	*18*
Student N	*49*	*39.1, 9.1*	*39 F, 9 M*	*S*	*24*	*25*	*49*	*41*
Total *N*	68	41.7, 9.6	48–56 F, 11–19 M	n/a	36	31	68	59

[a] Information not available; [b] One respondent did not answer this question.

As would be expected, students were consistently younger than practitioners ($p < 0.001$ for the difference in their ages, using an independent-samples *t*-test, with $t(64) = 3.8$). As for the gender of the attendees, even if all missing cases were men, there is still a significant preponderance of women ($p = 0.001$ using the Binomial test with a test proportion of 0.5). Again, for CAM practitioners, this would be expected [33].

Details of the treatments received are summarised in Supplementary Materials Table S1.

3.2. *Research Question 1: Fulfilment of Expectation*

3.2.1. Overall Patterns of Expectation

Although individuals' responses varied considerably, overall there were clear patterns of the relationships between the counts of expected and experienced "Y", "N", and "DK" change scores, shown in Figure 2 as "N→DK", etc.

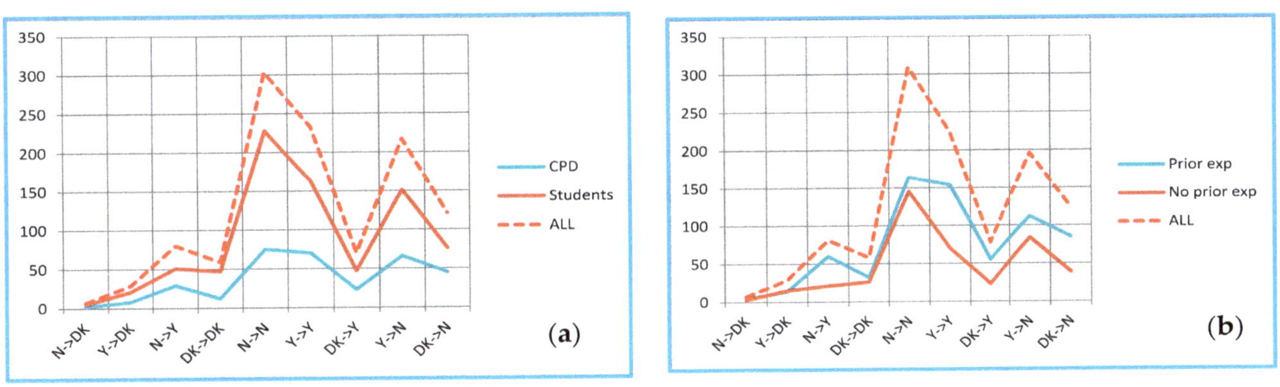

Figure 2. Relationships between counts of expected and experienced "Yes" (Y), "No" (N), and "Don't know" (DK) change scores: (**a**) CPD and student subgroups; (**b**) Subgroups of those with prior or no prior experience of EA/TENS.

Thus the expectations of change, whether negative or positive, were confirmed (N→N and Y→Y) more often than other combinations, the next most common combination being expected changes that were not confirmed in practice. DK→N also outnumbered DK→Y. (Similar patterns were found for the earlier versions of the questionnaires, $EXPre_{32}$ and $EXPost_{32}$ [28]). Furthermore, in each cohort except for the Brighton CPD group, significantly more respondents showed confirmatory scores than would be expected by chance ($p \leq 0.001$, using the Binomial test with a test proportion of 0.25, i.e., based on N→N and Y→Y, but ignoring the DK→DK responses).

When all items were considered together, there were positive linear correlations between items expected to change and experienced as changing (r = 0.869), and also between those not expected to change and not experienced as changing (r = 0.722). There were negative correlations between items not expected to change and those experienced as changing (r = 0.727) and vice versa (r = 0.832).

Only in one cohort (Brighton, $N = 11$) were expectations less often confirmed than not (for Y→N, but not N→Y).

Comparing the results for CPD and students, only for DK→N was the difference between these two subgroups significant ($p = 0.018$).

Those with prior experience of EA/TENS showed rather more N→Y and Y→Y scores than those without prior experience ($p < 0.001$). Differences between these two subgroups were also significant for DK→Y ($p = 0.002$) and DK→N ($p = 0.001$).

For increases (i) and decreases (d), there were no significant differences between when expectations of change were confirmed (i→i or d→d) or not (i→d or d→i) ($p > 0.05$). However, counts of each of these four combinations were higher for those with prior experience of EA/TENS than for those without prior experience, as indicated in Supplementary Materials Figure S1 (see also p 9 below).

When all the items were considered together, there were positive linear correlations between items expected to increase and experienced as increasing (r = 0.750), and also between those expected to decrease and experienced as decreasing (r = 0.916). These correlations were driven by increases in Relaxation, Tingling and Warmth, and by decreases in Being stressed, Pain and Tension. If these were removed from the analysis, the apparent linearity was no longer evident (r = 0.446 and r = 0.173, respectively).

There was no indication that respondents who tended to answer one way to the $EXPre_{20}$ questionnaire (as "increasers", "i", or "decreasers", "d" [29]) were likely to answer the same way to the $EXPost_{20}$ questionnaire ($p > 0.05$).

3.2.2. Patterns of Expectation for Individual Questionnaire Items

Counts of the various change responses for individual items were made. The highest counts for the various $EXPre_{20}$/$EXPOst_{20}$ combinations are shown in Supplementary Materials Table S3. For DK→DK and DK→N, two items were tied in first position, and for Y→DK, three items.

Items above the third quartile for Y→Y were Tingling (count 40), Relaxation (20), Pain and Tension (16), and Warmth (15), all of which were included in EXP_{32} (although not among the Y→Y items above the third quartile there). The third quartile N→N items in EXP_{20} were Cheerfulness (26), Clarity and Heaviness (23), Sleepiness (22), and Being spaced out (21). Again, although included in EXP_{32}, they did not occur in the third quartile EXP_{32} N→N items. The case for DK→DK is similar.

Expected/experienced increases and decreases are shown in Supplementary Materials Table S4.

The results for Tingling and Tension are in line with those in the previous table. Those for Relaxation (inc→dec) and Pain (dec→inc) are somewhat surprising (but involve only small numbers).

3.3. Research Question 2: Individual Questionnaire Items—Expectations of Change, Increase and Decrease

3.3.1. Changes/No Changes and Increases/Decreases Most and Least Expected

Questionnaire item counts were ranked and the results were tabulated. Those above the third quartile (75th percentile, in the "top five") are shown in Table 2.

Table 2. Changes/no changes and increases/decreases most and least expected. Items listed are for the whole sample. Subgroups in which the listed items did not occur are shown in the "not sub" columns.

Change Most *Expected*	**Not Sub**	**No Change Least** *Expected*	**Not Sub**	**Change Least** *Expected*	**Not Sub**	**No Change Most** *Expected*	**Not Sub**
Tingling *	-	Tingling	-	Cheerfulness	-	Cheerfulness	-
Relaxation *	n	Warmth	s	Being spaced out	-	Being spaced out	-
Tension *	c	Inner bodily flow	c	Sensory acuity	-	Heaviness	c
Pain	-	Relief	n	Sleepiness	s, n	Sleepiness	n
Relief	c, n	Relaxation	-	Clarity	c, n	Clarity	-
Increase Most *Expected*	**Not Sub**	**Decrease Least** *Expected*	**Not Sub**	**Increase Least** *Expected*	**Not Sub**	**Decrease Most** *Expected*	**Not Sub**
Tingling	-	Cheerfulness	-	Being stressed	-	**Pain**	-
Relaxation	-	Aliveness	-	Pain	-	**Tension**	-
Warmth	c	Wellbeing	-	Cheerfulness	-	Being stressed	-
Relief	c, n	Warmth	-	Tension	n	Heaviness	-
Wellbeing	s, n	(5 tied items †)	-	Heaviness	c, p	Sleepiness	c

Key: c = CPD; s = students; p = prior experience of EA/TENS; n = no prior experience of EA/TENS. Items in bold are those for which the most agreement occurred for "change" as well as for either "increase" or "decrease".
* Agreement with results for EXPre$_{32}$ [27]; † Clarity, Inner bodily flow, Mental energy, Mental focus, Sensory acuity.

3.3.2. Correlations between Items Expected to Change/Not Change, or Increase/Decrease

There is evidently some correspondence between items most expected to change and those least expected not to change (three items in common) and vice versa (four items in common). Taking all items into account, there was a strong negative linear correlation between those expected to change and those not expected to change (r = −0.893).

There is less correspondence between those items most expected to increase and those least expected to decrease (two items in common), and more between those items most expected to decrease and those least expected to increase (four items in common). Compared with expectations of change, there was a relatively small negative correlation between items expected to increase and those expected to decrease (r = −0.510).

3.4. *Research Question 2: Individual Questionnaire Items—Experiences of Change, Increase and Decrease*

3.4.1. Changes/No Changes and Increases/Decreases Most and Least Experienced

Questionnaire item counts were ranked and the results were tabulated. Those above the third quartile (75th percentile, in the "top five") are shown in Table 3. In addition, respondents were asked explicitly to asterisk changes they "noticed most" (see Appendix B-2). Only 16 did so (12 students, 4 practitioners), with 42 items asterisked between them (1–8 items per respondent, mode 2). The numbers of asterisked items are included (in parentheses) in Table 3. Other items asterisked but not above the third quartiles (not included in Table 3) were Aliveness (1), Being spaced out (2), Calmness (3), Heaviness (2), Inner bodily flow (1), Mental energy (1), and Sleepiness (4). Wellbeing was the only item not asterisked.

Here there is a similar degree of agreement between greater experience of change and lesser experience of no change (four items in common), and between greater experience of no change and lesser experience of change (four items in common). Taking all item counts into consideration, there was a negative linear correlation between those experienced as changing and not changing (r = −0.944). This was stronger than the correlation for the expected items.

Apart from Calmness and Sleepiness (asterisked three and four times), and Relief (asterisked twice), there is agreement between those items for which changes were most *often* experienced and those experienced with most *intensity* ("noticed most", and asterisked three times or more).

Table 3. Changes/no changes and increases/decreases most and least experienced. Items listed are for the whole sample. Subgroups in which the listed items did not occur are shown in the "not sub" columns.

Change Most *Experienced*	**Not Sub**	**No change Least** *Experienced*	**Not Sub**	**Change Least** *Experienced*	**Not Sub**	**No change Most** *Experienced*	**Not Sub**
Tingling (3)	-	Tingling (3)	-	Mental focus (2)	n	Intestinal rumblings * (2)	-
Relaxation * (6)	-	Pain (4)	p	Intestinal rumblings (2)	-	Sensory acuity (0)	-
Warmth (4)	-	Relief (2)	-	Sensory acuity (0)	-	Being stressed (0)	s,n
Pain (4)	s,p	Relaxation (6)	-	Cheerfulness (1)	-	Clarity (1)	-
Tension * (3)	c	Warmth (4)	n	Clarity (1)	-	Mental focus (2)	c,n
Increase Most *Experienced*	**Not Sub**	**Decrease Least** *Experienced*	**Not sub**	**Increase Least** *Experienced*	**Not Sub**	**Decrease Most** *Experienced*	**Not Sub**
Tingling	-	Sensory acuity	-	Mental focus	-	**Tension**	-
Relaxation	-	Inner bodily flow	-	Being stressed	-	**Pain**	-
Warmth	-	Warmth	-	Tension	n	Being stressed	-
Being spaced out	c,n	Mental focus	n	Sensory acuity	p	Aliveness	-
Calmness	c,n	(6 tied items †)	-	Intestinal rumblings	n	Heaviness	n

Key: c = CPD; s = students; p = prior experience of EA/TENS; n = no prior experience of EA/TENS. Numbers in square brackets indicate the numbers of an item asterisked as "most noticed" by respondents. Items in bold are those for which the most agreement occurred for "change" as well as for either "increase" or "decrease". * Agreement with results for $EXPre_{32}$ [27]; † Being spaced out, Calmness, Cheerfulness, Clarity, Intestinal rumblings, Tingling.

3.4.2. Correlations between Items Most/Least Experienced as Increasing/Decreasing

There is some correspondence between those items most experienced as increasing and those least experienced as decreasing (three items in common), but less between those items most experienced as decreasing and those least experienced as increasing (two items in common). There was a very weak negative correlation between items experienced as increasing and those experienced as decreasing ($r = -0.358$).

3.4.3. Ratios of "Yes"/"No" and "Increase"/"Decrease" Score Counts

Significance of the ratios of "Yes"/"No" and "increase"/"decrease" score counts are shown in Supplementary Materials Table S2, together with the sign of the difference between the counts.

Only for "Cheerfulness" was there a significant Expected/Not expected change ratio in both the $EXPre_{20}$ and $EXPost_{20}$. In contrast, 12 items (60%) showed a significant increased/decreased ratio in both $EXPre_{20}$ and $EXPost_{20}$. For all these 12 items, increases outnumbered decreases (whether expected or experienced).

3.5. Research Question —Differences in Response Patterns between Respondent Subgroups

3.5.1. Drop-outs, i.e., Those Not Completing the EXPost20 Questionnaire

Nine respondents did not complete the $EXPost_{20}$ questionnaire. Eight of these (more than expected) had no prior experience of EA/TENS, and were also students ($p = 0.039$ each, using the ratio test).

3.5.2. Those with and without Prior Experience of EA or TENS

Overall, similar numbers had (36) and had not (31) had prior experience of EA/TENS, with proportionally more in the practitioner/CPD cohorts having prior experience (however, this was a nonsignificant difference).

3.5.3. Prior Experience and Expectation

For no single $EXPre_{20}$ item was the Binomial test for those expecting a change significant. "Tingling" was the only item significant ($p = 0.025$) for those not expecting a change (none of those without prior experience expected no change in this item). Those who did expect a change in "Tingling" were divided almost equally between those with prior experience (28) and those without (27). For all $EXPre_{20}$ items taken together, however, the expectation of change and the expectation of increase approached significance for the 0.54 test proportion (and would have been significant had group sizes been equal).

Significantly more of those with prior experience were uncertain whether an increase or decrease was expected ($p = 0.023$; $p = 0.001$ for test proportion 0.50).

3.5.4. Practitioner and Student Expectation

No significant differences in expectation of change/no change were found between students and practitioners. Practitioners expected fewer decreases than students ($p = 0.024$), and were less likely to report uncertainty in their expectation of increase or decrease ($p = 0.003$). No differences were significant for any individual item.

3.5.5. Practitioner and Student Questionnaire Responses

Across all questionnaire items in $EXPre_{20}$, practitioners recorded 142 "yes" responses (106 increases, 26 decreases), 111 "no" responses, and 78 no-expectation responses. Students recorded 419 "yes" responses (294 increases, 104 decreases), 314 "no" responses, and 187 no-expectation responses.

Across all questionnaire items in $EXPost_{20}$, practitioners recorded 126 "yes" responses (72 increases, 17 decreases), 189 "no" responses, and 22 no-expectation responses. Students recorded 264 "yes" responses (202 increases, 50 decreases), 458 "no" responses, and 74 no-expectation responses.

Unspecified "yes" responses in both cases were those where neither increase nor decrease was indicated.

Across all responses in $EXPre_{20}$ there was no significant difference in the distribution between practitioners and students ($p > 0.05$). Similarly, there was no significant difference with respect to the direction of change ("increase" or "decrease"). Across all responses in $EXPost_{20}$, again the distributions were not significantly different when missing data responses were excluded ($p > 0.05$). In subsequent analyses (other than in Section 3.5 below), "don't know" (DK) and missing data responses were disregarded.

3.5.6. Ratios of "Yes" and "No" Counts in Questionnaire Responses

Ratios of "Yes"/"No" and "increase"/"decrease" counts are shown in Tables 4 and 5, respectively.

Table 4. Ratios of "Yes" and "No" counts for EXP_{20}.

EXP_{20}	Y/N (Pre)	Y/N (Post)	Y (Post/Pre)	N (Post/Pre)
CPD	1.28 ** (n.s.)	0.67 **	0.89 (n.s.)	1.70 **
Student	1.33 **	0.58 **	0.63 **	1.46 **
Total	1.32 **	0.60 **	0.70 **	1.52 **

** $p < 0.001$ (Binomial test, test ratio 0.50).

Table 5. Ratios of "increase" and "decrease" counts for EXP_{20}.

Subgroup	Inc/Dec (Pre)	Inc/Dec (Post)	Inc (Post/Pre)	Dec (Post/Pre)
CPD	4.07 **	4.24 **	0.68 *	0.65 (n.s.)
Student	2.83 **	4.04 **	0.69 **	0.48 **
Total	3.08 **	4.09 **	0.69 **	0.52 **

* $p = 0.001$; ** $p < 0.001$

All the $EXPre_{20}$ count ratios, except for the practitioner $EXPre_{20}$ "Yes/No" ratio and the practitioner $EXPost_{20}/EXPre_{20}$ "Yes" ratio, are significantly different from 1 ($p < 0.001$).

Obvious patterns are also that "Yes" responses outnumber "No's" in $EXPre_{20}$, but "No" responses outnumber "Yes" responses in $EXPost_{20}$, and that "No" responses in $EXPost_{20}$ outnumber those in $EXPre_{20}$, but that "Yes" responses in $EXPre_{20}$ outnumber those in $EXPost_{20}$. (Similar results were found for $EXPre_{32}$ and $EXPost_{32}$ [28]).

Again, all count ratios are significantly different from 1 ($p < 0.001$) except for the practitioner $EXPost_{20}/EXPre_{20}$ "increase" ratio ($p = 0.001$) and the practitioner "decrease" ratio (n.s.).

However, whereas the ratios of the change counts (Table 4) are quite dissimilar (median 1.76, interquartile range [IQR] 0.67–4.05), the "increase"/"decrease" ratios (Table 5) are quite similar for both $EXPre_{20}$ and $EXPost_{20}$, as are the $EXPost_{20}/EXPre_{20}$ ratios for both "increase" and "decrease" (median 1.09, IQR 0.66%–1.36%).

3.6. Research Question 4—Associations between Different Items and Exploratory Cluster Analysis

3.6.1. Associations between Pairs of Items

Cramer's V was used as a simple method of assessing how closely the different items were associated, based on the categorical scores ("Y" or "N") allocated by the respondents. Low values of V (<0.3) were ignored ($V \geq 0.3$ is considered by Cohen to indicate a medium level of association, and $V \geq 0.5$ a high level [34]). Figure 3 shows how frequently each item appeared in item pairs with a medium or high level of Cramer's V.

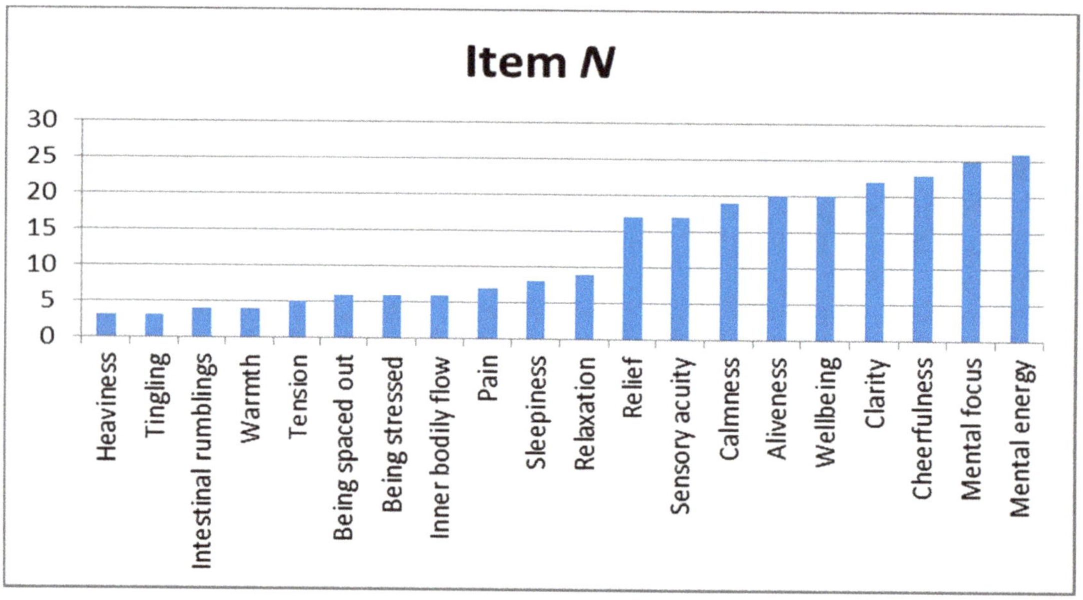

Figure 3. Number of times each item appeared in item pairs with a medium or high level of Cramer's V.

Using Cramer's V, there was a higher percentage (with a higher average V) of items showing significant $EXPre_{20}$-$EXPre_{20}$ associations than of items with significant $EXPre_{20}$-$EXPost_{20}$ or $EXPost_{20}$-$EXPost_{20}$ associations.

There are two subgroups of items here: a lower one (mean occurrence rate 5.5, range 3–9) and an upper one (mean occurrence rate 21.0, range 17–26). Of the $EXPre_{20}$-$EXPre_{20}$ pairs, 24 of 35 (68.6%) consisted of items only in the upper subgroup, of the $EXPost_{20}$-$EXPost_{20}$ pairs, 28 of 46 (60.9%), and of the $EXPre_{20}$-$EXPost_{20}$ pairs, 31 of 46 (67.4%).

3.6.2. Cluster Analysis

Numbers of estimated clusters using Jaccard's index, Sokal and Sneath's index 5, and Ward's method are shown in Supplementary Materials Table S5. Items in the clusters obtained using the different methods were compared, and those for which there was the most agreement were selected.

A comparison between Cramer's V and Ward's proximities showed no obvious relationship between the two measures overall. However, in both $EXPre_{20}$ and $EXPost_{20}$ two clusters stood out from all the others, having the highest mean V and lowest mean proximity. These could be considered as clusters for "Relaxation" and "Alertness". The values of mean Ward proximities (W) and Cramer's V for the two clusters suggest that "Alertness" was the more robust of the two (Supplementary Materials Table S6). Other possible clusters were "Relief" and "Bodily sensation", but there was less agreement between $EXPre_{20}$ and $EXPost_{20}$ on the items included.

If the data was split by subgroup (CPD vs. student respondents, or with vs. without prior experience of EA/TENS), no combinations of items appeared in corresponding clusters for all four subgroups. In the $EXPre_{20}$ responses, the Calmness/Relaxation dyad did not appear in any cluster for those with no prior experience of EA/TENS, and in the $EXPost_{20}$ responses only in the student subgroup. In the $EXPre_{20}$ responses, the triad of Aliveness, Cheerfulness, and Mental focus appeared together in a cluster for all subgroups except for that of students, and that of Cheerfulness, Mental energy, and Mental focus in a cluster for all but the subgroup with prior experience of EA/TENS. In the $EXPost_{20}$ responses, the dyad of Aliveness and Mental energy and the tetrad of Cheerfulness, Clarity, Mental focus, and Sensory acuity appeared together (albeit in separate clusters) for all subgroups except for those with no prior experience of EA/TENS. Subgroup analysis was not carried out for the $EXPre_{20}$ and $EXPost_{20}$ items taken together.

4. Discussion

4.1. Respondents

The pattern evident in those respondents who only filled out the $EXPre_{20}$ and not the $EXPost_{20}$ questionnaire suggests that those who did not complete the second questionnaire (predominantly students) had not really become more interested in EA/TEAS after the course than they were before attending. This could reflect a failure of teaching skill on the part of the instructor, or a lack of openness to something outside the normal ("traditional") curriculum among students, for whom this was an obligatory session (whereas the CPD respondents signed up for their sessions because of an interest in what was being taught). In addition, some of the students will have left the session early to ensure they were able to catch their usual transport home.

Practitioners tended to have somewhat more prior experience of the EA and TENS modalities than students. Given that the students were all enrolled in "traditional" acupuncture training courses, this was to be expected, even if the difference between the practitioners and students did not reach significance in this respect.

Somewhat surprisingly, six of the 36 respondents who had prior experience of EA/TENS expected no change in "Tingling", whereas none of the 31 without such prior experience expected no change in "Tingling". Electricity is commonly associated with a "Tingling" feeling [8].

Those with no prior experience of EA/TENS showed less uncertainty in their expectations of increases or decreases in feelings than those who did have prior experience. Real life clinical experience may soften the certainty of preconceptions.

4.2. Questionnaire Items—Overall Patterns

Overall, students and practitioners scored the questionnaires in a similar way. In particular, whereas more respondents expected feelings to change than did not expect them to, fewer respondents actually experienced changes in feelings (cf [28]). Thus there were fewer $EXPost_{20}$ than $EXPre_{20}$ "Yes" responses, but more "No" responses.

In contrast, more "increases" than "decreases" were both expected and experienced (with a slightly higher ratio of "increases" to "decreases" in $EXPost_{20}$ than $EXPre_{20}$). As there were fewer "Yes" counts following treatment than before, the $EXPost_{20}/EXPre_{20}$ ratios for both "increases" and "decreases" were all <1.

4.3. Individual Questionnaire Items—Expectations of Change, Increase and Decrease

Some responses might be self-evident to anyone familiar with any complementary therapy: following a treatment, a change (increase) in relaxation or relief would be expected or hoped for, and also a change (decrease) in pain or tension.

Inner bodily flow (which might be expected on the basis of prior experience of or teachings on energy-based medicine [8], and could be interpreted by some respondents in terms of electrical current flow) was considered less likely to change or increase by those with prior experience. Heaviness and Sleepiness were both among those items considered least likely to change AND those items likely to decrease. Calmness and Heaviness were considered likely to change by CPD respondents, but less so by the students.

4.4. Individual Questionnaire Items—Experiences of Change, Increase and Decrease

The changes most commonly experienced (Pain, Relaxation, Tension, Tingling, Warmth) were similar to those expected (Pain, Relaxation, Relief, Tension, Tingling), with Relaxation, Tingling, and Warmth among the items most often increasing, and Pain and Tension among those most often decreasing. There was overall agreement between those items for which changes were most *often* experienced and those experienced with most *intensity* ("noticed most").

Sleepiness was among the items most experienced as not changing for the (CPD/no prior experience) respondents, Heaviness for the (student/no prior experience) respondents, and Calmness and Mental focus for all those with no prior experience. Conversely, Relief was among the items most experienced as changing for the CPD and no prior experience respondents. The no prior experience subgroup therefore appears to have had a different experience of what did and did not change than the others.

Of the 12 items showing significantly more increases than decreases in both $EXPre_{20}$ and $EXPost_{20}$, all could be considered as "positive" in the sense of increasing with overall wellbeing rather than decreasing.

4.5. Fulfilment of Expectation

A key finding is that—as for the EXP_{32} questionnaires—expectations of change, whether negative or positive, were confirmed rather than not. Only in one cohort ($N = 11$) was this not the case.

Positive expectations of change were more marked among those with prior experience of EA/TENS than those without.

In contrast, expectations of increase or decrease were not fulfilled (rather than confirmed) by experience. However, there were significantly more counts of all four combinations of $EXPre_{20}$ and $EXPost_{20}$ "i" and "d" scores from respondents with prior experience of EA/TENS than from those without. Further study would be required to confirm these findings, as missing data rates were high (31 of 561, or 5.5%, for $EXPre_{20}$, and 49 of 390, or 12.6%, for $EXPost_{20}$).

That 10 out of the 59 (17%) respondents who completed both the $EXPre_{20}$ and $EXPost_{20}$ questionnaires reported a change in Being stressed, whereas they had expected not to, is concordant with the experienced decreases shown in Table 3 above (where "Being stressed" was included among the items above the third quartile). Eleven (19%) who were uncertain if they would experience a change in the feeling of Being stressed experienced no change, and 18 (31%) who expected a change in the feeling of tension experienced no change.

Nine of those who were uncertain if they would experience a change in warmth in fact did (it being one of the items most experienced as increasing, as shown in Table 3), whereas 11 (19%)

who were uncertain if they would experience a change in Intestinal rumblings also did not (this, like Sensory acuity and Mental focus, being an item that was least experienced as either increasing or decreasing, as shown in Table 3).

Taking Table 2, Table 3 and Tables S2–S4 together, the salient items are Relaxation, Tingling and Warmth, and Pain and Tension. Future research into the feelings elicited by EA and TEAS should at least take these into account (Cheerfulness also appears frequently in the Tables, but mostly because little change in this feeling was expected or experienced).

Associations were more evident between $EXPre_{20}$-$EXPre_{20}$ item pairs than between $EXPre_{20}$-$EXPost_{20}$ or $EXPost_{20}$-$EXPost_{20}$ pairs. Counts of items occurring in pairs with medium or high levels of Cramer's V showed that they fell into two groups, one of relatively low counts (range 3–9), and one with higher counts (range 17–26). Cluster analysis suggested the existence of two clusters for both $EXPre_{20}$ and $EXPost_{20}$ items, one which could be considered as indicating "Relaxation", and the other "Alertness". The latter appeared more robust; the two clusters considered together are redolent of the traditional acupuncture concepts of *yin* and *yang* [26].

Although there was no obvious relationship between Cramer's V and Ward's proximities, all but one of the items in the "Alertness" cluster were all in the higher count range for Cramer's V. In contrast, of the two items consistently occurring in the "Relaxation" cluster, the "Relaxation" item itself was in the lower count range (albeit at the top end of that range).

Further research using the EXP_{20} questionnaires should be conducted to replicate our findings and explore their application in different contexts, in particular in more rigorously designed clinical studies, and in relation to mainstream or CAM treatments other than EA. They could also be applied outside academic institutions, and even in everyday life situations. Such research should take into account the various issues flagged under "Limitations", described below.

5. Conclusions

Our main findings were that expectations of change, whether negative or positive, were confirmed rather than not, and that the changes most commonly experienced (Pain, Relaxation, Tension, Tingling, Warmth) were indeed similar to those expected (Pain, Relaxation, Relief, Tension, Tingling), with Relaxation, Tingling, and Warmth among the items most often increasing, and Pain and Tension among those most often decreasing. Cluster analysis suggested the existence of two primary clusters for both $EXPre_{20}$ and $EXPost_{20}$ items, one which could be considered as indicating "Relaxation" (consisting of the items Calmness and Relaxation), the other "Alertness" (Aliveness, Cheerfulness, [Clarity], Mental energy, Mental focus, and Sensory acuity).

It is hoped that the EXP_{20} questionnaires will be used by other researchers to replicate these findings, and also be developed further. It would be interesting, for example, to see whether results differ for men and women, and also whether different feelings are elicited by different types of acupuncture (in particular, sham acupuncture where significant debate exists surrounding the assumed inertia of the intervention [21,35,36]). They could perhaps also be used with outcome measures to explore whether "good responders" tend to experience complementary therapy treatments in a way that is different from those who respond less well.

5.1. Limitations

Attendees were not asked to provide information about their gender. Where available, this data was gathered retrospectively for each cohort, so that it is not possible to relate individuals' responses and their gender. Given the preponderance of women in the study (at least 68% and possibly as high as 81%), it is highly likely that our results are valid for women alone, but further research will be required to confirm that findings are valid for men as well as for women.

CPD attendees were not asked how many years they had been in practice. Differences between them could have impacted both the treatments they gave and their expectations and experiences of treatment effects. It would require a larger study to explore this factor.

CPD respondents attended these EA teaching sessions voluntarily, whereas the students did not. This may have had an impact on how seriously they took the task of completing the questionnaires. Nonetheless, this does not appear to have led to major differences between the C and S respondents (other than for Research question 1).

Because this study was conducted in teaching situations where attendees from different acupuncture training backgrounds were encouraged to explore the techniques of EA and TEAS for themselves, the treatments given were very heterogeneous. Beyond suggesting that it was good practice to obtain a *deqi* response before applying electrical stimulation through the needles, no attempt was made to control the needling technique or to change the methods of needling with which the attendees were already comfortable.

Furthermore, this is a small pilot study on participants familiar with acupuncture and the subjective sensations it may elicit. It is not known how far the results can be extrapolated to the wider population who are likely to be less familiar with such sensations, nor how they would be reflected in a purely clinical context.

A potential weakness in the test procedure concerns the contamination of responses to the later ($ExPost_{20}$) questionnaire. Small group discussion on the EA/TEAS techniques used was encouraged during the treatment exchange sessions before this questionnaire was administered, so that even though individuals completed it independently, their responses may have been somewhat influenced by others' comments. However, it is important to note that this effect is likely to be minimal since time was limited, the treatment/discussion groups were indeed small ($N = 3$ or 4), and the focus of the discussion was on the *technicalities* of EA/TEAS rather than on participants' subjective experience. Furthermore, although the "grain size" of the resulting $ExPost_{20}$ data may have been fairly coarse, it is highly unlikely that there was contamination *between* the small groups. In our view, despite the strong contrary opinion of our most rigorous anonymous reviewer, the results still support our conclusions regarding fulfillment of expectation, since: (A) the initial ($ExPre_{20}$) questionnaire was completed with no potential for contamination; (B) $ExPost_{20}$ was presented with a separately randomised question order, without recourse to $ExPre_{20}$ responses; (C) although there may conceivably have been contamination of responses within some of the small groups, it is highly unlikely that this was so consistent as to explain our findings; and (D) results were similar across the different cohorts. In other words, the experiences reported by the respondents were consistently in accord with and very likely influenced by their expectations (and not just their earlier reporting of expectations), and any within-group distortion was minimal.

Of course it must be kept in mind that the data analysed in the present study represent inherently subjective reports of feelings and experiences. There are therefore likely to be many factors contributing to the responses both to $ExPre_{20}$ and $ExPost_{20}$, the fine-grain investigation of which was not within the scope of this present study.

Finally, whereas most respondents were able to score most items for expected or experienced changes, there were more lacunae in the data for increases/decreases. Because of this missing data, the results for expected/experienced increases and decreases are less certain, and should be confirmed in further studies with more respondents.

Supplementary Materials:
Respondent cohorts, Table S2: Differences between score counts (change/no change, increase/decrease) for the $EXPre_{20}$ and $EXPost_{20}$ items, Table S3: Questionnaire items with the highest counts for the various "expected"/"experienced" combinations, Table S4: Questionnaire items with the highest counts for the various "increase" and "decrease" combinations, Table S5: Numbers of estimated clusters of $EXPre_{20}$, $EXPost_{20}$ and $EXPre_{20}$ *and* $EXPost_{20}$ items; Figure S1: Relationships between counts of expected and experienced increase (i) and decrease (d) scores.

Acknowledgments: To those who supported the development of these questionnaires, in particular Tony Steffert and Tim Watson; to Louise Percival, market research consultant, for her input on the questionnaire design; to Neil Spencer for the clarity of his teaching on statistics; to Ian Appleyard, Angie Hicks, Linda Johnson, and Deborah Woolf for providing descriptive data on the course participants at extremely short notice; to *Medicines'* anonymous reviewers for their very helpful critiques, and to all our participants. No funding was received for this project.

Author Contributions: D.F.M. proposed the pilot study as part of an ongoing research project, completed the Ethics application, collected and analysed the data, and wrote the first draft of this paper. L.S.M. and H.C.M. critiqued and rewrote this draft.

Appendix A. The original 32-item questionnaires, EXPre$_{32}$ and EXPost$_{32}$

A-1. EXPre$_{32}$

What do you expect from the electroacupuncture/TENS treatment you will receive today?

In one of the practical sessions today you will receive a session of electroacupuncture and/or TENS at one or two pairs of acupuncture points, such as LI-4 (Hegu) and ST-36 (Zusanli).

Do you expect to experience changes in any of the feelings listed below?

Instructions (please read carefully)

This questionnaire contains 32 statements about feelings.

For each feeling, ring the word/s that best represents your expectation of change in the feeling in your own case (this change may be an increase or a decrease):

Make sure that you ring the word/s in the correct column.

Please be as honest and accurate as you can throughout. Respond to each statement as if it were the only one. That is, don't worry about being 'consistent' in your responses. There are no 'correct' or 'incorrect' answers. Answer according to your own expectation, rather than how you think 'most acupuncturists' would answer.

I expect to experience a change in the feeling of ...

Feeling	**Yes**, I expect to experience a change in this feeling	**No**, I do not expect to experience a change in this feeling	**I don't know** if I expect to experience a change in this feeling
1. Aliveness	Yes	No	Don't know
2. Being at ease	Yes	No	Don't know
3. Being blue or down in the dumps	Yes	No	Don't know
4. Being in control	Yes	No	Don't know
5. Being spaced- out	Yes	No	Don't know
6. Calmness	Yes	No	Don't know
7. Cheerfulness	Yes	No	Don't know
8. Clarity	Yes	No	Don't know
9. Connectedness with others	Yes	No	Don't know
10. Contentment	Yes	No	Don't know
11. Excitement	Yes	No	Don't know
12. Heaviness	Yes	No	Don't know
13. Hunger	Yes	No	Don't know
14. Inner bodily awareness	Yes	No	Don't know

15. Inner bodily flow	Yes	No	Don't know
16. Intestinal rumblings	Yes	No	Don't know
17. Mental energy	Yes	No	Don't know
18. Mental focus	Yes	No	Don't know
19. Nervousness	Yes	No	Don't know
20. Pain	Yes	No	Don't know
21. Peacefulness	Yes	No	Don't know
22. Physical vitality	Yes	No	Don't know
23. Receptivity	Yes	No	Don't know
24. Relaxation	Yes	No	Don't know
25. Restlessness	Yes	No	Don't know
26. Sensory acuteness	Yes	No	Don't know
27. Sleepiness	Yes	No	Don't know
28. Suppleness	Yes	No	Don't know
29. Tension	Yes	No	Don't know
30. Tingling	Yes	No	Don't know
31. Warmth or coolness	Yes	No	Don't know
32. Worry	Yes	No	Don't know

If you have any comments you would like to make on this questionnaire, you can include them here:

A-2. EXPost$_{32}$

What did you experience from the standardised electroacupuncture/TENS treatment you will receive today?

Did you experience changes in any of the feelings listed below?

Instructions (please read carefully)

This questionnaire contains 32 statements about feelings.

For each feeling, ring the word/s that best represents the change in feeling you experienced in your own case (this change may have been an increase or a decrease):

Make sure that you ring the word/s in the correct column.

Please be as honest and accurate as you can throughout . Respond to each statement as if it were the only one. That is, don't worry about being 'consistent' in your responses. There are no 'correct' or 'incorrect' answers. Answer according to what you experienced, rather than how you think 'most acupuncturists' would answer.

I experienced a change in the feeling of ...

Feeling	**Yes**, I experienced a change in this feeling	**No**, I did not experience a change in this feeling	**I don't know** if I experienced a change in this feeling
1. Aliveness	Yes	No	Don't know
2. Being at ease	Yes	No	Don't know
3. Being blue or down in the dumps	Yes	No	Don't know
4. Being in control	Yes	No	Don't know

5. Being spaced- out	Yes	No	Don't know
6. Calmness	Yes	No	Don't know
7. Cheerfulness	Yes	No	Don't know
8. Clarity	Yes	No	Don't know
9. Connectedness with others	Yes	No	Don't know
10. Contentment	Yes	No	Don't know
11. Excitement	Yes	No	Don't know
12. Heaviness	Yes	No	Don't know
13. Hunger	Yes	No	Don't know
14. Inner bodily awareness	Yes	No	Don't know
15. Inner bodily flow	Yes	No	Don't know
16. Intestinal rumblings	Yes	No	Don't know
17. Mental energy	Yes	No	Don't know
18. Mental focus	Yes	No	Don't know
19. Nervousness	Yes	No	Don't know
20. Pain	Yes	No	Don't know
21. Peacefulness	Yes	No	Don't know
22. Physical vitality	Yes	No	Don't know
23. Receptivity	Yes	No	Don't know
24. Relaxation	Yes	No	Don't know
25. Restlessness	Yes	No	Don't know
26. Sensory acuteness	Yes	No	Don't know
27. Sleepiness	Yes	No	Don't know
28. Suppleness	Yes	No	Don't know
29. Tension	Yes	No	Don't know
30. Tingling	Yes	No	Don't know
31. Warmth or coolness	Yes	No	Don't know
32. Worry	Yes	No	Don't know

Please asterisk (*) those changes you noticed most.

If you have any comments you would like to make on this questionnaire, you can include them here:

Appendix B. The revised 20-item questionnaires, $EXPre_{20}$ and $EXPost_{20}$.

B-1. $EXPre_{20}$

Instructions

	Yes	**No**
First, please tell us if you have received EA or TEAS before		

There are twenty FEELINGS listed on the following page which we would like you to consider carefully.

We would like to know if you expect any of these feelings to <u>increase</u> or <u>decrease</u> for you personally in response to the standardised EA or TEAS treatment that you will receive today.

This will be at points such as LI-4 (Hegu) and ST-36 (Zusanli).

Please remember there are no right or wrong answers. Consider each feeling in isolation and answer as honestly and accurately as possible according to your own personal expectations.

For each feeling, <u>circle</u> the word or abbreviation that best represents your expectation of change in the feeling in your own case.

Do make sure that you put your circle in the **correct row** and **column**.

Relative to how you feel NOW, during or immediately following EA/TEAS do you expect to experience any change AT ALL in the feeling of ...

Feeling	**Expect** to experience a change	**Not expect** to experience a change	**Don't know** / can't say	If **Yes**, expect feeling to **INCREASE**	If **Yes**, expect feeling to **DECREASE**
Relaxation	Yes	No	DK/CS	Inc	Dec
Aliveness	Yes	No	DK/CS	Inc	Dec
Sleepiness	Yes	No	DK/CS	Inc	Dec
Tingling	Yes	No	DK/CS	Inc	Dec
Pain	Yes	No	DK/CS	Inc	Dec
Relief	Yes	No	DK/CS	Inc	Dec
Calmness	Yes	No	DK/CS	Inc	Dec
Being stressed	Yes	No	DK/CS	Inc	Dec
Inner bodily flow	Yes	No	DK/CS	Inc	Dec
Intestinal rumblings	Yes	No	DK/CS	Inc	Dec
Mental focus	Yes	No	DK/CS	Inc	Dec
Mental energy	Yes	No	DK/CS	Inc	Dec
Being spaced out	Yes	No	DK/CS	Inc	Dec
Warmth	Yes	No	DK/CS	Inc	Dec
Heaviness	Yes	No	DK/CS	Inc	Dec
Wellbeing	Yes	No	DK/CS	Inc	Dec
Clarity	Yes	No	DK/CS	Inc	Dec
Cheerfulness	Yes	No	DK/CS	Inc	Dec
Tension	Yes	No	DK/CS	Inc	Dec
Sensory acuity	Yes	No	DK/CS	Inc	Dec

Do you have anything else you would like to add?

B-2. EXPost$_{20}$

Instructions

There are twenty FEELINGS listed on the following page which we would like you to consider carefully.

We would like to know if you experienced any changes in these feelings in response to the standardised EA or TEAS treatment that you received today.

Please remember there are no right or wrong answers. Consider each feeling in isolation and answer as honestly and accurately as possible according to your own personal experience.

For each feeling, circle the word or abbreviation that best represents what you experienced in your own case.

Do make sure that you put your circle in the **correct row** and **column**.

Please also asterisk (*) those 'Yes' changes you noticed most!

Relative to how you felt when you completed the earlier questionnaire, during or immediately following EA/TEAS did you experience a change in the feeling of …

Feeling	**Experienced** a change	**Not experienced** a change	**Don't know** / can't say	If **Yes**, experienced **INCREASE** in feeling	If **Yes**, experienced **DECREASE** in feeling
Pain	Yes	No	DK/CS	Inc	Dec
Inner bodily flow	Yes	No	DK/CS	Inc	Dec
Calmness	Yes	No	DK/CS	Inc	Dec
Clarity	Yes	No	DK/CS	Inc	Dec
Mental energy	Yes	No	DK/CS	Inc	Dec
Tension	Yes	No	DK/CS	Inc	Dec
Being spaced out	Yes	No	DK/CS	Inc	Dec
Being stressed	Yes	No	DK/CS	Inc	Dec
Warmth	Yes	No	DK/CS	Inc	Dec
Wellbeing	Yes	No	DK/CS	Inc	Dec
Heaviness	Yes	No	DK/CS	Inc	Dec
Mental focus	Yes	No	DK/CS	Inc	Dec
Sensory acuity	Yes	No	DK/CS	Inc	Dec
Aliveness	Yes	No	DK/CS	Inc	Dec
Relaxation	Yes	No	DK/CS	Inc	Dec
Tingling	Yes	No	DK/CS	Inc	Dec
Sleepiness	Yes	No	DK/CS	Inc	Dec
Cheerfulness	Yes	No	DK/CS	Inc	Dec
Intestinal rumblings	Yes	No	DK/CS	Inc	Dec
Relief	Yes	No	DK/CS	Inc	Dec

Don't forget to asterisk (*) those 'Yes' changes you noticed most!
If you have any comments you would like to make, you can include them here:

References

1. Mayor, D.F. What do we mean by the 'nonspecific' effects of acupuncture treatment? A survey of experienced acupuncture practitioners and researchers. *Eur. J. Orient. Med.* **2014**, *7*, 38–43.
2. Peters, D. (Ed.) *Understanding the Placebo Effect in Complementary Medicine: Theory, Practice and Research*; Churchill Livingstone: London, UK, 2001.
3. Caspi, O.; Bootzin, R.R. Evaluating how placebos produce change. Logical and causal traps and understanding cognitive explanatory mechanisms. *Eval. Health. Prof.* **2002**, *25*, 436–464. [CrossRef] [PubMed]
4. Walach, H.; Jonas, W.B. Placebo research: The evidence base for harnessing self-healing capacities. *J. Altern. Complement. Med.* **2004**, *10* (Suppl. 1), S103–S112. [CrossRef] [PubMed]
5. Salih, N.; Bäumler, P.I.; Simang, M.; Irnich, D. *Deqi* sensations without cutaneous sensory input: Results of an RCT. *BMC Complement. Altern. Med.* **2010**, *10*, 81. [CrossRef] [PubMed]
6. Kerr, C.E.; Shaw, J.R.; Conboy, L.A.; Kelley, J.M.; Jacobson, E.; Kaptchuk, T.J. Placebo acupuncture as a form of ritual touch healing: A neurophenomenological model. *Conscious. Cogn.* **2011**, *20*, 784–791. [CrossRef] [PubMed]
7. Warber, S.L.; Cornelio, D.; Straughn, J.; Kile, G. Biofield energy healing from the inside. *J. Altern. Complement. Med.* **2004**, *10*, 1107–1113. [CrossRef] [PubMed]
8. Mayor, D. Elemental souls and vernacular *qi*: Some attributes of what moves us. In *Energy Medicine East and West: A Natural History of qi*; Mayor, D., Micozzi, M.S., Eds.; Churchill Livingstone: Edinburgh, UK, 2011; pp. 24–47.
9. Lundeberg, T. To be or not to be: The needling sensation (*de qi*) in acupuncture. *Acupunct. Med.* **2013**, *31*, 129–131. [CrossRef] [PubMed]
10. Pacheco-López, G.; Engler, H.; Niemi, M.B.; Schedlowski, M. Expectations and associations that heal: Immunomodulatory placebo effects and its neurobiology. *Brain Behav. Immun.* **2006**, *20*, 430–446. [CrossRef] [PubMed]
11. Geers, A.L.; Wellman, J.A.; Fowler, S.L.; Rasinski, H.M.; Helfer, S.G. Placebo expectations and the detection of somatic information. *J. Behav. Med.* **2011**, *34*, 208–217. [CrossRef] [PubMed]
12. Vincent, C.A.; Richardson, P.H.; Black, J.J.; Pither, C.E. The significance of needle placement site in acupuncture. *J. Psychosom. Res.* **1989**, *33*, 489–496. [CrossRef]
13. Park, H.; Park, J.; Lee, H.; Lee, H. Does *deqi* (needle sensation) exist? *Am. J. Chin. Med.* **2002**, *30*, 45–50. [CrossRef] [PubMed]
14. Park, J.; Park, H.; Lee, H.; Lim, S.; Ahn, K.; Lee, H. *Deqi* sensation between the acupuncture-experienced and the naïve: A Korean study II. *Am. J. Chin. Med.* **2005**, *33*, 329–337. [CrossRef] [PubMed]
15. Kong, J.; Fufa, D.T.; Gerber, A.J.; Rosman, I.S.; Vangel, M.G.; Gracely, R.H.; Gollub, R.L. Psychophysical outcomes from a randomized pilot study of manual, electro, and sham acupuncture treatment on experimentally induced thermal pain. *J. Pain* **2005**, *6*, 55–64. [CrossRef] [PubMed]
16. Kong, J.; Gollub, R.; Huang, T.; Polich, G.; Napadow, V.; Hui, K.; Vangel, M.; Rosen, B.; Kaptchuk, T.J. Acupuncture de *qi*, from qualitative history to quantitative measurement. *J. Altern. Complement. Med.* **2007**, *13*, 1059–1070. [CrossRef] [PubMed]
17. Kim, Y.; Park, J.; Lee, H.; Bang, H.; Park, H.J. Content validity of an acupuncture sensation questionnaire. *J. Altern. Complement. Med.* **2008**, *14*, 957–963. [CrossRef] [PubMed]

18. White, P.; Bishop, F.; Hardy, H.; Abdollahian, S.; White, A.; Park, J.; Kaptchuk, T.J.; Lewith, G.T. Southampton needle sensation questionnaire: Development and validation of a measure to gauge acupuncture needle sensation. *J. Altern. Complement. Med.* **2008**, *14*, 373–379. [CrossRef] [PubMed]
19. Pach, D.; Hohmann, C.; Lüdtke, R.; Zimmermann-Viehoff, F.; Witt, C.M.; Thiele, C. German translation of the Southampton Needle Sensation Questionnaire: use in an experimental acupuncture study. *Forsch. Komplementmed.* **2011**, *18*, 321–326. [CrossRef] [PubMed]
20. Yu, D.T.; Jones, A.Y.; Pang, M.Y. Development and validation of the Chinese version of the Massachusetts General Hospital Acupuncture Sensation Scale: An exploratory and methodological study. *Acupunct. Med.* **2012**, *30*, 214–221. [CrossRef] [PubMed]
21. Bauml, J.; Xie, S.X.; Farrar, J.T.; Bowman, M.A.; Li, S.Q.; Bruner, D.; DeMichele, A.; Mao, J.J. Expectancy in real and sham electroacupuncture: Does believing make it so? *J. Natl. Cancer Inst. Monogr.* **2014**, *2014*, 302–307. [CrossRef] [PubMed]
22. Judge, A.; Cooper, C.; Arden, N.K.; Williams, S.; Hobbs, N.; Dixon, D.; Günther, K.P.; Dreinhoefer, K.; Dieppe, P.A. Pre-operative expectation predicts 12-month post-operative outcome among patients undergoing primary total hip replacement in European orthopaedic centres. *Osteoarthr. Cartil.* **2011**, *19*, 659–667. [CrossRef] [PubMed]
23. Kongsted, A.; Vach, W.; Axø, M.; Bech, R.N.; Hestbaek, L. Expectation of recovery from low back pain: A longitudinal cohort study investigating patient characteristics related to expectations and the association between expectations and 3-month outcome. *Spine* **2014**, *39*, 81–90. [CrossRef] [PubMed]
24. Vîslă, A.; Constantino, M.J.; Newkirk, K.; Ogrodniczuk, J.S.; Söchting, I. The relation between outcome expectation, therapeutic alliance, and outcome among depressed patients in group cognitive-behavioral therapy. *Psychother. Res* **2016**, 1–11. [CrossRef]
25. Roccia, L.; Rogora, G.A. [Acupuncture and relaxation]. *Minerva Med.* **1976**, *67*, 1918–1920. [PubMed]
26. Wang, R.R. Yinyang (Yin-Yang). Internet Encyclopedia of Philosophy: A Peer-Reviewed Academic Resource. Available online: http://www.iep.utm.edu/yinyang/ (accessed on 26 February 2017).
27. Mayor, D.F. (Ed.) *Electroacupuncture: A Practical Manual and Resource*; Churchill Livingstone: Edinburgh, UK, 2007.
28. Mayor, D.; Steffert, T. Expectation and Experience of 'Nonspecific' Feelings Elicited by Acupuncture: Developing and Piloting a Set of Questionnaires. In Proceedings of the British Medical Acupuncture Society (BMAS) and Portuguese Medical Acupuncture Society (PMAS) Autumn Meeting, Porto, Portugal, 27–29 September 2013; Available online: http://www.qeeg.co.uk/electroacupuncture/eaq1.htm or http://f1000research.com/posters/1094397 (accessed on 17 October 2015).
29. Steffert, T.; Mayor, D. Mood changes in response to electroacupuncture treatment in a classroom situation. Personality type, emotional intelligence and prior acupuncture experience, with an exploration of Shannon entropy, response style and graphology variables. In Proceedings of the 19th International Acupuncture Research Symposium, London, UK, 25 March 2017.
30. Mayor, D.F. Expectation and experience of 'nonspecific' (whole person) feelings elicited by acupuncture: Content validity of a set of questionnaires. *Ger. J. Acupunct. Relat. Tech.* **2014**, *57*, 14–19. [CrossRef]
31. Hierarchical Cluster Analysis Measures for Binary Data. IBM Knowledge Center, 2011. Available online: http://www-01.ibm.com/support/knowledgecenter/SSLVMB_20.0.0/com.ibm.spss.statistics.help/cmd_cluster_measure_binary.htm (accessed on 16 October 2015).
32. Spencer, N. *Cluster Analysis seminar. Statistical Services and Consultancy Unit*; University of Hertfordshire: Hatfield, UK, 2015.
33. Keshet, Y.; Simchai, D. The 'gender puzzle' of alternative medicine and holistic spirituality: A literature review. *Soc. Sci. Med.* **2014**, *113*, 77–86. [CrossRef] [PubMed]
34. Gravetter, F.J.; Wallnau, L.B. *Study Guide: Essentials of Statistics for the Behavioral Sciences*, 6th ed.; Thomson/Wadsworth: Belmont, CA, USA, 2008.
35. Lund, I.; Lundeberg, T. Are minimal, superficial or sham acupuncture procedures acceptable as inert placebo controls? *Acupunct. Med.* **2006**, *24*, 13–15. [CrossRef] [PubMed]
36. Lundeberg, T.; Lund, I.; Sing, A.; Näslund, J. Is placebo acupuncture what it is intended to be? *Evid. Based Complement. Alternat. Med.* **2011**, *2011*, 932407. [CrossRef] [PubMed]

7

Evaluation of the Effectiveness of Acupuncture in the Treatment of Knee Osteoarthritis

Joana Teixeira [1], Maria João Santos [1], Luís Carlos Matos [2] and Jorge Pereira Machado [1,3,*]

1 ICBAS- Institute of Biomedical Sciences Abel Salazar, University of Porto, 4050-313 Porto, Portugal; joanabcteixeira@gmail.com (J.T.); mjrs.mtc@gmail.com (M.J.S.)
2 Faculdade de Engenharia da Universidade do Porto, Rua Dr. Roberto Frias, s/n 4200-465 Porto, Portugal; lcmatos@fe.up.pt
3 LABIOMEP—Porto Biomechanics Laboratory, University of Porto, 4200-450 Porto, Portugal
* Correspondence: jmachado@icbas.up.pt

Abstract: Background: Osteoarthritis is a widespread chronic disease seen as a continuum of clinical occurrences within several phases, which go from synovial inflammation and microscopic changes of bone and cartilage to painful destructive changes of all the joint structures. Being the most common joint disease, it is the leading cause of disability in working individuals above 50 years of age. In some cases, conventional treatments produce just a mild and brief pain reduction and have considerable side-effects. Contemporary Traditional Chinese Medicine (TCM) is a model of systems biology based on a logically accessible theoretical background. It integrates several therapeutic approaches, among them acupuncture, which has shown effective results in the treatment of knee and hip osteoarthritis, minimizing pain, improving functionality and consequently leading to a better quality of life. **Methods:** The present case study included two patients with clinical signs of osteoarthritis and diagnosis of medial pain, as defined by the Heidelberg Model of TCM. Over 6 weeks, those patients were treated with acupuncture, with a frequency of one session a week. The sessions lasted for thirty minutes and were based on the needling of 4 local acupoints. Before and after each session, pain and mobility assessments were performed. **Results:** The results were positive, with significant reduction of pain and increased knee joint flexion amplitude and mobility. **Conclusion:** Acupuncture was effective as an alternative or complementary treatment of knee osteoarthritis, with high levels of improvement within a modest intervention period.

Keywords: osteoarthritis; acupuncture; Heidelberg Model of Traditional Chinese Medicine

1. Introduction

Osteoarthritis is a chronic degenerative joint disease demonstrating articular cartilage damage and leading to disabling pain and joint dysfunction [1]. Clinically, osteoarthritis is characterized by pain, typically with gradual onset that worsens over time, swollen joint caused by synovitis, morning stiffness, crackling bone, muscle atrophy, narrowing of the intra-articular space, osteophyte formation, subchondral bone sclerosis and cyst formation [2].

Osteoarthritis of the knee is a multifactorial disease, whose etiology includes generalized systemic disease (e.g., gout, rheumatoid arthritis), constitutional factors (e.g., age, gender and genetics) and also biomechanical factors (e.g., joint damage, muscle weakness, overweight and obesity) [3]. The higher incidence and severity in females is related to hormonal status. Fluctuations of sex hormone levels in young females and loss of ovarian sex hormone production due to menopause in older ones contribute to the observed differences in gender prevalence [4,5].

The treatment of knee osteoarthritis may be categorized as either conservative or surgical. Conservative treatment may include medication, manual and physical therapies, medially directed patellar taping, walking aids, thermal agents, weight loss, Tai Chi practice, swimming, water aerobics, and resistance exercises. The American College of Rheumatology recommends most of the previous non-pharmacological approaches in the initial treatment of this disease [6]. Nevertheless, common interventions involve the use of analgesics, anti-inflammatories and infiltrations with corticosteroids. Pharmacological intervention may include the use of glucosamine, glucosamine with chondroitin, chondroitin, acetaminophen, oral and topical NSAIDs, tramadol, and intraarticular corticosteroid injections, intraarticular hyaluronate injections, duloxetine, and opioids [7]. Physiotherapy, occupational therapy and psychomotor rehabilitation may help controlling pain and improving joint function, restoring quality of life [6,8]. Surgical treatment, which can be divided into joint-preserving, such as arthroscopy and osteotomy (femoral or tibial), and joint-replacing procedures, such as partial and total arthroplasties, should be indicated in cases without symptom relief after conservative approaches [9].

Although conventional approaches, either pharmacological and surgical have been reported as successful, side effects such as toxicity manifestations, complications involving anesthesia, infection, osteoligamentous surgery-induced injuries are issues that cannot be ignored [1]. In this scenario, acupuncture comes as an alternative therapeutic approach in knee osteoarthritis conditions, showing good results in pain reduction and rehabilitation of motor abilities, improving functionality and quality of life, either when used as a stand-alone therapy or together with other procedures [7,10–19].

Nowadays, acupuncture is accepted among the Portuguese medical community with regard to its mechanisms of action as a medical procedure, with its analgesic and anti-inflammatory effects recognized a long time ago by the World Health Organization, and is considered superior to placebo in published randomized controlled trials [20]. Indeed, this integration requires a science-based approach supported by controlled research. Nevertheless, even with studies corroborating its benefits, there is still a great debate within the scientific community with regard to its mechanisms of action and therapeutic methodology [21–23].

Eastern and Western therapeutic approaches and anatomical and physiological views of the knee region are considerably different. In TCM, the knee is sustained by the liver (hepatic) and by the conduits that pass through this region; namely, the stomach, gallbladder and bladder, known as the *yang* conduits, and the liver, kidney and Spleen, known as the *yin* conduits [24–26]. These conduits are involved in the neurovegetative patterns of that anatomical region acting on the knee joint, nerves, and being responsible for the normal functioning of the knee processes [25]. The most common form of knee pain, known in TCM as center or medial pain, is characterized by a localized pain in the medial part of the knee that the Spleen conduit passes through [27]. Although many other acupoints could be used in the treatment of this condition [17], the approach based on the Heidelberg Model of TCM involves supporting the Centre by the simultaneous stimulation of specific acupoints from the Spleen and Stomach conduits, which belong to the Phase Earth, in order to promote orthopathy [26].

In this case study, conducted with two patients suffering from knee osteoarthritis with constant pain, the research team aimed to evaluate the effectiveness of acupuncture as a treatment procedure, using a protocol based on the needling of just 4 local acupoints to treat pain and increase joint mobility.

2. Materials and Methods

The patients considered in this study were selected according to the following inclusion and exclusion criteria.

Inclusion criteria: clinical signs of osteoarthritis and diagnosis of medial pain, as defined by Heidelberg Model of TCM, knee pain, mobility commitment and impairment in daily living activities, such as going up and down stairs.

Exclusion criteria: pregnancy and lactation, psychiatric or neurological disorders, presence of inflammatory autoimmune disease, history of substance abuse.

2.1. Sample Characterization

Subject A—A female of 46 years old, formerly a cook in a private hospital, currently unemployed, with acute pain in the knee and signs of osteoarthritis detected by imaging tests. Acupuncture was performed after a month of intense pain and loss of mobility. The patient used crutches during the rehabilitation period.

Subject B—A female of 56 years old, formerly a secretary, currently unemployed, suffering from internal and femoro-patellar gonarthrosis, was victim of a stairs accident in December 2010 and submitted to two surgical interventions in 2010 and 2012. The patient took medication and decided to start acupuncture after two years of constant pain and mobility problems.

A written informed consent from patients was required to proceed with the intervention.

2.2. Materials

Single-use sterilized acupuncture needles (25 mm length and 0.25 mm diameter) brand Tewa, Goniometer, and Portuguese pain assessment scale.

2.3. Methodology

The intervention consisted of 6 thirty-minute acupuncture sessions with a frequency of one session a week. The degree of pain was evaluated before and after the treatment by using the numeric pain rating scale, which is a single-dimensional instrument to assess pain intensity at rest or with activity. This scale is frequently used in adults with chronic pain due to rheumatic diseases, and is scored by choosing a number between 0 (no pain) and 10 (extreme pain or other label) to rate current pain intensity [28]. The mobility range tests were performed with a Goniometer at the beginning and 10 min after each session.

The acupuncture treatments were performed by a qualified TCM practitioner and the points used in this study were: St34 *Liang Qiu* (S34 *Monticulus Septi*), St36 *Zu San Li* (S36 *Vicus Tertius Pedis*), Sp9 *Yin Ling Quan* (L9 *Fons Tumuli Yin*) and Sp10 *Xue Hai* (L10 *Mare xue*) (acupoints denomination according to the Heidelberg Model of TCM is quoted between bracelets).

3. Results

As shown in Figures 1 and 2, subjects A and B reported clear improvements in their condition, with pain reduction along the acupuncture treatment (pain scores dropped from 9.5 to 2 and from 9 to 1 in subjects A and B, respectively). These good results allowed them to stop taking conventional medication for pain. The analgesic effect of acupuncture has been often reported by other authors. This effect can be induced both by a local stimulation of the tissue, thus resulting in the release of inflammatory related substances, vasodilatation and the increase of serotonin and immune cells, as well as by a hypothalamus activation and related endorphins release [29].

Although some studies point to pain relief in patients suffering from osteoarthrosis, the effects on articular mobility are unclear, probably due to different types of therapeutic methodologies [16,30]. As standardization is a key issue in research, protocols must control a wide range of variables, such as the acupuncture technique, the intervention protocol, the duration of the treatment, the selected acupoints, just to mention a few. It is easy to find studies in which a vast selection of acupoints and different stimulations were used in the treatment of knee osteoarthritis. Some used a combination of 9 to 10 local and distal points from several conduits such as Stomach, Spleen, Gall Bladder, Kidney, Urinary Bladder, Liver, Large Intestine, and the *xiyan* extraordinary acupoint, as well as a combination of manual and electrical stimulation [19,31–35]. In these studies, the duration of the intervention and the frequency of the sessions also varied between 2 and 12 weeks with one or two sessions a week. In fact, methodological standardization is a hard task, not only because, in some cases, there is no consensus between practitioners and their diagnosis, but also because each patient has a specific homeostatic imbalance and physiological compensation when submitted to the same stimulus [36].

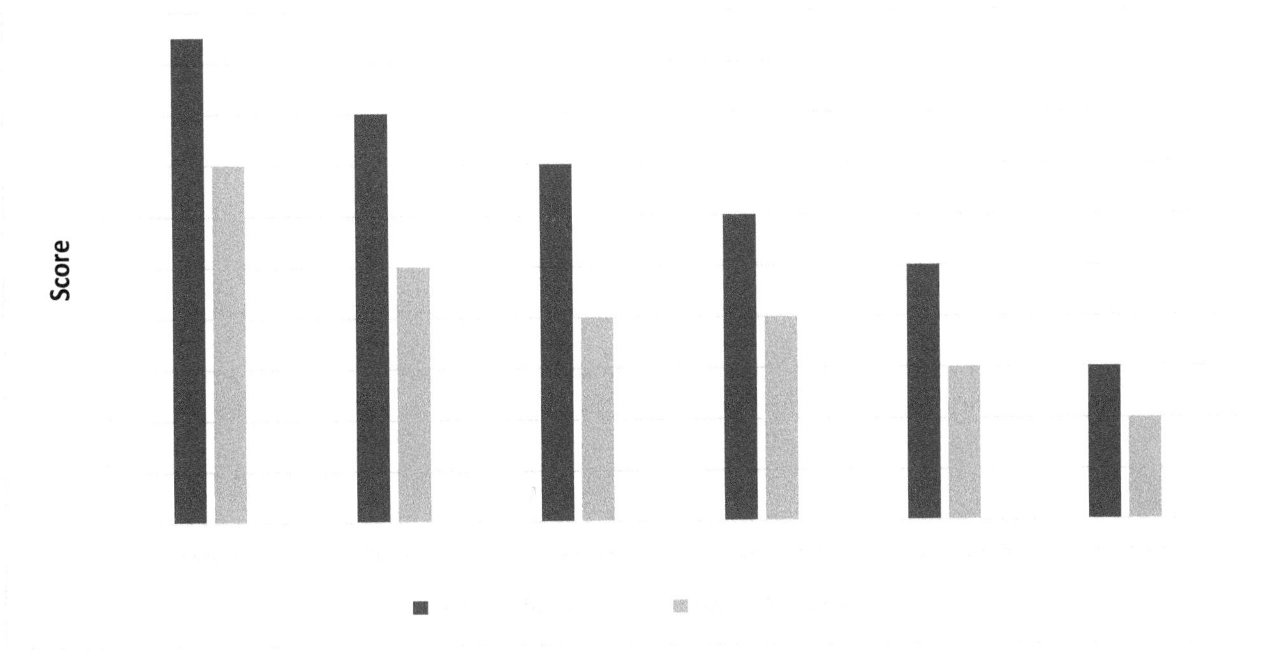

Figure 1. Assessment of pain per session, subject A.

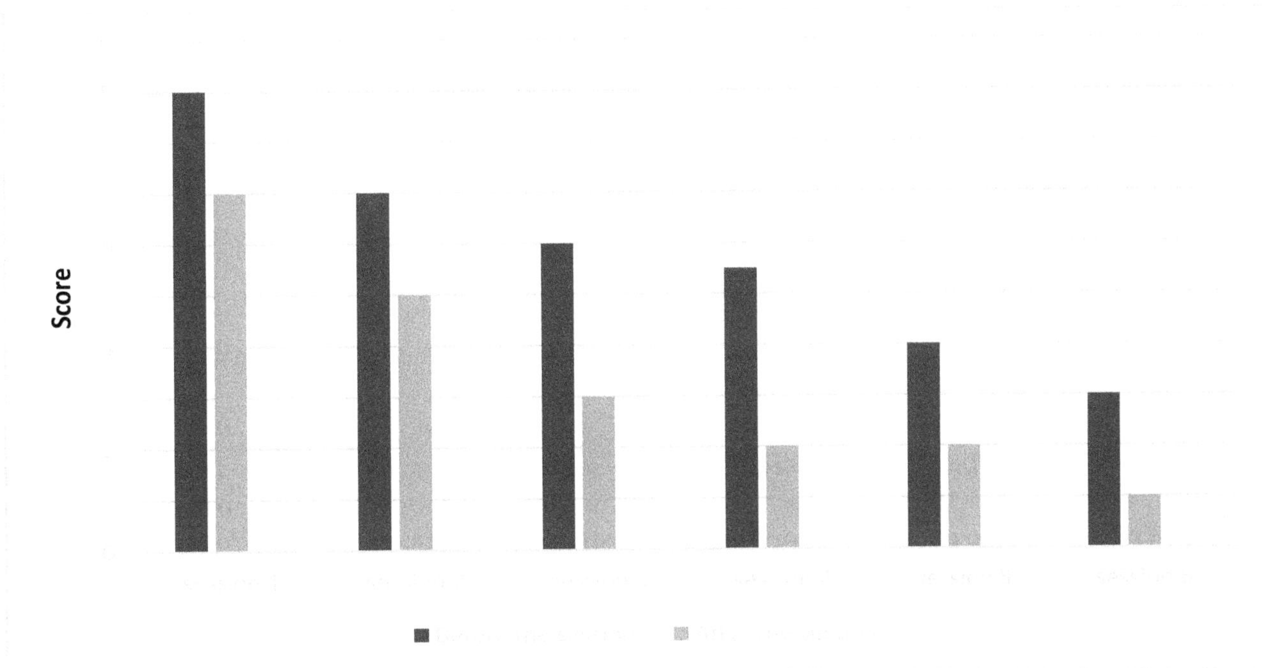

Figure 2. Assessment of pain per session, subject B.

In our study, Subjects A and B presented an increase in mobility and range of motion following treatment. The degree of knee flexion raised up from 45° with pain to 160° without pain to subject A and from 90° to 160° to subject B (Table 1). In this process, subject A abandoned the use of crutches.

Table 1. Knee joint flexion amplitude before and after acupuncture sessions.

Session	Subject A		Subject B	
	Before	**After**	**Before**	**After**
1st	45°	90°	90°	110°
2nd	60°	110°	110°	120°
3rd	90°	140°	110°	130°
4th	110°	155°	125°	140°
5th	140°	160°	130°	155°
6th	155°	160°	140°	155°

The improvement percentages for pain and knee joint flexion amplitude per session, considering each session initial and final scores, along the experimental period are shown in Figure 3.

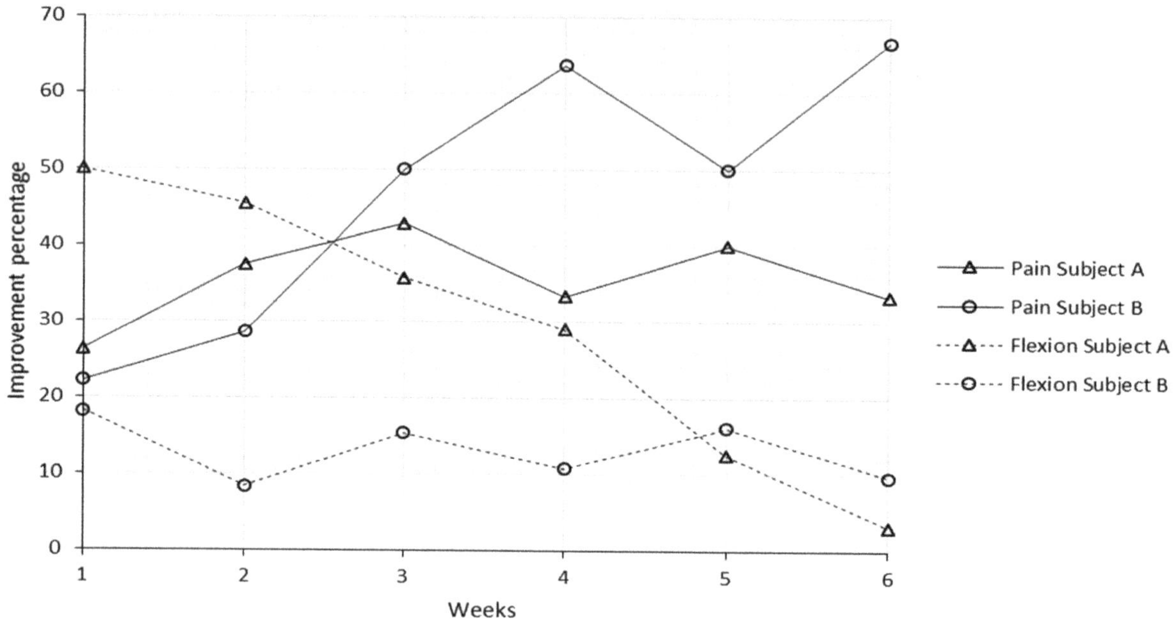

Figure 3. Improvement percentages for pain and knee joint flexion amplitude per session, considering each session initial and final scores, along the experimental period.

Regarding pain, Subject A experienced an increasing tendency in the improvement percentage per session from week 1 to 3, and from this point on, this tendency stopped rising. The average improvement percentage per session for Subject A was 36%, and the overall improvement at the end of the experimental period reflecting the initial to final evaluation, was 79%. In the case of Subject B, with the exception of week 5, the improvement per session was always higher than the week before, with an average of 47% and overall improvement of 89%. One week after each treatment, Subjects A and B had average regressions on pain of 19% and 29%, respectively, taking into account the previous evaluation and the evaluation before the acupuncture session.

With regard to knee joint flexion, the condition of Subject A in the beginning of the experimental period was worse than Subject B. Subject A experienced an improvement of 50% immediately after the first session. The following weeks, a decreasing tendency was noticed as knee flexion, before each session, tended to be higher as a result of the patient's response to the treatment. The average per-session and overall improvement percentages were 29% and 72% for Subject A and 13% and 42% for Subject B. Considering that Subject B's condition was better, the improvements per session were not as high as Subject A, and remained almost stable along the experimental period. Regressions one week after each session were also noticed in knee flexion amplitude, with scores falling on average 17% and 6%, for Subjects A and B, respectively.

The overall analysis of pain and knee flexion improvements presented in this case study is highly satisfactory. High improvement percentages, an average of 84% for pain and 57% for join flexion mobility, were achieved within a modest intervention period, 6 weeks, with just one session a week, and with a reduced number of needled acupoints, compared to most of the treatment protocols used in other studies. Knee flexion mobility per session (an average of 21%) was higher than the outcomes reported in similar studies (9% [30] and 16% [37]). Although the beneficial effects of acupuncture are shown here in just two patients, and the small sample can skew results, our study supports the thesis that acupuncture can be used as an effective therapeutic tool in the treatment of knee osteoarthritis.

4. Conclusions

Contemporary understanding of TCM considers it as a model of systems biology with a holistic therapeutic approach, in which the diagnosis is key to achieving positive results. Thus, systematized science-based analysis and decisions, both of the pathological condition and therapeutic intervention, are required to validate the results obtained by the use of acupuncture as a therapeutic tool. In our study, within the framework of the Heidelberg Model of TCM, we found that acupuncture was effective in the treatment of knee osteoarthritis with significant pain relief and improvement in knee joint mobility and range in 2 subjects whose initial presentation was characterized by extreme pain, scored 9.5 and 9, as well as reduced joint flexion amplitude, 45° and 90°. The overall pain relief, considering the whole intervention period, was 79% and 89% for subject A and B, respectively. With regard to mobility and range of motion, positive results were also found with considerable improvements in the knee flexion angle from 45° to 160° in subject A (an improvement of 72%), and 90° to 155° in subject B (an improvement of 42%). Although regressions, both in pain and joint flexion mobility, were noticed one week after each treatment, the improvements in each session were high enough to overcome this issue, allowing for maintenance of the recovery with increasing tendency along the experimental period.

In addition to concluding that acupuncture was effective as a therapeutic tool with high levels of recovery when compared with similar published studies, it is important to mention that these results were achieved within a modest intervention period, 6 weeks, with just one session a week, and with a reduced number of needled acupoints, compared to most of the treatment protocols used in other studies, and doesn't require electrical stimulation. Our outcomes are a good example of a successful intervention that can contribute to the debate about methodological standardization of acupuncture in the treatment of knee osteoarthrosis.

We are aware of the limitations of this study and suggest a follow up study with a statistically representative sample.

Acknowledgments: We would like to thank to everyone that somehow contributed to this study.

Author Contributions: J.T. conceived, designed and performed the experiments, analyzed the data, and wrote the first version of the paper. M.J.S. oversaw the experimental process and revised the paper. L.C.M. and J.P.M. participated in conceiving the study, interpreting data and revising the paper.

References

1. Crawford, D.C.; Miller, L.E.; Block, J.E. Conservative management of symptomatic knee osteoarthritis: A flawed strategy? *Orthop. Rev.* **2013**, *5*, e2. [CrossRef] [PubMed]
2. Langworthy, M.J.; Saad, A.; Langworthy, N.M. Conservative treatment modalities and outcomes for osteoarthritis: The concomitant pyramid of treatment. *Phys. Sportsmed.* **2010**, *38*, 133–145. [CrossRef] [PubMed]

3. Silverwood, V.; Blagojevic-Bucknall, M.; Jinks, C.; Jordan, J.; Protheroe, J.; Jordan, K. Current evidence on risk factors for knee osteoarthritis in older adults: A systematic review and meta-analysis. *Osteoarthr. Cartil.* **2015**, *23*, 507–515. [CrossRef] [PubMed]
4. Boyan, B.D.; Hart, D.A.; Enoka, R.M.; Nicolella, D.P.; Resnick, E.; Berkley, K.J.; Sluka, K.A.; Kwoh, C.K.; Tosi, L.L.; O'Connor, M.I.; et al. Hormonal modulation of connective tissue homeostasis and sex differences in risk for osteoarthritis of the knee. *Biol. Sex Differ.* **2013**, *4*, 3. [CrossRef] [PubMed]
5. Pereira, D.; Peleteiro, B.; Araujo, J.; Branco, J.; Santos, R.; Ramos, E. The effect of osteoarthritis definition on prevalence and incidence estimates: A systematic review. *Osteoarthr. Cartil.* **2011**, *19*, 1270–1285. [CrossRef] [PubMed]
6. Hochberg, M.C.; Altman, R.D.; April, K.T.; Benkhalti, M.; Guyatt, G.; McGowan, J.; Towheed, T.; Welch, V.; Wells, G.; Tugwell, P. American college of rheumatology 2012 recommendations for the use of nonpharmacologic and pharmacologic therapies in osteoarthritis of the hand, hip, and knee. *Arthritis Care Res.* **2012**, *64*, 465–474. [CrossRef]
7. Newberry, S.J.; FitzGerald, J.; SooHoo, N.F.; Booth, M.; Marks, J.; Motala, A.; Apaydin, E.; Chen, C.; Raaen, L.; Shanman, R. *Treatment of Osteoarthritis of the Knee: An Update Review*; Report No. 17-EHC011-EF; AHRQ (US Agency for Healthcare Research and Quality): Rockville, MD, USA, 2017.
8. Alshami, A.M. Knee osteoarthritis related pain: A narrative review of diagnosis and treatment. *Int. J. Health Sci.* **2014**, *8*, 85–104. [CrossRef]
9. Hussain, S.; Neilly, D.; Baliga, S.; Patil, S.; Meek, R. Knee osteoarthritis: A review of management options. *Scott. Med. J.* **2016**, *61*, 7–16. [CrossRef] [PubMed]
10. Yue, J. Treatment of 78 patients with knee osteoarthritis by acupuncture, moxibustion, and tuina. *World J. Acupunct. Moxibustion* **2015**, *25*, 53–56. [CrossRef]
11. Mavrommatis, C.I.; Argyra, E.; Vadalouka, A.; Vasilakos, D.G. Acupuncture as an adjunctive therapy to pharmacological treatment in patients with chronic pain due to osteoarthritis of the knee: A 3-armed, randomized, placebo-controlled trial. *Pain* **2012**, *153*, 1720–1726. [CrossRef] [PubMed]
12. Fu, M.; Zhang, Z. Knee osteoarthritis treated with acupuncture based on syndrome differentiation: A randomized controlled trial. *World J. Acupunct. Moxibustion* **2012**, *22*, 11–17. [CrossRef]
13. Corbett, M.S.; Rice, S.J.C.; Madurasinghe, V.; Slack, R.; Fayter, D.A.; Harden, M.; Sutton, A.J.; MacPherson, H.; Woolacott, N.F. Acupuncture and other physical treatments for the relief of pain due to osteoarthritis of the knee: Network meta-analysis. *Osteoarthr. Cartil.* **2013**, *21*, 1290–1298. [CrossRef] [PubMed]
14. Hou, P.-W.; Fu, P.-K.; Hsu, H.-C.; Hsieh, C.-L. Traditional chinese medicine in patients with osteoarthritis of the knee. *J. Tradit. Complement. Med.* **2015**, *5*, 182–196. [CrossRef] [PubMed]
15. Selfe, T.K.; Taylor, A.G. Acupuncture and osteoarthritis of the knee: A review of randomized, controlled trials. *Fam. Community Health* **2008**, *31*, 247–254. [CrossRef] [PubMed]
16. Ezzo, J.; Hadhazy, V.; Birch, S.; Lao, L.; Kaplan, G.; Hochberg, M.; Berman, B. Acupuncture for osteoarthritis of the knee: A systematic review. *Arthritis Rheumatol.* **2001**, *44*, 819–825. [CrossRef]
17. Mc Neill, S.; Fullen, B.M. Acupuncture for osteoarthritis of the knee: Common points and treatment parameters used. *Physiotherapy* **2015**, *101*, e968–e969. [CrossRef]
18. Witt, C.M.; Jena, S.; Brinkhaus, B.; Liecker, B.; Wegscheider, K.; Willich, S.N. Acupuncture in patients with osteoarthritis of the knee or hip: A randomized, controlled trial with an additional nonrandomized arm. *Arthritis Rheumatol.* **2006**, *54*, 3485–3493. [CrossRef] [PubMed]
19. Manyanga, T.; Froese, M.; Zarychanski, R.; Abou-Setta, A.; Friesen, C.; Tennenhouse, M.; Shay, B.L. Pain management with acupuncture in osteoarthritis: A systematic review and meta-analysis. *BMC Complement. Altern. Med.* **2014**, *14*, 312. [CrossRef] [PubMed]
20. World Health Organization. *Acupuncture: Review and Analysis of Reports on Controlled Clinical Trials*; World Health Organization: Geneva, Switzerland, 2002.
21. Soh, K.-S. Bonghan circulatory system as an extension of acupuncture meridians. *J. Acupunct. Meridian Stud.* **2009**, *2*, 93–106. [CrossRef]
22. Zhou, W.; Benharash, P. Effects and mechanisms of acupuncture based on the principle of meridians. *J. Acupunct. Meridian Stud.* **2014**, *7*, 190–193. [CrossRef] [PubMed]
23. Cheng, K.J. Neurobiological mechanisms of acupuncture for some common illnesses: A clinician's perspective. *J. Acupunct. Meridian Stud.* **2014**, *7*, 105–114. [CrossRef] [PubMed]

24. Frank Brazkiewicz, H.J.G. *Conduit-(Channel) System, Acupuncture Points, Basic*; Heidelberg School of Chinese Medicine: Heidelberg, Germany, 2009.
25. Greten, H. *Understanding Tcm—Scientific Chinese Medicine—The Heidelberg Model*; Heidelberg School of Chinese Medicine: Heidelberg, Germany, 2008.
26. Greten, H.J. *Clinical Subjects, Scientific Chinese Medicine, the Heidelberg Model*; Heidelberg School of Chinese Medicine: Heidelberg, Germany, 2008.
27. Sousa, C.; Gonçalves, M.; Machado, J.; Greten, H. Treating musculoskeletal pain with traditional chinese medicine techniques—A short review. *Exp. Pathol. Health Sci.* **2016**, *8*, 25–28.
28. Hawker, G.A.; Mian, S.; Kendzerska, T.; French, M. Measures of adult pain: Visual analog scale for pain (vas pain), numeric rating scale for pain (nrs pain), mcgill pain questionnaire (mpq), short-form mcgill pain questionnaire (sf-mpq), chronic pain grade scale (cpgs), short form-36 bodily pain scale (sf-36 bps), and measure of intermittent and constant osteoarthritis pain (icoap). *Arthritis Care Res.* **2011**, *63*, S240–S252.
29. Audette, J.F.; Bailey, A. *Integrative Pain Medicine: The Science and Practice of Complementary and Alternative Medicine in Pain Management*; Springer: Berlin/Heidelberg, Germany, 2008.
30. Karner, M.; Brazkiewicz, F.; Remppis, A.; Fischer, J.; Gerlach, O.; Stremmel, W.; Subramanian, S.V.; Greten, H.J. Objectifying specific and nonspecific effects of acupuncture: A double-blinded randomised trial in osteoarthritis of the knee. *Evid. Based Complement. Altern. Med. eCAM* **2013**, *2013*, 427265. [CrossRef] [PubMed]
31. Berman, B.M.; Lao, L.; Langenberg, P.; Lee, W.L.; Gilpin, A.M.; Hochberg, M.C. Effectiveness of acupuncture as adjunctive therapy in osteoarthritis of the kneea randomized, controlled trial. *Ann. Intern. Med.* **2004**, *141*, 901–910. [CrossRef] [PubMed]
32. Tukmachi, E.; Jubb, R.; Dempsey, E.; Jones, P. The effect of acupuncture on the symptoms of knee osteoarthritis-an open randomised controlled study. *Acupunct. Med.* **2004**, *22*, 14–22. [CrossRef] [PubMed]
33. Vas, J.; Méndez, C.; Perea-Milla, E.; Vega, E.; Panadero, M.D.; León, J.M.; Borge, M.Á.; Gaspar, O.; Sánchez-Rodríguez, F.; Aguilar, I. Acupuncture as a complementary therapy to the pharmacological treatment of osteoarthritis of the knee: Randomised controlled trial. *BMJ* **2004**, *329*, 1216. [CrossRef] [PubMed]
34. Witt, C.; Brinkhaus, B.; Jena, S.; Linde, K.; Streng, A.; Wagenpfeil, S.; Hummelsberger, J.; Walther, H.; Melchart, D.; Willich, S. Acupuncture in patients with osteoarthritis of the knee: A randomised trial. *Lancet* **2005**, *366*, 136–143. [CrossRef]
35. White, A.; Tough, L.; Eyre, V.; Vickery, J.; Asprey, A.; Quinn, C.; Warren, F.; Pritchard, C.; Foster, N.E.; Taylor, R.S.; et al. Western medical acupuncture in a group setting for knee osteoarthritis: Results of a pilot randomised controlled trial. *Pilot Feasibility Stud.* **2016**, *2*, 10. [CrossRef] [PubMed]
36. Cardoso, R.; Lumini-Oliveira, J.; Santos, M.J.; Ramos, B.; Machado, J.; Greten, H. Effect of acupuncture on delayed onset muscle soreness: Series of case studies. *Exp. Pathol. Health Sci.* **2016**, *8*, 85–92.
37. Liu, Y.-H.; Wei, I.-P.; Wang, T.-M.; Lu, T.-W.; Lin, J.-G. Immediate effects of acupuncture treatment on intra-and inter-limb contributions to body support during gait in patients with bilateral medial knee osteoarthritis. *Am. J. Chin. Med.* **2017**, *45*, 23–35. [CrossRef] [PubMed]

8

The Effects of Yin, Yang and Qi in the Skin on Pain

James David Adams, Jr.

University of Southern California, School of Pharmacy, 1985 Zonal Avenue, Los Angeles, CA, 90089-9121, USA; jadams@usc.edu

Academic Editors: Gerhard Litscher and William Chi-shing Cho

Abstract: The most effective and safe treatment site for pain is in the skin. This chapter discusses the reasons to treat pain in the skin. Pain is sensed in the skin through transient receptor potential cation channels and other receptors. These receptors have endogenous agonists (yang) and antagonists (yin) that help the body control pain. Acupuncture works through modulation of these receptor activities (qi) in the skin; as do moxibustion and liniments. The treatment of pain in the skin has the potential to save many lives and improve pain therapy in most patients.

Keywords: pain; skin; topical; liniment; acupuncture; transient receptor potential cation channels

---

1. Introduction

The ancient Chinese concepts of yin, yang and qi have been explained in modern scientific terms [1]. Yin is cold, wet and diminishes blood flow. Yang is hot, dry and increases blood flow. Yin can also be represented by an antagonist that decreases pain and inflammation by inhibiting a receptor, such as a transient receptor potential cation channel (TRP). Yang can be represented by an agonist that decreases pain and inflammation by increasing the activity of a receptor, such as an opioid receptor. Qi is the flow of signal transduction mechanisms that occurs in cells because of the actions of agonists and antagonists. When qi flows well, these signal transduction mechanisms result in less pain and inflammation. A balance of yin and yang is necessary for qi to flow well. Signal transduction mechanisms may influence yin and yang by altering the transcription or activation of TRP or other receptors. There is a pain cycle that starts in the skin, travels to the brainstem and brain, and returns to the skin [2]. This pain cycle can magnify pain if left unchecked. The pain cycle is caused when yin and yang are not in balance and qi does not flow correctly in the skin.

The gate control theory of pain presents the pain cycle in terms of the brainstem rather than the skin [3]. In this theory, pain is sensed in the brain not the skin, and can be modified by non-painful sensations in the skin, such as rubbing the skin after a painful incident. This theory contends that inhibitory interneurons in the brainstem can suppress the transmission of pain signals into the brain. The gate control theory is useful, but does not take into account the many pain sensors in the skin and the fact that the signals from these pain sensors can be modified in the skin [2]. The fact that the skin is involved in pain sensation is obvious, since injection of a local anesthetic into the skin causes analgesia near the site of injection. The current paper proposes a modification of the gate control theory in which the skin is involved in sensing and modifying pain signals. The brainstem can modify pain signals. The brain is responsible for processing and modifying pain signals.

It is well known that ice packs decrease pain and swelling soon after an injury. Later, heat packs may be applied in order to decrease pain and swelling. How do ice and heat work? They work through TRPs that are sensitive to cold and heat. Initial TRP activation by cold or heat results in TRP deactivation that causes pain relief and decreases inflammation. TRPs are the most abundant pain receptors in the body. They are located in the plasma membranes of many cells of the body and are sensitive to heat, cold, pain, mechanical stimulation and other stimuli. They are abundant in the skin where they are located in the terminals of sensory afferent neurons [2]. TRP activation causes pain. TRPs are unusual receptors in that activation by an agonist may cause them to deactivate. This can lead to pain relief for much longer than expected. TRPs are channels that allow calcium and other positive ions to enter sensory neurons. Excessive calcium permeability can cause apoptosis of sensory terminals. This causes long term pain relief until nerve terminals can be regenerated [4]. TRPs are also involved in inflammation in the skin and other sites in the body [2].

2. TRP Diversity and Neuronal Populations

There are at least 28 different TRPs in the skin (Table 1), most of which are pain receptors [5]. In other words, these receptors are activated by painful stimuli and transmit these pain stimuli to the brain. There is no evidence of tolerance to the analgesia produced by inhibiting or deactivating TRPs. The body makes agonists and antagonists for these receptors which are derived from arachidonic acid and other fats. There are transient receptor potential cation channel vanilloid receptors, TRPV1–6, that can be inhibited by plant derived compounds such as capsaicin and some monoterpenoids [5]. Several TRPV receptor subtypes are activated by heat. As heat is applied, the receptors are initially activated, then deactivated resulting in channel closing and analgesia. TRPV receptors respond to endocannabinoids, endovanilloids, cannabinoids, hydroperoxyeicosatetraenoic acid (HPETE) and hydroxyeicosatetraenoic acid (HETE) [5]. Mechanical stimuli, such as pressure on the skin, can also activate some vanilloid channels such as TRPV4. There is one transient receptor potential cation channel ankyrin receptor, TRPA1, which can be inhibited by some monoterpenoids, other plant derived compounds, arachidonic acid and some prostaglandins. TRPA1 also responds to cold and mechanical stimuli. There are transient receptor potential cation channel canonical receptors, TRPC1–7, that are inhibited by hyperforin and other compounds. TRPC5 is activated by low temperature. TRPC1 and 6 are activated by mechanical stretch. Transient receptor potential cation channel melastatin receptors, TRPM1–8, are inhibited by monoterpenoids such as menthol and by fats such as sphingosine. TRPM1, 2, 3, 4 and 5 are activated by heat. TRPM8 is activated by cold. The transient receptor potential cation channel polycystin receptors, TRPP1–3, may be inhibited by diterpenes such as triptolide. TRPP1 and 2 are mechanosensitive channels. The transient receptor potential cation channel mucolipin receptors, TRPML1–3, respond to protons.

Table 1. Skin Pain Receptors.

Receptor	Agonist	Antagonist
TRPV1–6	Heat, monoterpenoids, endocannabinoids, endovanilloids, capsaicin	Dynorphins, adenosine, resolvins
TRPA1	Cold, prostaglandins	Monoterpenoids, resolvins
TRPC1–7	Diacylglycerol	-
TRPM1–8	Heat, cold, steroids, menthol	-
TRPP1–3	Mechanical stress, calcium	-
TRPML1–3	Protons	-
CB1–2	Cannabinoids, endocannabinoids	-
EP1–4	Prostaglandins	-
Lipoxin A4 receptor and others	Lipoxins	-
Resolvin D1 receptor and others	Resolvins	-
H1, H3, H4	Histamine	Antihistamines
5-HT1AR, 5-HT2AR, 5-HT3R	Serotonin	Methysergide
BLTR1-2	Leukotriene B4	-
MOR, KOR, DOR, NOP	Enkephalins, endorphins, dynorphins, nociceptin, fentanyl	-
B1-2	Bradykinins	-
P2 receptors	ATP	-
N-type calcium channels	-	Gabapentin, ziconotide
Voltage gated ion channels	Aconitine, delphinine	Local anesthetics
NMDA, AMPA, Kainate	Glutamate	Ketamine, ibogaine

TRPV—transient receptor potential cation channel vanilloid, TRPA—transient receptor potential cation channel ankyrin, TRPC—transient receptor potential cation channel canonical, TRPM—transient receptor potential cation channel melastatin, TRPP—transient receptor potential cation channel polycystin, TRPML—transient receptor potential cation channel mucolipin, CB—cannabinoid receptor, EP—prostaglandin receptor, H—histamine receptor, 5-HTR—serotonin receptor, BLTR—leukotriene receptor, MOR—mu opioid receptor, KOR—kappa opioid receptor, DOR—delta opioid receptor, NOP—nociception receptor, B—bradykinin receptor, P2—adenosine triphosphate (ATP) receptor, NMDA—N-methyl-D-aspartate receptor, AMPA—alpha-amino-3-hydroxy-5-methyl-4-isoxazolepropionic acid receptor.

TRPs are found in non-overlapping populations of nerve terminals in the skin [6]. Many of these receptors also are found in endothelial and dendritic cells and are involved in dermatitis. Since these receptors are found in non-overlapping neuron populations, this makes pain treatment complex. For instance, if a menthol liniment is applied to the skin, it may not inhibit all of the neuronal terminals in the area, and may not adequately relieve pain. It is important to use a liniment that inhibits as many skin TRPs as possible in order to get pain relief, which may involve multiple monoterpenoids [7–9].

3. Other Skin Receptors Involved in Pain

The skin contains a variety of receptors involved in pain [10]. TRP receptors are the most abundant and varied. There are cannabinoid receptors, CB1 and CB2, which are involved in inflammation and pain sensation in the skin [11]. Cannabinoids are also agonists for several TRPs and cause an initial activation of the receptors followed by deactivation. There are skin lipoxin receptors that cause pain [12]. There are skin resolvin receptors that decrease pain [12]. Resolvins also inhibit TRPA1, TRPV3 and TRPV4. There are opioid receptors in the skin [13]. Opioid peptides such as the enkephalins are also made in the skin [13]. Fentanyl patches are used to treat pain and stimulate opioid receptors by direct application to the skin. Other pain receptors in the skin include bradykinin receptors, histamine receptors, serotonin receptors, adenosine triphosphate (ATP) receptors, prostaglandin receptors, *N*-type calcium channels, voltage gated sodium channels and glutamate receptors [10]. Voltage gated sodium channels are inhibited by local anesthetics and result in pain inhibition in the skin [10]. All of these receptors are involved in causing and relieving pain. All of these receptors have endogenous agonists and antagonists that are involved in pain and analgesia. Pain occurs when the production of these endogenous compounds is out of balance and causes too much stimulation of pain receptors.

4. Interactions of Pain Receptor Responses

The activation of one pain receptor can potentiate the activity of other pain receptors in the skin. This interaction greatly increases pain, in other words increases the improper flow of qi in the skin. TRPC5 activity is potentiated by Gq coupled G-protein coupled receptor (GPCR) activation [2], such as by glutamate, serotonin, histamine, muscarine and angtiotensin II receptors. TRPM2 is potentiated by receptor activation that involves the formation of cyclic-adenosine diphosphate (ADP) ribose, such as by muscarinic receptors [2]. Bradykinin receptor activation potentiates TRPA1 activity [2]. TRPC channels are activated by phospholipase C [14]. Several receptors activate phospholipase C, such as muscarinic, histaminergic, serotonergic, glutamatergic and muscarinic. Interactions of these pain receptors alter qi in the skin such that pain is magnified.

5. Skin Cyclooxygenase-2

Cyclooxygense-2 (COX2) is the main source of prostaglandins. As mentioned before, prostaglandins cause pain by interacting with prostaglandin receptors and TRPs. They also potentiate TRPV1 activity by increasing protein kinase A and C activity [2]. COX2 activity increases in the skin in chronic pain conditions [15]. This induction of skin COX2 makes pain worse and ensures that pain will continue until COX2 activity decreases. It is not known how skin COX2 is induced in chronic pain. Nonsteroidal anti-inflammatory agents (NSAIDS) are used to inhibit both COX1 and COX2 in the treatment of pain. These oral or injected agents do not penetrate adequately into the skin to inhibit skin COX2 [2]. On the other hand, topical sesquiterpenes are known to penetrate the skin and may inhibit COX2 or decrease the expression of COX2 in the skin [7,8]. Topical preparations can be superior to oral or injected preparations for pain treatment.

6. Moxibustion and Skin Yin, Yang and Qi

Moxibustion involves heating the skin at specific acupuncture points to relieve pain [16]. Application of heat for several seconds causes the deactivation of some TRPs [5]. This diminishes pain by decreasing the activity of skin sensory neurons. The heat sensitive TRPs are discussed above. By using a yang influence, heat, moxibustion reestablishes the proper flow of qi that comes from TRPs in sensory neurons and decreases pain.

7. Acupuncture and Skin Yin, Yang and Qi

Acupuncture causes an initial activation of several different TRPs by causing an initial pain sensation and a mechanical stimulation. Several TRPs are activated by pain and mechanical stimuli as discussed above. The continued application of the acupuncture needle for more than several seconds, may cause these channels to deactivate and relieve pain. As discussed before, the application of too much yin (antagonist) or yang (agonist) to TRPs, causes them to shut down. This relieves pain by allowing qi (signal transduction) to flow correctly. It has been suggested that mast cell degranulation involves TRPV2 activation and that acupuncture may increase this process [17]. Mast cell degranulation is important in skin inflammation, irritation and pain. In addition, electroacupuncture was shown to decrease the expression of TRPV1 [13]. COX2 expression can also be diminished by acupuncture [18–21], which is important in the treatment of chronic pain conditions. Since acupuncture is applied to the skin, it inhibits the expression of skin COX2 [21]. It has been known for centuries that acupuncture is useful in the treatment of acute and chronic pain. TRP inhibition and decreased COX2 expression may be involved in this pain relief.

8. The Superiority Pain Treatment in the Skin

The most popular treatments for pain are oral medications such as NSAIDS and opioids. These agents are given in large doses and cause many toxic reactions. NSAIDS cause 100,000 ulcers in the US every year that result in 10,000 deaths. NSAIDS also cause kidney damage and clotting problems that lead to stroke and heart attack. COX1 is the major source of thromboxane. COX2 is the major source of prostaglandins. The prostaglandin, prostacyclin (PGI2) can inhibit clotting. It is possible that inhibition of COX2 in platelets leads to excess thromboxane, inadequate PGI2 and clotting. NSAIDS alter the balance of arachidonic acid metabolites, including prostaglandins and lipoxins, such that drug toxicity occurs. Opioids cause tolerance, addiction and toxicity that leads to 14,000 deaths in the US every year. Opioid medicines alter the balance of natural opioid proteins in the body, including enkephalins and dynorphins, preventing the ability of the body to stop pain.

The gate control theory of pain supports the use of oral medications to treat pain, since the theory contends that pain is sensed in the brain and can be modified in the brainstem. The gate control theory has led to the overuse of oral pain medications and the many deaths discussed above.

In contrast, acupuncture is a safe treatment. Various liniments are available to treat pain by topical application [7–9]. These liniments are applied where they are needed, work quickly, and are very effective and safe.

9. Endovanilloids, Endocannabinoids and Arachidonic Acid Metabolites

The body has the ability to stop pain through a number of mechanisms (Table 1). The opioid peptides are important, including endorphins, enkephalins and dynorphins. They are produced in the brain and skin, work at opioid receptors in the brain and skin and are effective [10]. Several other compounds are made in the skin to either cause or inhibit pain sensed in the skin.

Endovanilloids work through deactivation of vanilloid receptors, the TRPV channels [22]. Several endovanilloids are made from arachidonic acid such as 15-hydroperoxyeicosatetraenoic acid (15-HPETE) made by 15-lipoxygenase, 12-HPETE made by 12-lipoxygenase, anandamide, and *N*-arachidonoyldopamine. 5-Lipoxygenase makes 5-HPETE, and leukotriene B4 that are both endovanilloids [23,24]. Other endovanilloids are not made from arachidonic acid and include *N*-oleoyldopamine, palmitoylethanolamide and the resolvins.

Lipoxins are trihydroxy-eicosatetraenoic acids made from arachidonic acid by 15-lipoxygenase and cause pain. They bind to several receptors such as, lipoxin A_4 receptor, ALX/formyl peptide receptor 2, and resolvin D1 receptor [10]. Lipoxins also may act through stimulation of TRPV1 to cause pain [12]. They are made in very small amounts, where they are needed and are cleared quickly. They are balanced by the resolvins that inhibit pain.

Resolvins are trihydroxy-eicosapentaenoic acids made from omega-3 fatty acids by 15-lipoxygenase and COX2 [25]. Resolvins interact with several receptors, at least one of which is responsible for relieving pain. These receptors are resolvin D1 receptor, resolvin E1 receptor, G protein coupled receptor 32, lipoxin A_4 receptor, chemokine like receptor 1 (also called chemerin receptor 23, ChemR23) and leukotriene B4 receptor [10]. Resolvins inhibit TRPA1, TRPV3 and TRPV4 which also relieves pain. One of the consequences of COX2 inhibition is that resolvin synthesis is inhibited, which alters the ability of the body to decrease pain.

Endocannabinoids include anadamide (made by phospholipase D), *N*-arachidonoyldopamine and 2-arachidonoylglycerol and interact with CB1 and CB2. Both of these receptors are found on sensory neurons in the skin and are involved in pain relief induced by cannabinoids and endocannabinoids [26]. It should be pointed out that although the endocannabinoids appear to be agonists for TRPV1, plant derived cannabinoids also interact with TRPV2, TRPV3, TRPV4, TRPA1 and TRPM8. It has been proposed that TRPV1 activity can be modulated through CB1 or CB2 activation by endocannabinoids [26].

All of these yin and yang influences alter the flow of qi. When qi flows correctly, pain is relieved. When qi flows incorrectly, pain occurs and may be magnified. Pain treatment should reestablish the proper balance of yin and yang. When the body is in balance, the body can heal itself [27,28].

10. Conclusions

In general, the inhibition of COX enzymes decreases prostaglandin and resolvin synthesis and shifts the metabolism of arachidonic acid to the lipoxygenase pathways. The synthesis of lipoxins and hepoxilins, mediators of pain and inflammation, may increase. Hepoxilins are made by 12-lipoxygenase [29]. However, the synthesis of several endocannabinoids and endovanilloids may increase, which decreases pain and inflammation.

There are several endogenous compounds that that come from omega-3 fatty acids through docosahexaenoic acid such as protectins and maresins. Protectins are antiapoptotic and anti-inflammatory [30]. Protectins are made by 17-lipoxygnease. Maresins are anti-inflammatory, analgesic and are made by macrophage 12-lipoxygenase [31]. The effects of COX inhibition on these compounds is not known.

The consequences of systemic inhibition of COX2 in the body are only now being understood. When orally active COX2 inhibitors, such as valdecoxib, were first released, thousands of patients experienced angina, heart attacks and other clotting issues. This may be due to inhibition of platelet COX2 that throws off the balance of PGI_2 and thromboxanes, leading to clotting. Valdecoxib was removed from the US market in April of 2005. Since that time, clinical trials and meta-analyses have shown that all orally active or injected COX2 or nonselective COX inhibitors cause strokes, heart attacks and other clotting issues. Since July of 2015, the FDA requires the labels of all NSAIDS to indicate the increased risk of excess clotting. It is not known if inhibition of skin COX2 increases the risk of clotting. However, acupuncture inhibits skin COX2 and has been shown to not alter blood clotting [32].

TRP inhibition provides analgesia. Many TRP receptors are involved in this analgesia. It is important to inhibit as many types of TRP receptors as possible to provide effective pain relief, such as by using several monoterpenoids at the same time. Acupuncture and moxibustion provide pain relief, at least in part, through inhibition of TRP receptors.

The skin is a complex organ and is the major pain sensing organ. Many receptors that sense pain are found in the skin and are involved in the pain cycle that can magnify pain. These receptors interact with each other through signal transduction pathways. These pathways can be used to decrease sensitivity to pain such as by acupuncture, the application of cold, heat or topical preparations. This approach to pain treatment is safer and can be more effective than the use of oral or injected drugs.

Acknowledgments: The author is grateful to Gerhard Litscher for the invitation to write this review.

Author Contributions: All of this work was performed solely by James David Adams, Jr.

References

1. Adams, J.; Lien, E. The traditional and scientific bases for traditional Chinese medicine: Communication between traditional practitioners, physicians and scientists. In *Traditional Chinese Medicine Scientific Basis for Its Use*; Adams, J., Lien, E., Eds.; The Royal Society of Chemistry: Cambridge, UK, 2013; pp. 1–10.
2. Moran, M.M.; McAlexander, M.A.; Bíró, T.; Szallasi, A. Transient receptor potential channels as therapeutic targets. *Nat. Rev. Drug Discov.* **2011**, *10*, 601–620. [CrossRef] [PubMed]
3. Melzack, R.; Wall, P. Pain mechanisms: A new theory. *Science* **1965**, *150*, 971–979. [CrossRef] [PubMed]
4. Adams, J. Apoptosis is critical to pain control. *Open J. Apoptosis* **2013**, *2*, 23–24. [CrossRef]
5. Premkumar, L. Transient receptor potential channels as targets for phytochemicals. *ACS Chem. Neurosci.* **2014**, *5*, 1117–1130. [CrossRef] [PubMed]
6. Basbaum, A.I.; Bautista, D.M.; Scherrer, G.; Julius, D. Cellular and molecular mechanisms of pain. *Cell* **2009**, *139*, 267–284. [CrossRef] [PubMed]
7. Adams, J. The use of California sagebrush (*Artemisia californica*) liniment to control pain. *Pharmaceuticals (Basel)* **2012**, *5*, 1045–1053. [CrossRef] [PubMed]

8. Fontaine, P.; Wong, V.; Williams, T.J.; Garcia, C.; Adams, J. Chemical composition and antinociceptive activity of California sagebrush (*Artemisia californica*). *J. Pharmacogn. Phytother.* **2013**, *5*, 1–11.
9. Garcia, C.; Adams, J. *Healing with Medicinal Plants of the West—Cultural and Scientific Basis for Their Use*; Abedus Press: La Crescenta, CA, USA, 2012.
10. Adams, J.; Wang, X. Control of pain with topical plant medicines. *Asian Pac. J. Trop. Biomed.* **2015**, *5*, 930–935. [CrossRef]
11. Rani Sagar, D.; Burston, J.; Woodhams, S.; Chapman, V. Dynamic changes to the endocannabinoid system in models of chronic pain. *Philos. Trans. R. Soc. Lond. B Biol. Sci.* **2012**, *367*, 3300–3311. [CrossRef] [PubMed]
12. Serhan, C. Pro-resolvin lipid mediators are leads for resolution physiology. *Nature* **2014**, *510*, 92–101. [CrossRef] [PubMed]
13. Bigliardi, P.; Tobin, D.; Gaveriaux-Ruff, C.; Bigliardi-Qi, M. Opioids and the skin—where do we stand? *Exp. Dermatol.* **2009**, *18*, 424–430. [CrossRef] [PubMed]
14. Yue, Z.; Xie, J.; Yu, A.; Stock, J.; Du, J.; Yue, L. Role of TRP channels in the cardiovascular system. *Am. J. Physiol. Heart Circ. Physiol.* **2015**, *308*, H157–H182. [CrossRef] [PubMed]
15. Ma, W.; Quirion, R. Does COX2 dependent PGE2 play a role in neuropathic pain? *Neurosci. Lett.* **2008**, *437*, 165–169. [CrossRef] [PubMed]
16. Wang, M. Huang di nei jing and the treatment of low back pain. In *Traditional Chinese Medicine Scientific Basis for Its Use*; Adams, J., Lien, E., Eds.; The Royal Society of Chemistry: Cambridge, UK, 2013; pp. 17–47.
17. Zhang, D.; Spielmann, A.; Wang, L.; Ding, G.; Huang, F.; Gu, Q.; Schwarz, W. Mast cell degranulation induced by physical stimuli involves the activation of transient receptor potential channel TRPV2. *Physiol. Res.* **2012**, *61*, 113–124. [PubMed]
18. Zhang, Z.; Wang, C.; Gu, G.; Li, H.; Zhao, H.; Wang, K.; Han, F.; Wang, G. The effects of electroacupuncture at the ST36 (Zusanli) acupoint on cancer pain and transient receptor potential vanilloid subfamily 1 expression in Walker 256 tumor bearing rats. *Anesth. Analg.* **2012**, *114*, 879–885. [CrossRef] [PubMed]
19. Kim, J.; Shin, K.; Na, C. Effect of acupuncture treatment on uterine motility and cyclooxygenase-2 expression in pregnant rats. *Gynecol. Obstet. Investig.* **2000**, *50*, 225–230. [CrossRef]
20. Kim, J.; Na, C.; Hwang, W.; Lee, B.; Shin, K.; Pak, S. Immunohistochemical localization of cyclooxygenase-2 in pregnant rat uterus by Sp-6 acupuncture. *Am. J. Chin. Med.* **2003**, *31*, 481–488. [CrossRef] [PubMed]
21. Lee, J.; Jang, K.; Lee, Y.; Choi, Y.; Choi, B. Electroacupuncture inhibits inflammatory edema and hyperalgesia through regulation of cyclooxygenase synthesis in both peripheral and central nociceptive sites. *Am. J. Chin. Med.* **2006**, *34*, 981–988. [CrossRef] [PubMed]
22. Van der Stelt, M.; Di Marzo, V. Endovanilloids putative ligands of transient receptor potential vanilloid 1 channels. *Eur. J. Biochem.* **2004**, *271*, 1827–1834. [CrossRef] [PubMed]
23. Meves, H. Arachidonic acid and ion channels: An update. *Br. J. Pharmacol.* **2008**, *155*, 4–16. [CrossRef] [PubMed]
24. Mazini, S.; Meini, S. Involvement of capsaicin sensitive nerves in the bronchomotor effects of arachidonic acid and melittin: A possible role for lipoxin A4. *Br. J. Pharmacol.* **1991**, *103*, 1027–1032. [CrossRef]
25. Serhan, C.; Hong, S.; Gronert, K.; Colgan, S.; Devchand, P.; Mirick, G.; Moussignac, R. Resolvins a family of bioactive products of omega-3 fatty acid transformation circuits initiated by aspirin treatment that counter proinflammation signals. *J. Exp. Med.* **2002**, *196*, 1025–1037. [CrossRef] [PubMed]
26. Caterina, M. TRP channel cannabinoid receptors in skin sensation, homeostasis and inflammation. *ACS Chem. Neurosci.* **2014**, *5*, 1107–1116. [CrossRef] [PubMed]
27. Adams, J. Preventive medicine and the traditional concept of living in balance. *World J. Pharmacol.* **2013**, *2*, 73–77. [CrossRef]
28. Adams, J. *The Balanced Diet for You and the Planet*; Abedus Press: La Crescenta, CA, USA, 2014.
29. Mrsny, R.; Gewirtz, A.; Siccardi, D.; Savidge, T.; Hurley, B.; Madara, J.; McCormick, B. Identification of hepoxilin A3 in inflammatory events: A required role in neutrophil migration across intestinal epithelium. *Proc. Natl. Acad. Sci. USA* **2004**, *101*, 7421–7426. [CrossRef] [PubMed]
30. Serhan, C.; Gotlinger, K.; Hong, S.; Lu, Y.; Siegelman, J.; Baer, T.; Yang, R.; Colgan, S.; Petasis, N. Anti-inflammatory actions of neuroprotection D1/protectin D1 and its natural stereoisomers: Assignments of dihydroxy containing docosatrienes. *J. Immunol.* **2006**, *176*, 1848–1859. [CrossRef] [PubMed]

31. Serhan, C.; Dalli, J.; Karamnov, S.; Choi, A.; Park, C.; Xu, Z.; Ji, R.; Zhu, M.; Petasis, N. Macrophage proresolving mediator maresin 1 stimulates tissue regeneration and controls pain. *FASEB J.* **2012**, *26*, 1755–1765. [CrossRef] [PubMed]
32. Berqqvist, D. Vascular injuries caused by acupuncture: A systematic review. *Int. Angiol.* **2013**, *32*, 1–8.

9

Why We Need Minimum Basic Requirements in Science for Acupuncture Education

Narda G. Robinson

Department of Clinical Sciences, Colorado State University, Fort Collins, CO 80526, USA; narda@onehealthsim.org

Academic Editors: Gerhard Litscher and William Chi-shing Cho

Abstract: As enthusiasm for alternatives to pharmaceuticals and surgery grows, healthcare consumers are turning increasingly to physical medicine modalities such as acupuncture. However, they may encounter obstacles in accessing acupuncture due to several reasons, such as the inability to locate a suitable practitioner, insufficient reimbursement for treatment, or difficulty gaining a referral due to perceived lack of evidence or scientific rigor by specialists. Claims made about a range of treatment paradigms outstrip evidence and students in acupuncture courses are thus led to believe that the approaches they learn are effective and clinically meaningful. Critical inquiry and critical analysis of techniques taught are often omitted, leading to unquestioning acceptance, adoption, and implementation into practice of approaches that may or may not be rational and effective. Acupuncture education for both licensed physicians (DOs and MDs) and non-physicians needs to include science (i.e., explanation of its effects based on contemporary explanations of biological processes), evidence, and critical thinking. Erroneous notions concerning its mechanisms such as moving "stuck Qi (Chi)" or "energy" with needles and that this energy stagnates at specific, tiny locations on the body called acupuncture points invite errors in methodologic design. For example, researchers may select sham and verum point locations that overlap considerably in their neural connections, leading to nonsignificant differences between the two interventions. Furthermore, attributing the effects of acupuncture to metaphorical and arcane views of physiology limits both acceptance and validation of acupuncture in both research and clinical settings. Finally, the content and quality of education and clinical exposure across acupuncture programs varies widely, with currently no minimum basic educational requirements in a scientific methodology. Considering the pressures mounting on clinicians to practice in an evidence-based and scientific manner that also demonstrates cost-effectiveness, acupuncture schools and continuing medical education (CME) courses should provide their students a strong foundation in rational approaches supported by research.

Keywords: acupuncture; education; evidence-based

---

1. Introduction

Today, acupuncture, especially in the West, spans a broad continuum [1]. At one pole sit the strictly scientific practitioners, i.e., those that eschew the myriad metaphors and metaphysical, mystical mechanisms so long associated with this form of medicine. At the other end reside acupuncturists content to view their practice as the manipulation and management of subtle energy circuits, relying on subjective observations of the patient that then determine both diagnosis and treatment.

The majority of physician acupuncturists likely land somewhere between these two ends of the spectrum, practicing a panoply of techniques that have greater and lesser degrees of scientific backing. Acupuncture coursework may focus more fully on one or a few approaches, whether neuroanatomic or myofascial trigger point therapy (i.e., the scientific methods) or Traditional Chinese Medicine, microsystems, Five Phases (or Five Elements), and more (largely abstract, metaphorical, irrational, or otherwise unscientific approaches). What physician acupuncturists learn in a given course stems more from the intellectual and philosophical proclivities of the course director(s) rather than agreed-upon standards profession-wide. Thus, in North America, acupuncture education for physicians has existed, for the most part, on its own in CME programs [2] or acupuncture schools [3] apart from coursework consisting of the "mainstream" of medicine, leading to, in some cases, markedly different standards and expectations for curricula and graduates.

With course content depending solely on the determination of each individual course director, students in that program sign up not only to learn "acupuncture" but in effect are brought into the fold of one or more systems with premises they may or may not agree. That is, should a medical practitioner find the approaches of neuroanatomic acupuncture and trigger point therapy more attractive because they rest on biomedical principles, that individual needs to select carefully a course of study that aligns with those ideals. Otherwise, one could find oneself in a program that espouses what he or she might consider pseudoscience, i.e., explaining acupuncture mechanisms metaphysically rather than through analysis of the actual, tangible, readily identifiable structures involved [4,5]. This divergence sets up a dichotomy within the profession: some practice in accordance with scientific principles and others based on abstract explanations. However, even if a physician seeks a purely scientific acupuncture education, s/he must learn a broad array of philosophies and techniques, some based on abstract and metaphorical approaches, in order to become board certified in medical acupuncture, as reflected in the recommended readings for the American Board of Medical Acupuncture board certification examination [6].

Whereas physicians typically spend years in medical school and postgraduate programs and then add acupuncture as CME, certified acupuncturists typically spend years in school learning acupuncture and herbal treatment medicine [7]. However, most programs that train certified or licensed acupuncturists (L.Ac.'s) teach that acupuncture works, at least in part, by moving energies and eliminating "pathogenic factors" such as metaphorical wind, damp, heat, and cold. Their qualifying examination (i.e., that offered by the National Certification Commission for Acupuncture and Oriental Medicine or NCCAOM) reflects this. It also includes testing on clinical examination methods [8] such as tongue and pulse diagnosis that have low interrater reliability and little proven validity as diagnostic tools [9,10]. Considering that healthcare decisions made by acupuncturists rely heavily on the subjective assessment by the practitioner, relying on arcane and unproven methods to differentiate between health and disease puts patients at risk medically and financially if limited resources lead to ineffective or harmful treatments.

While current medical diagnostic approaches can also have some subjectivity and inter-rater differences, the assessments made involve actual anatomical structures such as trigger points [11] that are palpated or otherwise analyzed, not abstract inferences concerning organ function based on the appearance of the tongue or the quality of the pulse.

2. Overview

In postgraduate medicine programs, one assumes that academic educators regularly undergo self-examination and question whether requirements for postgraduate training, licensure, and specialty education are meeting the intended objectives [12]. As techniques develop and evidence accrues, needs for certain types of knowledge or skills may change. Furthermore, in most other courses of study, a student may safely assume that the premises and content within a CME course are valid, tested, and reliable. This does not necessarily apply to acupuncture, given the wide variation in content one might find, ranging from a discussion of the neuroanatomy and neurophysiology of acupuncture to what some might call "superstition", i.e., processes that contradict natural science.

In such instances, uncertainty about the veracity of the techniques taught put the learner, no matter how earnest, at a clear disadvantage. She or he may have mistakenly assumed that by definition a continuing medical education program, especially one approved for CME credits, would be quality controlled for rational content and substantiation. While it is wise to think critically about any course content, most physicians attending conventional CME courses do not find themselves needing to do further research on their own in order to determine whether what they learned defied rational explanation and evidential support. With acupuncture, they do, at least for now where training programs offer such widely divergent methodologies.

Currently, patients seeking care even from board-certified physician acupuncturists could receive treatment ranging from rational and evidence-informed methodologies (such as neuroanatomic acupuncture or trigger point therapy) or approaches that have no scientific basis and little to no evidence of effectiveness. This uncertainty places them in a vulnerable position, i.e., assuming and expecting a level of care in accordance with contemporary biomedicine as well as a fair expectation of a beneficial clinical outcome. Approaches practiced by certified acupuncturists typically involve Traditional Chinese Medicine (TCM) philosophies and practices—also unscientific. Remaining unaware and, in some cases, uninterested in the actual anatomy of acupuncture and its underlying physiologic mechanisms of needling and related techniques hinders one's ability justify point selection and defend treatment techniques, even though this information is available [4].

Even if the practitioner believes that she or he is moving mysterious energies, acupuncture often has physiologic effects, thereby reaffirming his or her belief that what was taught was real, but that faith is misplaced. For example, microsystems approaches such as scalp, hand, and ear acupuncture have many followers and some research, but the premises upon which they rest are fundamentally flawed and unsupported by evidence. No matter what one believes in terms of special "maps" of the body on the surface of the head, hand, or ear, acupuncture stimulation leads to physiologic changes that can be therapeutic. Does that mean that the topography of the ear actually contains an implied inverted fetus somewhere encoded into its tissue? No. It merely indicates that the cranial and upper cervical nerves that supply the ear cause myriad physiologic changes when stimulated.

Despite there being a clear, neuroanatomic description of the neural supply of the ear and reflex connections through the brainstem that explain how auricular point stimulation neuromodulates vagal pathways as well as evidence that does not support the theory of a highly specific functional map on the ear [13], the majority of practitioners of auricular acupuncture cling to unfounded notions that the auricular acupuncture diagrams are accurate and reliable [14]. This leads to inconsistent results in research and in the practice of auricular acupuncture [13]. Unless and until a standardized auricular acupuncture map [15] becomes available and is based on systematic analysis of the physiologic and anatomic outcomes of point stimulation rather than opinion and voting [16], current "ear maps" are no more reliable than other fanciful, imagined maps as in scalp acupuncture [17–19], Korean hand acupuncture [20], foot reflexology, and iridology.

Problems plaguing auricular acupuncture, if resolved, could facilitate its integration into conventional settings such as the emergency department [21,22] and drug detoxification settings [23].

2.1. Is There a Better Way?

There is another option. Insights into the anatomy and physiology of acupuncture have grown to where there is no longer any need to rely on metaphysical ideations regarding how acupuncture works. Having certification programs institute a minimum basic requirement for scientific content and critical thinking skills, all would ensure that practitioners certified by that group could describe and defend their scientific acupuncture techniques to colleagues, insurers, and institutions. They would also become better researchers and advocates for the profession. As stated by Ning and Lao, "The most critical challenge in acupuncture research is the selection of controls and the design of appropriate sham needling [24]." Designing higher quality studies mandates that the researchers have a clear picture of what constitutes an acupuncture point and how the structures affiliated with that site produce the physiologic effects classically attributed to that site's activation.

2.2. *Proposed Curricular Content*

In which ways, specifically, could acupuncture schools and CME programs ensure that training protects the public by graduating highly qualified acupuncturists with a strong background in science and evidence that can provide safe, efficacious, and cost-effective health care [25]? What information and strategies should acupuncture providers learn that would give them the ability to discern between rational and irrational approaches, whether in their work as clinicians, researchers, or educators? How can acupuncture education evolve so that training is "based on rigorous scientific evidence and a robust system of quality assurance [25]"?

To begin with, acupuncture students should learn about acupuncture history, become familiar with research milestones, and develop critical thinking skills that will show them how to assess the veracity and validity of acupuncture principles and practices. For example, instead of learning how to perform tongue and pulse "diagnosis" in preparation for determining the diagnosis and treatment approach as in Traditional Chinese Medicine (TCM), students should first learn to how to appropriately question and critique research on these highly unreliable measures. Before moving forward with adopting these skills, they need to understand that neither pulse nor tongue diagnosis has been validated as a reliable method by which to determine health or pathology in a patient [26,27]. At least by recognizing the high level of subjectivity in these tools, acupuncturists have the opportunity to introduce caution in the judgments they make. Treatment follows diagnosis. As such, if the diagnostic techniques are neither reliable nor valid, the veracity of a patient assessment and the effectiveness of treatment come into question.

Acupuncturists also need to become acquainted with Western (scientific) medical acupuncture [26], its rational premise, and methods of diagnosis and treatment that include and rely heavily upon appropriate, well established analyses as well as myofascial palpation.

The anatomical segment of the minimum basic requirement in science would include in-depth study of point anatomy as well as discussions about how the structures at each point relate to the physiologic effects one expects to see based on clinical experience and/or research-based evidence.

For clinical applications, students would learn the central tenets of neuromodulation [28,29] and connective tissue effects [30] as the basis of acupuncture, continue with a critical examination of acupuncture research methodologies and flaws, and proceed into a science-based, evidence-informed review of a scientific approach to the gamut of medical conditions and clinical challenges effectively treated by acupuncture. They would be able to differentiate scientific medical acupuncture from other forms of acupuncture [26].

2.3. *Encouraging Better-Designed Acupuncture Research*

In order to best serve patients and make the best use of healthcare dollars and resources [31], acupuncture practitioners need factual and reliable information on which to base their care and inform their patients or clients of the relative merit of various options. This information comes from rigorous, scientific research. However, the same problems that plague acupuncture practice (i.e., outmoded or imagined mechanisms of action, methods of diagnosis that lack validity and reliability, unsubstantiated premises of treatment) also plague acupuncture research. New standards have been developed [32], but problems remain.

Furthermore, the lack of distance between verum and sham input effects and the inclusion of primitive, folkloric diagnostic methods, lay the acupuncture profession open to criticism from skeptical observers who claim that acupuncture is a "theatrical placebo" [33,34]. Graduates of acupuncture educational programs should be well-equipped to respond to critics that dismiss acupuncture as nothing more than placebo with facts from the latest research [35,36]. Most practitioners of acupuncture, whether MDs, DOs, or LAcs, would not feel confident building a strong, science based defense at this time.

3. Conclusions

Requiring a solid foundation in the science and evidence of acupuncture does not make the approach any less of an art. Rather, a clinician who recognizes and addresses the multifaceted nature of neural and connective tissue interrelationships is working with active and anatomically identifiable structures rather than ethereal energies that may not even exist.

References

1. Kalauokalani, D.; Cherkin, D.C.; Sherman, K.J. A comparison of physician and nonphysician acupuncture treatment for chronic low back pain. *Clin. J. Pain.* **2005**, *21*, 406–411. [CrossRef] [PubMed]
2. American Board of Medical Acupuncture. ABMA Approved Training Programs. Available online: http://dabma.org/programs (accessed on 6 September 2016).
3. Acupuncture Today. Acupuncture Schools. Available online: http://www.acupuncturetoday.com/schools/ (accessed on 6 September 2016).
4. Robinson, N.G. *Interactive Medical Acupuncture Anatomy*; Teton NewMedia: Jackson, WY, USA, 2016.
5. Cheng, K.J. Neuroanatomical characteristics of acupuncture points: Relationship between their anatomical locations and traditional clinical indications. *Acupunct. Med.* **2011**, *29*, 289–294. [CrossRef] [PubMed]
6. American Board of Medical Acupuncture Website. Recommended Readings for the ABMA Board Certification Examination. Available online: http://dabma.org/documents/EXAM_RECOMMENDED.pdf (accessed on 25 July 2016).
7. Council of Colleges of Acupuncture and Oriental Medicine. Know Your Acupuncturist. Available online: http://www.ccaom.org/downloads/CCAOM_KnowYourAcu.pdf (accessed on 25 July 2016).
8. NCCAOM® Study Guide for Diplomate in Acupuncture Certification, 2016. Available online: http://www.nccaom.org/forms-and-applications/ (accessed on 25 July 2016).
9. O'Brien, K.A.; Abbas, E.; Zhang, J.; Guo, Z.-X.; Luo, R.; Bensoussan, A.; Komesaroff, P.A. Understanding the reliability of diagnostic variables in a Chinese Medicine examination. *J. Altern. Complement. Med.* **2009**, *15*, 727–734.
10. Zhang, G.G.; Lee, W.L.; Lao, L.; Lee, W.L.; Handwerger, B.; Berman, B. The variability of TCM pattern diagnosis and herbal prescription on rheumatoid arthritis patients. *Altern. Ther. Health Med.* **2004**, *10*, 58–63. [PubMed]
11. Gerwin, R.D. Diagnosis of myofascial pain syndrome. *Phys. Med. Rehabil. Clin. N. Am.* **2014**, *25*, 341–355. [CrossRef] [PubMed]
12. Freeman, B.D. Is it time to rethink postgraduate training requirements for licensure? *Acad. Med.* **2016**, *91*, 20–22. [CrossRef] [PubMed]
13. He, W.; Want, X.; Shi, H.; Shang, H.; Li, L.; Jing, X.; Zhu, B. Auricular acupuncture and vagal regulation. *Evid.-Based Complement. Altern. Med.* **2012**. [CrossRef] [PubMed]
14. Robinson, N.G. Personal communication with medical acupuncturists at the 2016 American Academy of Medical Acupuncture Annual Symposium during Dr. Robinson's afternoon neuroanatomic acupuncture workshop presentation. Unpublished work, 2016.
15. Litscher, G.; Rong, P.J. Auricular acupuncture. *Evid.-Based Complement. Altern. Med.* **2016**. [CrossRef] [PubMed]
16. Rong, P.J.; Zhao, J.J.; Wang, L.; Zhou, L.Q. Analysis of advantages and disadvantages of the location methods of international auricular acupuncture points. *Evid.-Based Complement. Altern. Med.* **2016**. [CrossRef] [PubMed]
17. Liu, Z.; Guan, L.; Wang, Y.; Xie, C.L.; Lin, X.M.; Zheng, G.Q. History and mechanism for treatment of intracerebral hemorrhage with scalp acupuncture. *Evid.-Based Complement. Altern. Med.* **2012**. [CrossRef] [PubMed]
18. Rezvani, M.; Yaraghi, A.; Mohseni, M.; Fathimoghadam, F. Efficacy of Yamamoto New Scalp Acupuncture versus Traditional Chinese acupuncture for migraine treatment. *J. Altern. Complement. Med.* **2014**, *20*, 371–374. [CrossRef] [PubMed]

19. Zheng, G.Q.; Zhao, Z.M.; Wang, Y.; Gu, Y.; Li, Y.; Chen, X.M.; Fu, S.P.; Shen, J. Meta-analysis of scalp acupuncture for acute hypertensive intracerebral hemorrhage. *J. Altern. Complement. Med.* **2011**, *17*, 293–299. [CrossRef] [PubMed]
20. Ochi, J.W. Korean hand therapy for tonsillectomy pain in children. *Int. J. Pediatr. Otorhinolaryngol.* **2015**, *79*, 1263–1267. [CrossRef] [PubMed]
21. Tsai, S.L.; Fox, L.M.; Murakami, M.; Tsung, J.W. Auricular acupuncture in emergency department treatment of acute pain. *Ann. Emerg. Med.* **2016**. [CrossRef] [PubMed]
22. Ushinohama, A.; Cunha, B.P.; Costa, L.O.; Barela, A.M.; Freitas, P.B. Effect of a single session of ear acupuncture on pain intensity and postural control in individuals with chronic low back pain: A randomized controlled trial. *Braz. J. Phys. Therapy* **2016**. [CrossRef] [PubMed]
23. Wu, S.L.Y.; Leung, A.W.N.; Yew, D.T.W. Acupuncture for detoxification in treatment of opioid addiction. *East Asian Arch. Psychiatry* **2016**, *26*, 70–76. [PubMed]
24. Ning, Z.; Lao, L. Acupuncture for pain management in evidence-based medicine. *J. Acupunct. Meridian Stud.* **2015**, *8*, 270–273. [CrossRef] [PubMed]
25. Jiang, J.; Peng, W.; Gu, T.; King, C.; Yin, J.K. Critical review of data evaluation in teaching clinics of Traditional Chinese Medicine outside China: Implications for education. *Explore* **2016**, *12*, 188–195. [CrossRef] [PubMed]
26. White, A.; Editorial board of acupuncture in medicine. Western medical acupuncture: A definition. *Acupunct. Med.* **2009**, *27*, 33–35. [PubMed]
27. Hua, B.; Abbas, E.; Hayes, A.; Ryan, P.; Nelson, L.; O'Brien, K. Reliability of Chinese medicine diagnostic variables in the examination of patients with osteoarthritis of the knee. *J. Altern. Complement. Med.* **2012**, *18*, 1028–1037. [CrossRef] [PubMed]
28. Da Silva, M.A.; Dorsher, P.T. Neuroanatomic and clinical correspondences: acupuncture and vagus nerve stimulation. *J. Altern. Complement. Med.* **2014**, *20*, 233–240. [CrossRef] [PubMed]
29. Takahashi, T. Mechanism of acupuncture on neuromodulation in the gut—A review. *Neuromodulation* **2011**, *14*, 8–12. [CrossRef] [PubMed]
30. Langevin, H.M.; Churchill, D.L.; Cipolla, M.J. Mechanical signaling through connective tissue: A mechanism for the therapeutic effect of acupuncture. *FASEB J.* **2001**, *15*, 2275–2282. [CrossRef] [PubMed]
31. Zhang, F.; Kong, L.L.; Zhang, Y.Y.; Li, S.C. Evaluation of impact on health-related quality of life and cost effectiveness of Traditional Chinese Medicine: A systematic review of randomized clinical trials. *J. Altern. Complement. Med.* **2012**, *18*, 1108–1120. [CrossRef] [PubMed]
32. STRICTA. Standards for Reporting Interventions in Controlled Trials of Acupuncture. Available online: http://www.stricta.info/ (accessed on 25 July 2016).
33. DC's Improbable Science Blog. Acupuncture Is a Theatrical Placebo: The End of a Myth. 30 May 2013. Available online: http://www.dcscience.net/2013/05/30/acupuncture-is-a-theatrical-placebo-the-end-of-a-myth/ (accessed on 17 June 2016).
34. Want, S.M.; Harris, R.E.; Lin, Y.C.; Gan, T.J. Acupuncture in 21st century anesthesia: Is there a needle in the haystack? *Anesth. Analg.* **2013**, *116*, 1356–1359.
35. Deng, S.; Zhao, X.; Du, R.; He, S.; Wen, Y.; Huang, L.; Tian, G.; Zhang, C.; Meng, Z.; Shi, X. Is acupuncture no more than a placebo? Extensive discussion required about possible bias. *Exp. Ther. Med.* **2015**, *10*, 1247–1252. [CrossRef] [PubMed]
36. Lundeberg, T.; Lund, I.; Naslund, J.; Thomas, M. The Emperor's sham—Wrong assumption that sham needling is sham. *Acupunct. Med.* **2008**, *26*, 239–242. [CrossRef] [PubMed]

10

Acupuncture and Lifestyle Myopia in Primary School Children—Results from a Transcontinental Pilot Study Performed in Comparison to Moxibustion

Xiaojuan Shang [1], Luquan Chen [1,*], Gerhard Litscher [1,2,3,4,*], Yanxia Sun [3], Chuxiong Pan [3], Cun-Zhi Liu [4], Daniela Litscher [2] and Lu Wang [1,2,3]

1 Department of Traditional Chinese Medicine, Beijing Tongren Hospital, Capital Medical University, Beijing 100730, China; joy_shang@hotmail.com (X.S.); lu.wang@medunigraz.at (L.W.)
2 TCM Research Center Graz, Research Unit of Biomedical Engineering in Anesthesia and Intensive Care Medicine, and Research Unit for Complementary and Integrative Laser Medicine, Medical University of Graz, 8036 Graz, Austria; daniela.litscher@medunigraz.at
3 Department of Anesthesiology, Beijing Tongren Hospital, Capital Medical University, Beijing 100730, China; sun00017@gmail.com (Y.S.); pandedao@126.com (C.P.)
4 Department of Acupuncture and Moxibustion, Dongfang Hospital Affiliated to Beijing University of Chinese Medicine, Beijing 100078, China; lcz623780@126.com
* Correspondence: chenluquan@hotmail.com (L.C.); gerhard.litscher@medunigraz.at (G.L.);

Abstract: Background: Lifestyle risks for myopia are well known and the disease has become a major global public health issue worldwide. There is a relation between reading, writing, and computer work and the development of myopia. **Methods:** Within this prospective pilot study in 44 patients aged between 6 and 12 years with myopia we compared possible treatment effects of acupuncture or moxibustion. The diopters of the right and left eye were evaluated before and after the two treatment methods. **Results:** Myopia was improved in 14 eyes of 13 patients (15.9%) within both complementary methods. Using acupuncture an improvement was observed in seven eyes from six patients out of 22 patients and a similar result (improvement in seven eyes from seven patients out of 22 patients) was noticed in the moxibustion group. The extent of improvement was better in the acupuncture group ($p = 0.008$ s., comparison before and after treatment); however, group analysis between acupuncture and moxibustion revealed no significant difference. **Conclusions:** Possible therapeutic aspects with the help of evidence-based complementary methods like acupuncture or moxibustion have not yet been investigated adequately in myopic patients. Our study showed that both acupuncture and moxibustion can improve myopia of young patients. Acupuncture seems to be more effective than moxibustion in treating myopia, however group analysis did not prove this trend. Therefore, further Big data studies are necessary to confirm or refute the preliminary results.

Keywords: acupuncture; moxibustion; evidence-based complementary medicine; myopia; primary school children; lifestyle; computer; eye diseases

---

1. Introduction

Myopia has become a major global public health issue worldwide. Lifestyle risk factors are well known and summarized in recent publications [1–3]. It has been shown that there is a relation between reading and writing from a short distance and the development of myopia. Computer work is also responsible for this relationship [4–7].

The constantly increasing number of eye diseases, as a result of too intensive personal computer work, increases the need for adequate treatment methods. In this context evidence-based complementary methods like acupuncture and/or moxibustion could be potential starting points for early intervention of myopia, which is defined as more than equal to −0.50 diopter (D) [3].

The purpose of this study was to investigate complementary medical methods (acupuncture and moxibustion) in school children with mild or moderate myopia because conventional medical therapies do not show sufficient improvements [1–3]. Acupuncture and moxibustion are among the most important methods used clinically in myopia in school age in China. Since this is an invasive method (needle acupuncture) on the one hand and a non-invasive procedure (moxibustion) on the other hand, it is obvious to compare both methods in one study. The aim is also to find out whether the methods differ significantly in terms of a possible improvement of myopia or not.

Within this transcontinental (Asia-Europe) prospective study in 44 children with low (<−3.0 D) and medium (between −3.0 D and −6.0 D) myopia [3] we compared possible treatment effects of acupuncture or moxibustion for the first time. The measurements were performed at the Tongren Eye Hospital affiliated to Capital Medical University in Beijing, China and the analysis was performed at the Traditional Chinese Medicine (TCM) Research Center at the Medical University of Graz, Austria.

2. Materials and Methods

2.1. Patients

A total of 44 patients aged between 6 and 12 years, with a mean age ± SD of 9.3 ± 1.4 years (27 female, 17 male) were treated either with acupuncture (group A) or with moxibustion (group B). The children suffer from mild-to-moderate myopia (−0.5 D to −4.25 D), and their lens-corrected vision was 100%. The average stature of the 44 subjects was 137.7 ± 9.4 cm (115–157 cm), and the average body weight was 33.2 ± 7.9 kg (21–53 kg). No person was under the influence of drugs. The treatments (needle acupuncture or moxibustion) were approved by the local ethics committee of the Tongren Hospital for treatment and research (EPU 5/2017) and performed in accordance with the recommendations of the Helsinki Declaration of the World Medical Association. Informed consent has been obtained from at least one of their parents.

Acupuncture treatment was used in group A, moxibustion in group B. Each group consisted of 22 patients. Age, sex, and basic demographic data are shown in Table 1.

Table 1. Demographic data of the 44 patients.

Parameter	Group A	Group B
	Acupuncture (*N* = 22)	**Moxibustion (*N* = 22)**
Age (years)	9.4 ± 0.9	9.3 ± 1.7
Sex (female, male)	14 f, 8 m	13 f, 9 m
Height (cm)	140.2 ± 6.8	137.2 ± 11.4
Weight (kg)	34.6 ± 8.0	31.8 ± 7.8
Treatment sessions	6.9 ± 1.7	9.1 ± 1.2

Randomization to one of the groups A or B has been done by an independent employee (medical doctor) from the Tongren Hospital using an envelope (group A, group B). The duration of one treatment (acupuncture or moxibustion) was 20 min. Altogether completion of 10 sessions was planned (~2 sessions per week) however not all participants could finish the examinations (compare treatment sessions in Table 1).

The following exclusion criteria were applied: (i) Less than −0.5 diopters; (ii) other eye diseases/disorders affecting visual acuity; (iii) secondary eye diseases (e.g., following diabetes); (iv) cardiologic, neurologic, nephrologic, hepatologic, hematologic, or psychiatric disorders; (v) chronic diseases requiring medication that must not be interrupted.

2.2. Treatment Methods

2.2.1. Acupuncture

All 22 patients in group A received needle acupuncture at traditional point locations (see Figures 1 and 2).

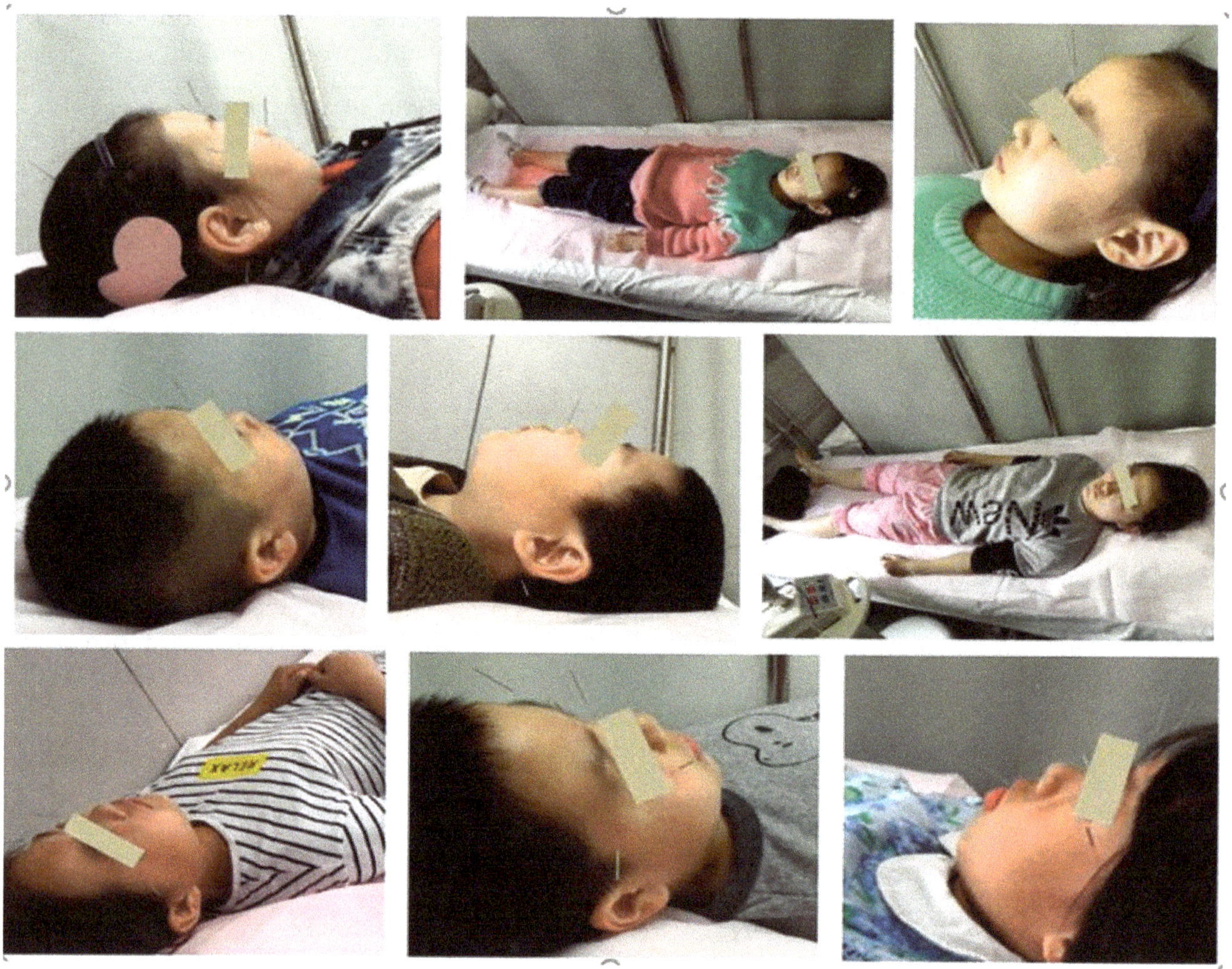

Figure 1. Acupuncture treatment in 22 young patients with myopia (group A).

After the patients lay down on a bed in a relaxed manner, the skin at the acupoint locations was disinfected with cotton which contains 75% alcohol. Disposable acupuncture needles (0.25 mm × 25 mm) were used. The needling method used is called mild reinforcing and attenuating, and was performed by inserting the needle at the appropriate depth. The angle of insertion was straight for the points on hands, body, and ankles, and oblique for the points on head, face, and neck. The depth of perpendicular needling was 25 mm, which of oblique is 15 mm. The needles were not stimulated and stayed in the body. After 20 min the needles were removed with dry cotton. An expert panel of acupuncturists from the Tongren Hospital in Beijing, China have reviewed and participated in the selection of the points. Acupuncture was always performed by the same highly experienced acupuncturist.

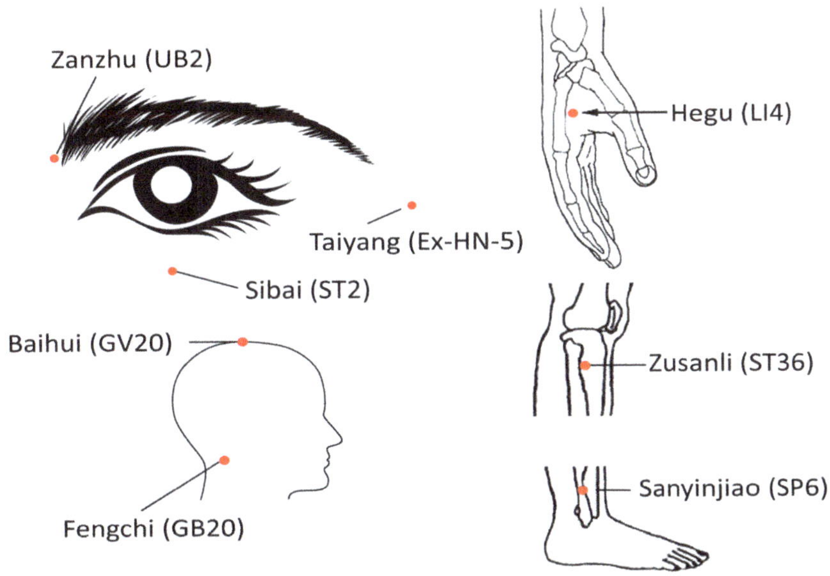

Figure 2. Acupuncture points for group A (acupuncture treatment). UB2 = Urinary Bladder 2; ST2 = Stomach 2; Ex-HN-5 = Extra Point Head/Neck 5; GV20 = Governing Vessel 20; GB20 = Gallbladder 20; LI4 = Large Intestine 4; ST36 = Stomach 36; SP6 = Spleen 6.

2.2.2. Moxibustion

For moxibustion treatment the patients sat down and closed their eyes. Then moxibustion on the forehead was performed for two minutes moving the stick in a horizontal direction (see Figure 3). Moxibustion was also performed around the eyes for duration of three minutes (moving the moxa in a horizontal direction for one minute, clockwise for one minute, vertical direction for one minute). Then sparrow-pecking Moxa on acupuncture points near the eyes (Ex-HN5, ST2 and UB2) was done for two minutes. This method is characterized by the ignited moxa stick being moved up and down over the point like a bird pecking or moving left and right, or circularly simultaneously. Acupressure was made on the same points simultaneously. In addition, moxibustion around the ears was made for two minutes moving the stick in vertical directions. Sparrow-pecking moxa on LI4 and simultaneous acupressure at the same point for one minute completed the Zhao's thunder-fire moxa (manufacturer: Chongqing Zhao's Thunder-fire Moxa Institute of Traditional Medicine, Chongqing, China) procedure. The points for moxibustion are shown in Figure 4.

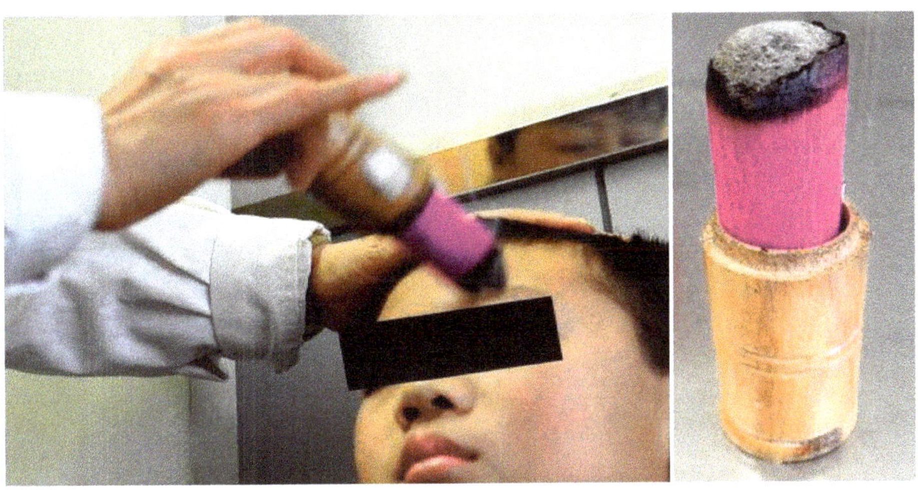

Figure 3. A part of the moxibustion treatment in 22 young patients with myopia (group B).

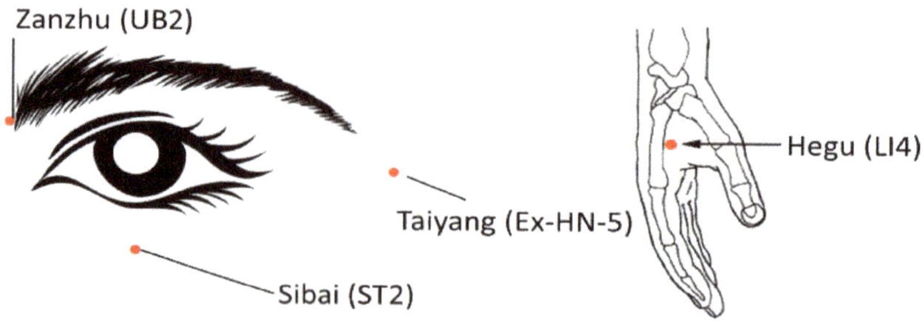

Figure 4. Points for group B (moxibustion treatment). UB2 = Urinary Bladder 2; Ex-HN-5 = Extra Point Head/Neck 5; ST2 = Stomach 2; LI4 = Large Intestine 4.

2.3. Evaluation Parameters

Axial lengths were observed before and after treatment with acupuncture or moxibustion. The diopters of the right (OD) and left (OS) eye were evaluated before and after the two treatment methods by a blinded assessor (medical doctor from Tongren Hospital). Compound tropicamide eye drops (0.5% tropicamide, 0.5% phenylephrine hydrochloride) were used before and after the last treatment session.

2.4. Statistical Analysis

The statistical analysis was carried out with the computer program SigmaPlot 14.0 (Systat Software, Chicago, IL, USA). Kruskal-Wallis One Way Analysis of Variance (ANOVA) on Ranks for group analysis and box plot analysis was used. In addition, paired t-tests before and after the treatments were carried out. The level of significance was set at $p < 0.05$. The original data can be found at the Department of Traditional Chinese Medicine & Acupuncture, Tongren Hospital affiliated to Capital Medical University, 100730 Beijing, China and at the TCM Research Center Graz, Medical University of Graz, 8036 Graz, Austria.

3. Results

All 44 patients finished at least five treatment session (mean sessions: 8.0 ± 1.8 (range: 5–10 treatments)). Due to time reasons, treatment in the children in Beijing was only possible during holiday time. Group analysis of the demographic data showed no statistical difference in age, sex, height, and weight. Acupuncture and moxibustion were accepted well and there were no side effects monitored by the medical doctors of the Tongren Hospital in any of the children. Table 2 demonstrates the mean ± SD of OD and OS from all patients and each from both groups (A and B) respectively.

Table 2. Diopters of the right (OD) and left (OS) eye before and after the two treatment methods (N = number of eyes).

N: Number of Eyes	Both Complementary Treatment Methods	Group A	Group B
		Acupuncture	Moxibustion
OD + OS before	-1.68 ± 1.03 ($N = 88$)	-1.57 ± 0.84 ($N = 44$)	-1.79 ± 1.18 ($N = 44$)
OD + OS after	$-1.67 \pm 1.08^{\#}$ ($N = 88$)	$-1.52 \pm 0.87^{**}$ ($N = 44$)	-1.81 ± 1.25 ($N = 44$)
OD before	-1.66 ± 1.03 ($N = 44$)	-1.53 ± 0.86 ($N = 22$)	-1.80 ± 1.20 ($N = 22$)
OD after	-1.72 ± 1.08 ($N = 4$)	-1.50 ± 0.88 ($N = 22$)	-1.80 ± 1.20 ($N = 22$)
OS before	-1.69 ± 1.03 ($N = 44$)	-1.60 ± 0.83 ($N = 22$)	-1.81 ± 1.20 ($N = 22$)
OS after	$-1.61 \pm 1.08^{*}$ ($N = 44$)	$-1.53 \pm 0.87^{+}$ ($N = 22$)	-1.71 ± 1.31 ($N = 22$)

$^{\#}$ $p = 0.011$; * $p = 0.002$; ** $p = 0.008$; $^{+}$ $p = 0.030$.

Altogether myopia was improved (diopters) in 14 eyes of 13 patients (15.9%) with both complementary methods. Using acupuncture, an improvement was observed in seven eyes from six patients out of 22 patients and a similar result (improvement in seven eyes from seven patients out of

22 patients) was noticed in the moxibustion group (group B). However the extent of the improvement was significantly different between the acupuncture (group A: $p = 0.008$) and the moxibustion (group B: No significance).

The results are graphically presented in Figure 5. The basic values before the treatment of both acupuncture and moxibustion are similar (see median values). Only needle acupuncture treatment changes the diopters in the sense of an improvement of myopic children significantly.

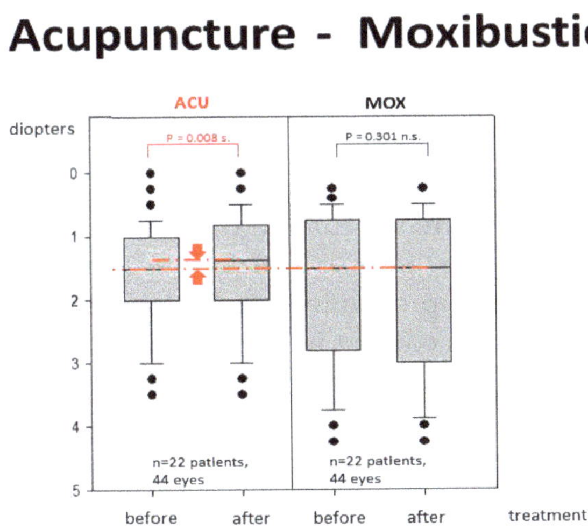

Figure 5. Box-plot of change in diopter values of all 44 subjects before and after treatment. The line in the box indicates the position of the median; the ends of the boxes define the 25th and 75th percentiles. The error bars show the 10th and 90th percentiles, and the dots represent "outliers". Note the significance ($p = 0.008$ s.) of the decrease in diopters after acupuncture treatment (left part).

In addition, a group analysis has been performed. The differences in the median values among the two treatment groups (acupuncture and moxibustion) was not great enough to exclude the possibility that the difference is due to random sampling variability; there was not a statistically significant difference ($p = 0.973$ n.s.) between the acupuncture and moxibustion group.

4. Discussion

A current literature analysis in the two databases PubMed and Cochrane Library regarding this important topic yielded the following results: up to now (1 June 2018) there are 28,106 published articles in PubMed under the search term "acupuncture" (11,464 at Cochrane Library). The term "myopia" provided 21,252 results in PubMed, and in Cochrane Library 1435 articles. The search term "personal computer" yielded 24,940 results in PubMed, and Cochrane Library 1905 published articles. The search with combined keywords yielded fewer results. The combined search terms "personal computer myopia", "personal computer acupuncture", and "acupuncture myopia personal computer" led to no results in Cochrane Library (in PubMed at least double-digit results, excluding "acupuncture myopia personal computer"). The only combined keyword which yielded more results in both databases was "acupuncture myopia". PubMed listed 46 articles, and in Cochrane Library 22 articles were found.

The result of the database analysis shows that until now there is very little research related to therapeutic aspects of eye diseases and screen handling. Therefore, new research like the present study is absolutely necessary. As already mentioned in the introduction, acupuncture or moxibustion could be possible starting points. The database analysis also clearly shows that acupuncture has already been used in myopia, but currently plays a very minor role in relation to PC-work induced disorders.

A study from Beijing which has been published in 2015 in PLoS One [2], deals with myopia in high school students. The title of the article is "*Prevalence and associated factors of myopia in high-school students in Beijing*". The authors came to the worrying result that students aged between 16 and 18 years have an 80% prevalence of myopia. They even speak of a 10% prevalence of severe myopia. When this generation which has grown up with PCs gets older, it will cause enormous costs for the health care system. Experts warn that myopia will win importance as a cause of visual impairment and blindness [2].

"*Acupuncture for teenagers with mild to moderate myopia: study protocol for a randomized controlled trial*" is the title of another important work. Especially the safety of acupuncture application in this field and its effectiveness should be investigated for a period of six months. Here is a brief excerpt from the study protocol: This randomized, parallel, blinded clinical trial will be conducted controlled. A total of 100 young people aged between seven and twelve years with mild to moderate myopia are recruited. The patients are randomized into two groups (control group and acupuncture group). Each group consists of 50 young people. In the acupuncture group, the five acupoints Zanzhu bilaterally, Tongziliao, Sibai, Muchuang and Hegu are stimulated daily for nine consecutive days. Then there is a one-day treatment break. Six of these treatment cycles are carried out continuously over a total of 60 days. After six months, a follow-up examination takes place. The primary endpoint is the determination of the diopter [8]. This is in context with our present study and also some acupoint are the same. The study could provide very interesting results. Another work that should be mentioned in the context of this discussion was written by Ming Yeung. According to this work, 3–4% of children are affected by tired eyes. Attention is drawn to a treatment with acupuncture. This method of treatment is according to the authors well tolerated by children and shows promising results [9].

In the following some important experiences from our own research should be mentioned briefly.

Myopia in children and adolescents up to the age of 21 is also well treatable with complementary medical methods. In adults, however, only little success has been recorded [10].

Our study has been performed as a transcontinental research pilot study. This means that two main research teams were involved; one team from Asia (Beijing, China) and one from Europe (Graz, Austria). Although it was a pilot study, the preliminary results are promising. The examinations showed that a total of 14 eyes of 13 patients out of 44 patients showed a significant improvement in myopia. The improvements were better with acupuncture than with moxibustion (comparison before and after treatment). The invasiveness of acupuncture seems to play a role over the non-invasiveness of moxibustion or acupressure.

However, the investigation has also limitations. Firstly, the sample size was very small and in the future sample size will be calculated according to rigorous methodology and considered in the improvement rate of this pilot study. Secondly, the average number of treatment sessions was lower in the moxibustion group than in the acupuncture group. Thirdly, because of ethical principles and actual clinical conditions in China, neither a control group of individuals who did not receive treatment nor a placebo group who received sham acupuncture was included. Fourthly, without a follow-up evaluation it would be difficult to determine if the treatment produces only temporary improvement or more clinically relevant long-term sustainable effects. Nevertheless, the scientific methodological guidelines were followed strictly through the trial, and the outcomes still showed meaningful and effective treatment corresponding to other previous publications.

5. Conclusions

In summary it can be stated that the enormously important topic screen handling, eye diseases, and possible therapeutic aspects with the help of acupuncture or moxibustion has not yet been investigated adequately from a scientific perspective, although some work (mainly from China) already exists. The problem, however, is not only interesting for Asia, also in the Western world ametropia [11] caused by screen handling will increase, as the scientific search and research of this work illustrates.

Our transcontinental pilot study showed that both acupuncture and moxibustion can improve mild and/or moderate myopia of young patients (6–12 years). Acupuncture seems to be more effective than moxibustion in treating myopia however at the moment we do not have conclusive explanations concerning the underling mechanisms of needle and thermal stimulation on myopia from a neurophysiological perspective.

Author Contributions: X.S., L.C., G.L., Y.S., C.P., C.-Z.L., D.L. and L.W. created the study design, X.S. and L.C. performed the measurements, G.L., D.L. and L.W. performed the data analyzes, G.L. designed the manuscript, and all authors (X.S., L.C., G.L., Y.S., C.P., C.-Z.L., D.L. and L.W.) participated in the discussion section and read the final manuscript.

Acknowledgments: Lu Wang and Gerhard Litscher are also visiting professors at the Capital Medical University, Beijing, China and G. Litscher is also guest professor at the Beijing University of Chinese Medicine in Beijing, China.

References

1. Wu, L.J.; Wang, Y.X.; You, Q.S.; Duan, J.L.; Luo, Y.X.; Liu, L.J.; Li, X.; Gao, Q.; Zhu, H.P.; He, Y.; et al. Risk factors of myopic shift among primary school children in Beijing, China: A prospective study. *Int. J. Med. Sci.* **2015**, *12*, 633–638. [CrossRef] [PubMed]
2. Wu, L.J.; You, Q.S.; Duan, J.L.; Luo, Y.X.; Liu, L.J.; Li, X.; Gao, Q.; Zhu, H.P.; He, Y.; Xu, L.; et al. Prevalence and associated factors of myopia in high-school students in Beijing. *PLoS ONE* **2015**, *10*. [CrossRef] [PubMed]
3. Zorena, K.; Gladysiak, A.; Slezak, D. Early intervention and nonpharmacological therapy of myopia in young adults. *J. Ophthalmol.* **2018**, *2018*. [CrossRef] [PubMed]
4. Holden, B.A.; Fricke, T.R.; Wilson, D.A.; Jong, M.; Naidoo, K.S.; Sankaridury, P.; Wong, T.Y.; Naduvilath, T.J.; Resnikoff, S. Global prevalence of myopia and high myopia and temporal trends from 2000 through 2050. *J. Ophthalmol.* **2016**, *123*, 1036–1042. [CrossRef] [PubMed]
5. Czepita, M.; Czepita, D.; Lubiński, W. The influence of environmental factors on the prevalence of myopia in Poland. *J. Ophthalmol.* **2017**, *2017*. [CrossRef] [PubMed]
6. Eye Problems through Screen Work. Available online: http://vorarlberg.orf.at/news/stories/2726280/ (accessed on 13 August 2015).
7. Le, Q.; Zhou, X.; Ge, L.; Wu, L.; Hong, J.; Xu, J. Impact of dry eye syndrome on vision-related quality of life in a non-clinic-based general population. *BMC Ophthalmol.* **2012**, *12*. [CrossRef] [PubMed]
8. Wang, Y.; Gao, Y.X.; Sun, Q.; Bu, Q.; Shi, J.; Zhang, Y.N.; Xu, Q.; Ji, Y.; Tong, M.; Jiang, G.L. Acupuncture for adolescents with mild-to-moderate myopia: Study protocol for a randomized controlled trial. *Trials* **2014**, *15*. [CrossRef] [PubMed]
9. Acupuncture Breakthrough for Treating Eye Condition. Available online: http://www.chinadaily.com.cn/hkedition/2010-06/15/content_9977403.htm (accessed on 15 June 2010).
10. Brucker, K. *Augen-Akupunktur: Sehstörungen Natürlich Heilen*; Georg Thieme Verlag: Stuttgart, Germany, 2001.
11. Disease and Injury Country Estimates. Available online: http://www.who.int/healthinfo/global_burden_disease/estimates_country/en/ (accessed on 12 February 2012).

11

Treatment of Sciatica Following Uterine Cancer with Acupuncture

Henry Xiao [1,*], Christopher Zaslawski [1], Janette Vardy [2,3] and Byeongsang Oh [1,2,4]

1 School of Life Sciences, University of Technology Sydney, Ultimo, NSW 2007, Australia; chris.Zaslawski@uts.edu.au (C.Z.); byeong.oh@sydney.edu.au (B.O.)
2 Sydney Medical School, University of Sydney, Camperdown, NSW 2006, Australia; janette.vardy@sydney.edu.au
3 Concord Cancer Centre, Concord Repatriation General Hospital, Concord, NSW 2137, Australia
4 Northern Sydney Cancer Centre, Royal North Shore Hospital, St Leonards, NSW 2065, Australia
* Correspondence: henry-xiao@outlook.com

Abstract: For women, gynaecological or obstetrical disorders are second to disc prolapse as the most common cause of sciatica. As not many effective conventional treatments can be found for sciatica following uterine cancer, patients may seek assistance from complementary and alternative medicine. Here, we present a case of a woman with severe and chronic sciatica secondary to uterine cancer who experienced temporary relief from acupuncture.

Keywords: uterine cancer; sciatica; acupuncture

---

1. Introduction

Uterine cancer (UC), also known as endometrial cancer, arises from the epithelium lining of the uterus [1]. The most common symptoms in women are abnormal uterine bleeding, vaginal discharge and nonspecific gastrointestinal symptoms [1]. On the other hand, the observed symptoms of the sciatica could be due to a number of factors, which we are unfortunately unable to confirm. However from a neuro-anatomical perspective, sciatica is generally caused by a disc herniation or spinal epidural abscess along the sciatic nerve, which anatomically contains fibres originating in the L4-S2 roots [1]. It is not uncommon for sciatica to result from the uterine tumour compressing the lumbosacral plexus, in particular the L4-L5 nerve roots [2]. The first reported case of this was in 1992 when a calcified degenerated myoma, suspected to be an ovarian tumour, induced sciatica by compressing the sciatic nerve in the lumbosacral plexus [3]. Uterine fibroids are another diagnostic consideration [4], and after pregnancy endometriosis is the most common cause of sciatica [2].

Acupuncture has been utilised to treat sciatic symptoms in China and in Western countries. Clinical trials have documented the effects of acupuncture on multiple cancer-related symptoms including pain, but the efficacy of acupuncture for managing cancer-related sciatic symptoms remains unclear [5]. Here, we report a case of acupuncture treating sciatica following uterine cancer.

2. Case Description

The patient was a 66-year-old female diagnosed with a stage III, type 2 endometrial cancer in late 2013. Her past medical history included type 2 diabetes diagnosed in 2012 (treated with oral hypoglycaemics), asthma (managed with inhalers), and arthritis in her foot (treated with Glucosamine hydrochloride/Chondroitin sulphate 500 mg/400 mg and Paracetamol 665 mg as required). In addition she described her difficulties with concentrating and memory for which she took ginkgo biloba 2000 mg (1–2 tablets a day).

The tumour was a serous, poorly differentiated, uterine adenocarcinoma that invaded more than 50% of the myometrial thickness, and involved the uterus and cervix. She was treated with a total abdominal hysterectomy and bilateral salpingo-oophorectomy. Post-operatively, she had 5 cycles of chemotherapy (Paclitaxel and Carboplatin), which was complicated by neutropenia and peripheral neuropathy. This was followed by 25 fractions of pelvic radiotherapy.

After surgery, although there were no recurrent symptoms of UC, the patient developed a dull pain down the left leg, radiating from the L5-S1 segments to the second toe. Standing and sitting exacerbated the pain. Before the tumour diagnosis, there were no sciatic symptoms. The sciatica therefore considerably impacted her quality of life.

In 2016, she was referred to the acupuncture clinic for individualised acupuncture treatments of her back and leg pain. The pain was described as a dull and radiating from the L5-S1 segments to her second toe, and had been present for three years. The patient attended 6 weekly sessions to have the acupuncture administered by a final year intern (HX) at a university-affiliated cancer centre that was supervised by a professional acupuncturist (BO). At each visit, the patient rated her pain from 0 to 10, with 0 being no pain and 10 being the worst conceivable pain. The patient initially reported a 3/10 pain at rest, worsening to 8/10 when she stood up or sat down.

The style of acupuncture conducted was Traditional Chinese Medicine. During the acupuncture treatment, a combination of local and distal points were needled to address the sciatica, as shown in Figure 1. Apart than the acupuncture, there were no other interventions. The Traditional Chinese Medicine (TCM) diagnosis was Qi Stagnation in the Gall Bladder Channel.

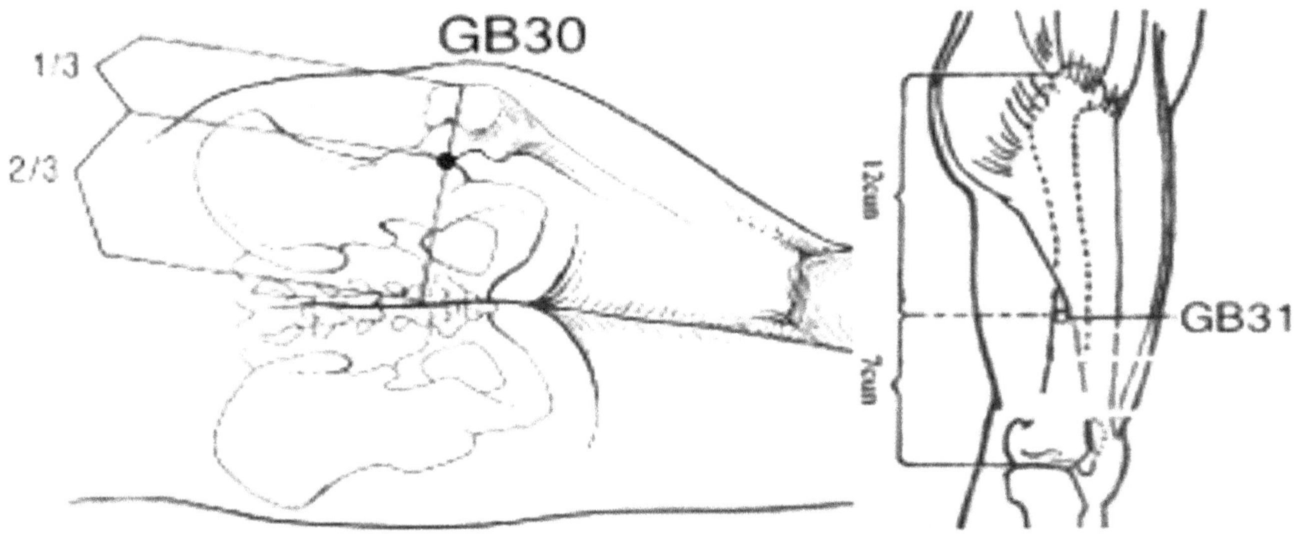

Figure 1. Acupuncture points GB30 and GB31.

With the patient lying on one side, the area was sterilised with an alcohol swab, the needles (30 and 0.12 mm gauge, Tempo J-Type Acupuncture Needles) were inserted at 90° until the patient experienced De Qi (a dull pressing and radiating sensation). The insertion for GB30 and GB31 for sciatica was 4–6 cm and 2–3 cm respectively [6] in the left hand side. The acupuncture points administered for her other signs and symptoms (e.g., shoulder pain, arthritis in her feet, poor concentration) were GB21, LI14, BL60, SP6, KD3 (first treatment), BL60, BL28, KD7, GB34, GB21 (second treatment), GB21, LU3, *Yintang*, LR3, *Erjian*, TE5 (third treatment), LI4, LI10, GB34, ST41, BL13, BL15, BL23 (fourth treatment), SP3, BL65, GB34, GV24, *Anmian* (fifth treatment), and GV20, LU7, GB34, LR3, KD6 (sixth treatment). The patient was left to rest for 30 min before the needles were removed.

After one treatment, the patient reported a decrease in pain intensity, rating her pain as 1/10 at rest and 5/10 when she stood up or sat down. After the second treatment, she reported further improvement in pain and she was able to perform most of her daily activities, including sitting and standing. She was able to perform stretching exercises such as Qigong without experiencing severe sciatic pain. The patient expressed improved mood and an interest in continuing acupuncture to address her other pain symptoms such as her arthritis in her feet, so that she would be able to participate in low impact exercises. Treatments in weeks 3–5 focused on her right shoulder pain and arthritis in her feet. The patient experienced little to no sciatica during this time. During the follow-up assessment at week 12, she presented with sciatica again, and rated the pain to be 2/10 at rest, worsening to 5/10 when she stood up or sat down.

3. Discussion

Sciatica is usually treated with non-steroidal anti-inflammatory drugs, but there is a lack of consensus regarding the efficacy of these drugs [7]. As a result, some patients turn to acupuncture for which there is some evidence of efficacy in treating painful symptoms associated with sciatica [8]. Acupuncture has been shown to be minimally invasive [9] and safe [10]. The treatment modality of acupuncture is based on the principles of TCM. The classic text, 'Song of Points for Miscellaneous Diseases' from 'The Glorious Anthology of Acupuncture and Moxibustion' written during the Ming Dynasty, in China, indicates that the acupuncture points of GB30, GB31 and LR2 were used for lumbar pain radiating down the leg [11].

In this report, we document the earliest case, to our knowledge, of potentially decreasing the intensity of sciatica following uterine cancer with acupuncture. After two treatment sessions, our patient provided feedback that her pain had improved. She reported that not only did she experience less sciatic pain, but the acupuncture also greatly improved her mood, contributing to better quality of life with family and friends. Furthermore, her newly managed pain opened her up to consider acupuncture for addressing other symptoms such as foot arthritis, which had been a secondary complaint. Nevertheless, she did not have complete relief from her sciatic pain at the sixth treatment, suggesting that chronic conditions may require a longer-term pain-management plan.

There are limitations to our case report. Firstly, there is a possibility of the synergistic effect of acupuncture with her pharmaceutical intervention; however, this had been stable and long term. The pharmaceutical intervention in this case refers to the patient's ongoing medications for type 2 diabetes, asthma, and foot arthritis. Furthermore, it may be that acupuncture plus lifestyle change could have improved the treatment efficacy. The very nature of a case report is that the clinical experience of only a single patient is presented; however, a testable hypothesis can be generated for future studies to investigate. Furthermore, the proximity between the tumour and sciatica events in the timeline leads to the conclusion that there could be a connection between the two. There exists the possibility that the patient's sciatic pain originated partially from a problem that was musculoskeletal in nature. To confirm the effect of acupuncture on sciatica following uterine cancer would require a much larger study, controlling for confounding factors and bias, including the placebo effect.

4. Conclusions

Sciatica following uterine cancer can be a debilitating condition with few successful treatments. Our case report documents how a woman with severe and persistent sciatica pain that could have been a result of her uterine cancer experienced considerable relief from acupuncture. This warrants further evaluation to determine the efficacy of acupuncture for sciatica following uterine cancer.

Author Contributions: H.X. drafted the article, J.V., C.Z. and B.O. revised it critically for important intellectual content. B.O. supervised the acupuncture clinic and all authors approved the final version to be published.

References

1. Goldman, L.; Schafer, A. *Goldman-Cecil Medicine*, 25th ed.; Elsevier Saunders: Philadelphia, PA, USA, 2016.
2. Al-Khodairy, A.W.; Bovay, P.; Gobelet, C. Sciatica in the female patient: Anatomical considerations, aetiology and review of the literature. *Eur. Spine J.* **2007**, *16*, 721–731. [CrossRef] [PubMed]

3. Acar, B.; Kadanali, S.; Acar, U. Rare gynecological condition causing sciatic pain. *Int. J. Gynecol. Obstet.* **1993**, *42*, 50–51. [CrossRef]
4. Bodack, M.P.; Cole, J.C.; Nagler, W. Sciatic neuropathy secondary to a uterine fibroid: A Case Report. *Am. J. Phys. Med. Rehabil.* **1999**, *78*, 157–159. [CrossRef] [PubMed]
5. Posadzki, P.; Moon, T.W.; Choi, T.Y.; Park, T.Y.; Lee, M.S.; Ernst, E. Acupuncture for cancer-related fatigue: A systematic review of randomized clinical trials. *Support. Care Cancer* **2013**, *21*, 2067–2073. [CrossRef] [PubMed]
6. Deadman, P.; Al-Khafaji, M.; Baker, K. *A Manual of Acupuncture*, 1st ed.; Journal of Chinese Medicine Publications: Hove, UK, 2001.
7. Machado, G.C.; Maher, C.G.; Ferreira, P.H.; Day, R.O.; Pinheiro, M.B.; Ferreira, M.L. Non-steroidal anti-inflammatory drugs for spinal pain: A systematic review and meta-analysis. *Ann. Rheum. Dis.* **2017**, *76*, 1269–1278. [CrossRef] [PubMed]
8. Fernandez, M.; Ferreira, P.H. Acupuncture for sciatica and a comparison with Western Medicine. *Br. J. Sports Med.* **2016**. [CrossRef]
9. Davison, B. Advanced techniques in musculoskeletal medicine & physiotherapy using minimally invasive therapies in practice. *Phys. Ther. Sport* **2016**, *21*, 94.
10. Patil, S.; Sen, S.; Bral, M.; Reddy, S.; Bradley, K.K.; Cornett, E.M.; Fox, C.J.; Kaye, A.D. The Role of Acupuncture in Pain Management. *Curr. Pain Headache Rep.* **2016**, *20*, 1–8. [CrossRef] [PubMed]
11. Gao, W. *The Glorious Anthology of Acupuncture and Moxibustion*, 1st ed.; Ming Dynasty; 1529.

12

A Population-Based Cohort Study on the Ability of Acupuncture to Reduce Post-Stroke Depression

Shuo-Ping Tseng [1], Yu-Ching Hsu [2,*], Ching-Ju Chiu [3,*] and Shang-Te Wu [4]

1. Department of Chinese Medicine, Tainan Municipal Hospital, Tainan 700, Taiwan; cfc54321@gmail.com
2. Department of Chinese Medicine, Tainan Hospital, Ministry of Health and Welfare, Tainan 701, Taiwan
3. Institute of Gerontology, College of Medicine, National Cheng Kung University, Tainan 701, Taiwan
4. Department of Internal Medicine and Neurology, Kuo General Hospital, Tainan 700, Taiwan; wst31853@yahoo.com.tw

* Correspondence: yuchinghsupro@gmail.com (Y.-C.H.); cjchiu@mail.ncku.edu.tw (C.-J.C.)

Academic Editors: Gerhard Litscher and William Chi-shing Cho

Abstract: Objective: Post-stroke depression (PSD) is common and has a negative impact on recovery. Although many stroke patients in Taiwan have used acupuncture as a supplementary treatment for reducing stroke comorbidities, little research has been done on the use of acupuncture to prevent PSD. Accordingly, our goal is to investigate whether using acupuncture after a stroke can reduce the risk of PSD. **Method:** This population-based cohort study examined medical claims data from a random sample of 1 million insured people registered in Taiwan. Newly diagnosed stroke patients in the period 2000–2005 were recruited in our study. All patients were followed through to the end of 2007 to determine whether they had developed symptoms of depression. A Cox proportional hazard model was used to estimate the relative risk of depression in patients after being diagnosed as having had a stroke, with a focus on the differences in those with and without acupuncture treatment. **Results:** A total of 8487 newly-diagnosed stroke patients were included in our study; of these, 1036 patients received acupuncture more than five times following their stroke, 1053 patients received acupuncture 1–5 times following their stroke and 6398 did not receive acupuncture. After we controlled for potential confounders (e.g., age, sex, insurance premium, residential area, type of stroke, length of hospital stay, stroke severity index, rehabilitation and major illness–related depression), we found that acupuncture after stroke significantly reduced the risk of depression, with a hazard ratio (HR) of 0.475 (95% CI, 0.389–0.580) in frequent acupuncture users and 0.718 (95% CI, 0.612–0.842) in infrequent acupuncture users, indicating that acupuncture may lower the risk of PSD by an estimated 52.5% in frequent users and 28.2% in infrequent users. **Conclusions:** After we controlled for potential confounders, it appears that using acupuncture after a stroke lowers the risk of depression. Additional strictly-designed randomized controlled trials are needed to better understand the specific mechanisms relating acupuncture to health outcomes.

Keywords: post-stroke depression; acupuncture

1. Introduction

Strokes are the third leading cause of death and the most common cause of complex disability in Taiwan [1]. Many medical complications of stroke are common and often lead to poor clinical outcomes, such as depression, known as post-stroke depression (PSD). PSD has a high prevalence and a negative impact on stroke patients' long-term survival and well-being [2]. Thus, it is important to reduce or prevent PSD in stroke survivors.

Many studies have evaluated various approaches to prevent PSD, including pharmacological therapy and psychotherapy. In some clinical trials, medicines such as Escitalopram and Duloxetine have shown some effectiveness in preventing PSD; however, most remedies had small treatment effect [3]. Other studies have also revealed that rehabilitation after a stroke may have positive effects in preventing PSD [4].

Traditional Chinese medicine (TCM) is classified as one form of complementary and alternative medicine (CAM) and is popular in Asian countries; for example, 52.7% of stroke patients receive both Chinese herbal remedies and acupuncture/traumatology treatment in Taiwan [5]. Some studies have reported that acupuncture may be effective in preventing PSD; however, such studies have so far been either too small or lacking big data analysis. If a case is to be made for the usefulness of acupuncture in relation to PSD, it is imperative to provide empirical evidence showing its positive effects on stroke patients' psychological well-being.

Potential confounders related to PSD have been explored, including gender (female) [6], disabilities, comorbidities [7], stroke severity [8], pre-stroke depression [9], cognitive impairment after stroke, dysphagia [10], incontinence [10], anxiety, and social isolation at follow-up [10]. In order to evaluate the preventive effect of acupuncture after subjects have been diagnosed as having had a stroke, a more rigorous study must be performed. In response, the main purpose of this study was to investigate whether acupuncture treatment after stroke attack reduces the risk of PSD after empirically controlling for covariates during the observation period.

2. Materials and Method

2.1. Source of Data

Our study used reimbursement claims data obtained from the National Health Insurance Research Dataset (NHIRD) in Taiwan. The NHIRD covers more than 99% of the population and has contracts with 97% of the hospitals and clinics in Taiwan [11]. The National Health Research Institute maintains and updates the NHIRD. The institute has publicly released a sub-dataset composed of claims data for 1,000,000 randomly selected insurance enrollees for research and administrative purposes. This random subgroup represents approximately 5% of the entire insured population in Taiwan. This sub-dataset, consisting of a longitudinal health insurance database for 2005 (LHID2005), was employed for this study after obtaining approval from the National Health Research Institute review committee. For data analysis, we retrieved information about patients' characteristics and medical care records by linking ambulatory care visit claims, in-patient expenditures by admissions, and the registry for beneficiaries. Secondary data were collected and administered by the Taiwan National Institute of Family Planning (now the Bureau of Health Promotion, BHP), and approved by their IRB. All data analyzed in this study were anonymized.

2.2. Participants and End-Point

Patients who were newly diagnosed with a stroke (ICD-9-CM codes: 430–434, 436–437) between 2000 and 2005 were included in this study. We excluded patients who had had a head injury before 2000 (N = 340); who had suffered from depression before their stroke (N = 1381); who were not insured or had died within 3 months of suffering the stroke (N = 256); had sought ambulatory care for depression within the first 3 months following their stroke (N = 58); or had not had an acupuncture interval for more than six months (N = 98). The study criteria, the exclusion criteria, and the follow-up procedure are presented in Figure 1.

In Taiwan, TCM doctors must finish a training course in Chinese medicine and acupuncture and pass the national examination before they are certified to practice and, thereafter, qualified for filing NHI claims for acupuncture reimbursement. We classified the stroke patients into two groups based upon their acupuncture use or non-use after their stroke: (1) acupuncture users: those who received six or more or 1–5 acupuncture treatments after being diagnosed with a stroke from 2000 to 2007 (respectively N = 1036, 12.21%; and, N = 1053, 12.41%); these were respectively called frequent and infrequent users; and (2) acupuncture non-users: those who were defined as reporting no acupuncture received after their stroke from 2000 to 2007 (N = 6398, 75.39%).

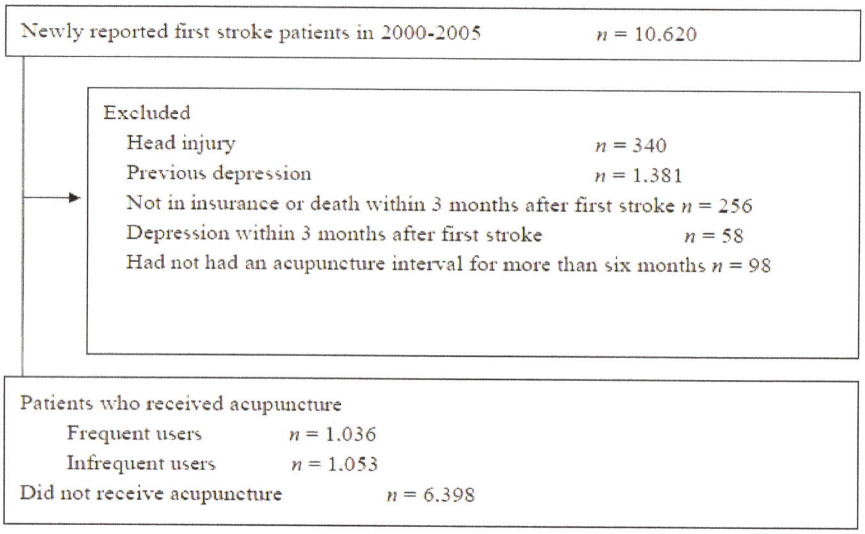

Figure 1. Flow chart showing details of subject recruitment from the National Health Insurance Research Dataset (NHIRD) of Taiwan for the years 2000 to 2005.

The Diagnostic and Statistical Manual (DSM) IV categorizes PSD as a "mood disorder due to a general medical condition (i.e., stroke)" with certain depressive features serving as specifiers, for example, major depressive-like episodes, manic features, or mixed features [12]. The patients were linked to the ambulatory care visit claims and inpatient expenditures by admissions claims during the years 2000–2007 to identify possible treatment for depression. The follow-up ended on the date of depression diagnosis (diagnosed according to ICD-9-CM code 296, 309, or 311, or A-code A212 or A219) in outpatient care or on the date of censoring, which was either the date of withdrawal (including death) from the NHI program or the date of the follow-up end (i.e., 31 December 2007).

2.3. Covariates

The covariates considered in our analysis include socio-economic factors and covariates related to stroke severity or progress. The socio-economic factors include gender, age, living area (categorized as "urban area", "satellite city", and "rural area") [13], and insurance premium (categorized as "<15,000 New Taiwan Dollars (NTD)", and "$\geq$15,000 NTD").

The covariates related to stroke severity or progress include type of stroke (categorized as hemorrhagic, occlusion or others (e.g., transient ischemic attack)), length of hospital stay, rehabilitation after stroke in 3 months, comorbidities that are correlated to depression or disability, such as cancer (ICD-9-CM code: 140–208), arthritis or rheumatism (ICD-9-CM code: 714.0, 729.0), chronic obstructive pulmonary disease (ICD-9-CM code: 490–496), peripheral arterial disease (ICD-9-CM code: 440–449), diabetes (ICD-9-CM code: 250) chronic kidney disease (ICD-9-CM: 585) and ranking according to the stroke severity index (SSI). The SSI is an index that estimates a stroke's severity by using six items listed in the hospitalization data in the NHI database [14], namely airway suction, bacterial sensitivity test, general ward stay, intensive care unit stay, nasogastric intubation, osmotherapy, and urinary catheterization.

2.4. Statistical Analysis

A chi-square test was used to compare differences in age, sex, residential area, insurance premium, type of stroke, length of hospital stay, and the aforementioned comorbidities between groups. A Kaplan–Meier analysis was performed for censored graft survival. To assess the independent effects of acupuncture on the risk of depression, we conducted a Cox proportional hazard regression analysis with age, sex, insurance premium, urbanization level, SSI, rehabilitation after stroke in three months, and selected comorbidities adjusted simultaneously in the model. We also adjusted the urbanization level to account for the urban rural difference in accessibility to medical care in Taiwan. All statistical analyses were performed using SAS (version 9.4, SAS Institute, Inc., Cary, NC, USA), in which a p-value < 0.05 was considered statistically significant.

3. Results

3.1. Sample Characteristics

Characteristics of the newly-diagnosed stroke patients based on whether they are acupuncture users or non-users are presented in Table 1. A total of 8487 newly-diagnosed stroke patients were included in our study, 1036 patients defined as higher acupuncture users, 1053 patients defined as lower acupuncture users and 6735 patients defined as acupuncture non-users after stroke diagnosis. According to Table 1, stroke patients who received frequent acupuncture treatment were, on average, younger, more likely to live in an urban area, of higher economic status, more likely to have had a hemorrhagic stroke, and had more hospitalization days compared to nonusers. Both frequent or infrequent acupuncture users also received more rehabilitation treatment than non-users. The three participating groups also had different comorbid diseases, including rheumatoid arthritis, peripheral arterial disease, diabetes or hypertension. However, other factors such as gender, comorbidities with myocardial infarction, cancer, chronic kidney disease, chronic obstructive pulmonary disease or head traumatic injury were not statistically different between frequent and infrequent users and non-users. It was found that patients not using acupuncture treatment had a higher chance of being diagnosed with PSD or withdrawal (including death) from the NHI program than those in both the frequent and infrequent acupuncture groups. Over a 7-year follow-up, 110 patients (10.62%) from the frequent acupuncture group, 177 patients (16.81%) from the infrequent acupuncture group and 1551 non-users (24.24%) developed PSD.

Table 1. Demographic characteristics between frequent, infrequent acupuncture users and non-users in patients using acupuncture with newly diagnosed strokes from the 1-million enrollee random sample of the National Health Insurance Research Database (NHIRD) from 2000 to 2007 in Taiwan.

Characteristic	Frequent Acupuncture Users [a] (N = 1036, 12.21%)	Infrequent Acupuncture Users [b] (N = 1053, 12.41%)	Acupuncture Non-Users [c] (N = 6398, 75.39%)	p Value
Female (%)	444 (42.86)	425 (40.36)	2622 (40.98)	0.378
Age of diagnosis (Mean ± SD)	61.28 ± 13.19	61.77 ± 13.59	66.21 ± 14.35	<0.001
Follow-up time (year) (Mean ± SD)	4.67 ± 1.78	4.82 ± 1.76	4.28 ± 1.87	<0.001
Living area (%)				<0.001
Urban area	307 (30.10)	275 (26.52)	1471 (23.45)	
Satellite city	303 (29.71)	305 (29.41)	1668 (26.59)	
Rural area	410 (40.20)	457 (44.07)	3133 (49.95)	
Insurance income ranks (%) [d,e]				<0.001
<15,000 NTD	320 (30.89%)	314 (29.82)	2379 (37.18%)	
≥15,000 NTD	716 (69.11%)	739 (70.18)	4019 (62.82%)	
Type of stroke				<0.001
hemorrhagic stroke	261 (25.19)	217 (20.61)	1288 (20.13)	
occlusion stroke	617 (59.56)	647 (61.44)	3923 (61.32)	
unknown	158 (15.25)	189 (17.95)	1187 (18.55)	
Hospitalization days				<0.001
≤7 days	458 (44.21)	536 (50.90)	3540 (52.20)	
8–14 days	253 (24.42)	298 (28.30)	1626 (25.52)	
15–21 days	111 (10.71)	74 (7.03)	541 (8.46)	
22–28 days	63 (6.08)	52 (4.94)	316 (4.94)	
≥28 days	151 (14.58)	93 (8.83)	575 (8.99)	
Comorbidities [f]				
Rheumatoid arthritis (%)	91 (8.78)	83 (7.88)	440 (6.88)	0.018
Peripheral arterial disease (%)	265 (25.58)	234 (22.22)	1216 (19.01)	<0.001

Table 1. *Cont.*

Characteristic	Frequent Acupuncture Users [a] (*N* = 1036, 12.21%)	Infrequent Acupuncture Users [b] (*N* = 1053, 12.41%)	Acupuncture Non-Users [c] (*N* = 6398, 75.39%)	*p* Value
Myocardial infarction (%)	50 (4.83)	54 (5.13)	278 (4.35)	0.312
Cancer (%)	152 (14.67)	173 (16.43)	919 (14.36)	0.400
Diabetes (%)	531 (51.25)	520 (49.38)	2989 (46.72)	0.003
Hypertension (%)	873 (84.27)	887 (84.24)	5160 (80.65)	<0.001
Chronic kidney diseases (%)	112 (10.81)	110 (10.45)	767 (11.99)	0.140
Chronic obstructive pulmonary diseases (%)	554 (53.47)	572 (54.32)	3592 (56.14)	0.070
Head traumatic injury (%)	23 (2.22)	31 (2.94)	231 (3.33)	0.055
Rehabilitation [g]	390 (37.64)	295 (28.02)	1126 (17.60)	<0.001
SSI (Mean ± SD) [h]	−0.16 ± 1.39	−0.35 ± 1.22	−0.14 ± 1.40	<0.001
Censor after stroke [i]				
Yes	110 (10.62)	177 (16.81)	1551 (24.24)	<0.001

Abbreviation: NHIRD = National Health Insurance Research Database; SD = standard deviation; NTD = New Taiwan Dollar. [a] Frequent acupuncture users: Subjects received six or more acupuncture treatments between 2000 and 2007 after stroke diagnosis; [b] Infrequent acupuncture users: Subjects received 1–5 acupuncture treatments between 2000 and 2007 after stroke diagnosis; [c] Acupuncture non-users: Subjects did not receive any acupuncture treatment between 2000 and 2007 after stroke diagnosis; [d] The income-related insurance payment category set by the Bureau of National Health Insurance in Taiwan; [e] 1 US $ = 30 NTD (New Taiwan Dollars); [f] Comorbidities = Medical illness, including rheumatoid arthritis, peripheral arterial disease, myocardial infarction, cancer, diabetes, hypertension, chronic kidney diseases, chronic obstructive pulmonary disease, and head traumatic injury, which are related to acupuncture use and depression; [g] Rehabilitation: had rehabilitation in the 3 months after stroke; [h] SSI = Stroke severity index; [i] Censor after stroke: Subjects sought ambulatory care for depression in outpatient care after stroke diagnosis between 2000 and 2005 or withdrew (including death) from the NHI program in 2000–2007.

3.2. Cox Proportional Hazard Regression Analysis

Figure 2 compares the Kaplan–Meier Survival Curves of depression between patients in the frequent and infrequent acupuncture treatment groups and the non-user group. As can be seen, patients with acupuncture treatment after stroke had a significantly lower risk of depression over the study period (p value for log-rank test ≤ 0.0001).

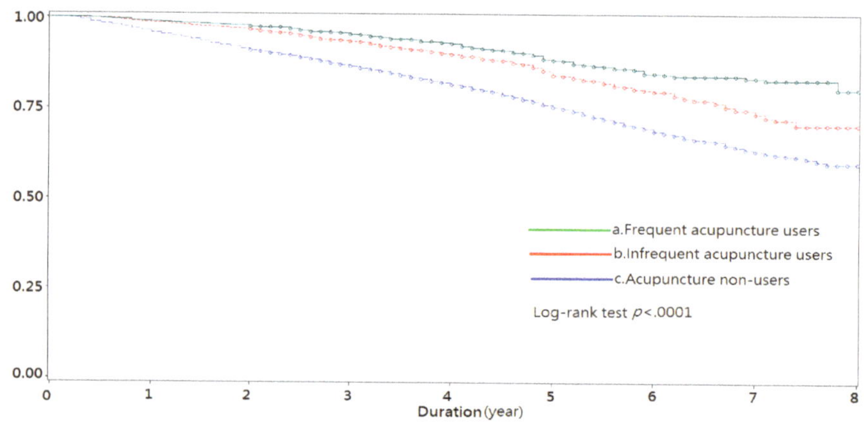

Figure 2. Kaplan–Meier Survival Curves of depression for comparing frequent acupuncture users, infrequent acupuncture users and non-users. a. Frequent acupuncture users: Subjects received six or more acupuncture treatments between 2000 and 2007 after stroke diagnosis; b. Infrequent acupuncture users: Subjects received 1–5 acupuncture treatments between 2000 and 2007 after stroke diagnosis; c. Acupuncture non-users: Subjects did not receive any acupuncture treatment between 2000 and 2007 after stroke diagnosis.

In Table 2, after controlling for potential confounders (e.g., age at diagnosis, gender, insurance premium level, living area, type of stroke, length of hospital stay, SSI, rehabilitation and major illness–related depression), acupuncture treatment after stroke appeared to significantly reduce the risk of PSD, with a hazard ratio (HR) of 0.475 (95% CI, 0.389–0.580) and 0.718 (95% CI, 0.612–0.842) for the frequent and infrequent acupuncture groups, respectively. In the multivariate analysis, females had a lower risk of depression than males (HR = 0.777; 95% CI, 0.705–0.856). Stroke patients with longer hospital stays, who are older, or have higher SSI tended to be at significantly greater risk of PSD after their stroke than the other patients in this study (HR = 1.098; 95% CI, 1.053–1.145; HR = 1.045; 95% CI, 1.040–1.050; HR = 1.210; 95% CI, 1.166–1.256, respectively). Comorbidity with myocardial infarction (HR =1.298; 95% CI, 1.080–1.559), cancer (HR = 1.423; 95% CI, 1.268–1.597), diabetes (HR = 1.136; 95% CI, 1.032–1.251), chronic kidney diseases (HR = 1.519; 95% CI, 1.345–1.715), chronic obstructive pulmonary disease (HR = 1.219; 95% CI, 1.097–1.355) or traumatic head injury (HR = 1.629; 95% CI, 1.335–1.988) also showed higher risk than those without these comorbidities. However, stroke patients living in urban areas, with peripheral arterial disease or hypertension had a lower risk of PSD after stroke diagnosis (HR = 0.836; 95% CI, 0.738–0.947; HR = 0.878; 95% CI, 0.781–0.986; HR = 0.844; 95% CI, 0.744–0.956, respectively). Meanwhile, economic status, rehabilitation, and presence of comorbid diseases with rheumatoid arthritis were not significantly more likely to be correlated with PSD risk. However, different risk of PSD development was found between hemorrhagic stroke and other types of stroke (HR = 0.796; 95% CI, 0.676–0.936). We further analyzed the effects of acupuncture treatment in developing PSD in hemorrhagic stroke and occlusion stroke (Table 3). The results suggest that occlusion-stroke patients receiving acupuncture treatment (either frequent or infrequent) would decrease the risk of developing PSD (HR = 0.499; 95% CI, 0.391–0.638; HR = 0.707; 95% CI, 0.578–0.865, respectively). In addition, patients with hemorrhagic stroke that received frequent acupuncture treatments appeared to minimize the risk of PSD (HR = 0.446; 95% CI, 0.283–0.702); however, those in the infrequent acupuncture group had no significant benefit over the non-users group (HR = 0.831; 95% CI, 0.577–1.196).

Table 2. Multivariable adjusted hazard ratios of covariates for depression.

Characteristic	Hazard Ratio [a]	p Value	95% CI	
Acupuncture users (ref: Acupuncture non-users [d])				
Frequent acupuncture users [b]	0.475	<0.001	0.389	0.580
Infrequent acupuncture users [c]	0.718	<0.001	0.612	0.842
Female	0.777	<0.001	0.705	0.856
Age of diagnosis	1.045	<0.001	1.040	1.050
Living area (ref: Rural area)				
Urban area	0.836	0.005	0.738	0.947
Satellite city	0.966	0.548	0.861	1.082
Insurance income (ref: <15,000 NTD) [e,f]				
≥15,000 NTD	1.082	0.128	0.978	1.198
Type of stroke (ref: unknown)				
hemorrhagic stroke	0.796	0.006	0.676	0.936
occlusion stroke	0.911	0.131	0.808	1.028
Hospitalization days [g]	1.098	<0.001	1.053	1.145
Comorbidities				
Rheumatoid arthritis	0.998	0.989	0.833	1.195
Peripheral arterial disease	0.878	0.029	0.781	0.986
Myocardial Infarction	1.298	0.005	1.080	1.559
Cancer	1.423	<0.001	1.268	1.597
Diabetes	1.136	0.009	1.032	1.251
Hypertension	0.844	0.008	0.744	0.956
Chronic kidney diseases	1.519	<0.001	1.345	1.715
Chronic obstructive pulmonary diseases	1.219	<0.001	1.097	1.355
Head traumatic injury	1.629	<0.001	1.335	1.988
Rehabilitation [h] (ref: no rehabilitation)	0.929	0.221	0.825	1.045
SSI i	1.210	<0.001	1.166	1.256

Abbreviation: SD = standard deviation; NTD = New Taiwan Dollar; CI = confidence interval; ref = reference. [a] Hazard ratio (95% confidence interval) was adjusted for all listed variables in the table; [b] Frequent acupuncture users: Subjects received six or more acupuncture treatments between 2000 and 2007 after stroke diagnosis; [c] Infrequent acupuncture users: Subjects received 1–5 acupuncture treatments between 2000 and 2007 after stroke diagnosis; [d] Acupuncture non-users: Subjects did not receive any acupuncture treatment between 2000 and 2007 after stroke diagnosis; [e] The income-related insurance payment category set by the Bureau of National Health Insurance in Taiwan; [f] 1 US $ = 30 NTD(New Taiwan Dollars); [g] Hospitalization days treated as continuous variable (≤7, 8–14, 15–21, 22–28 and ≥28 days); [h] Rehabilitation: had rehabilitation in the 3 months after stroke; [i] SSI = Stroke severity index.

Table 3. Multivariable adjusted hazard ratios of covariates for depression between hemorrhagic stroke and occlusion stroke.

Characteristic [e]	Hemorrhagic Stroke				Occlusion Stroke			
	Hazard Ratio [a]	*p* Value	95% CI		Hazard Ratio [a]	*p* Value	95% CI	
Acupuncture users (ref: Acupuncture non-users [d])								
Frequent acupuncture users [b]	0.446	<0.001	0.283	0.702	0.499	<0.001	0.391	0.638
Infrequent acupuncture users [c]	0.831	0.318	0.577	1.196	0.707	<0.001	0.578	0.865

Abbreviation: SD = standard deviation; NTD = New Taiwan Dollar; CI = confidence interval; ref = reference. [a] Hazard ratio (95% confidence interval) was adjusted for all listed variables in the table; [b] Frequent acupuncture users: Subjects received six or more acupuncture treatments between 2000 and 2007 after stroke diagnosis; [c] Infrequent acupuncture users: Subjects received 1–5 acupuncture treatments between 2000 and 2007 after stroke diagnosis; [d] Acupuncture non-users: Subjects did not receive any acupuncture treatment between 2000 and 2007 after stroke diagnosis; [e] Covariates including gender, age of diagnosis, living area, insurance income, hospitalization days, comorbidities (such as cancer, arthritis or rheumatism, chronic obstructive pulmonary disease, peripheral arterial disease, diabetes, chronic kidney disease), rehabilitation and the stroke severity index (SSI) were controlled.

4. Discussion

Our results indicate that using acupuncture after stroke diagnosis lowers the risk of PSD by an estimated 52.5% (1–0.475) in frequent acupuncture users and 28.2% (1–0.718) in infrequent acupuncture users. Applying acupuncture to treat stroke complications is common in Taiwan, and to our knowledge, our study is the first to investigate the effects of acupuncture in preventing PSD in a large population-based cohort. Within a 7-year observation period, the results indicate that recently-diagnosed stroke patients using acupuncture after being diagnosed were likely to have a lower risk of PSD. The overall risk reduction is estimated to be about 30.6%.

Strokes may increase vulnerability to the development of depression through a variety of neurobiological mechanisms. Three possible explanations for the association between physical illness and depression include a coincidental relationship; a negative mood reaction to the physical consequences of the stroke; and a neurotransmitter imbalance as a result of cerebral damage caused by the stroke [15]. Based on these PSD mechanisms, our hypothesis is that using acupuncture after a stroke might improve stroke complications and result in the prevention of PSD. Studies suggest that acupuncture after a stroke may improve problems with pain [16], spasticity [16], physical functions [17], quality of life [18] and cognitive functions [19]. Our findings seem to support the hypothesis that acupuncture reduces complications caused by a stroke and thus lowers the risk of PSD.

However, the short-term or long-term effects of using acupuncture to prevent PSD are unknown. To address this issue, a sensitivity analysis controlling for acupuncture over a three-month or six-month period after a stroke diagnosis was performed (table not shown). The results did not show that receiving acupuncture offered benefits in terms of depression symptoms. Nevertheless, the study did reveal that TCM-use benefited patients with higher depressive symptoms by attenuating their worsening [20]. These results suggest that the preventive effect from a continuous acupuncture treatment period may vary widely after a stroke. Further randomized control trials between short-term or long-term follow-up times are needed for verification.

In addition, our study also explored potential confounders related to PSD. Females have a lower risk of depression than males, and the overall risk reduction is estimated to be about 22.1% in our study. Although these findings are similar to those found in [4], other research has reported that female stroke patients have a higher risk of PSD. However, our findings that stroke patients with advanced age [21], greater stroke severity [8] and compounded comorbidities [7] have a higher risk of PSD are consistent with much of the related prior literature. Be that as it may, a summed measure of comorbidities may ignore potentially important relationships between diseases and PSD. For example, our study revealed that stroke patients comorbid with myocardial infarction (HR = 1.301), cancer (HR = 1.414), diabetes (HR = 1.139), chronic kidney diseases (HR = 1.518), chronic obstructive pulmonary disease (HR = 1.218) or head traumatic injury (HR = 1.658) are at higher risk than their counterparts without these comorbidities. Furthermore, stroke patients with peripheral arterial disease or hypertension have a lower risk of depression after stroke diagnosis, while comorbid rheumatoid arthritis is not significantly correlated with PSD. Meanwhile, the benefit of 3-months rehabilitation was evaluated after stroke diagnosis in a previous study [4], but those results do not correspond with ours. This might be due to the short-term and long-term ability of acupuncture or rehabilitation to prevent PSD being unknown. Accordingly, it is suggested that future research include these comorbid factors or the long-term effects of rehabilitation to further our understanding in this line of research. In addition, there was little evidence that compared the risk of PSD between occlusion-stroke and hemorrhagic stroke. Our study provided some information to fill this research gap. The results also indicated that patients, with occlusion-stroke or hemorrhagic stroke, who received frequent acupuncture treatments, may minimize the risk of PSD (HR = 0.446–0.499).

Our study has some strong points. One is that it is the first population-based study to investigate acupuncture's potential in preventing PSD based upon the real clinical conditions of stroke patients. A second is that acupuncture is a relatively low-cost treatment and, when performed by a TCM doctor, has none of the potential side effects associated with taking medicines. A third is that our study is an observational study based on reimbursement claims data obtained from the National Health Insurance Research Dataset (NHIRD). Compared to studies using questionnaires to detect depressive symptoms, our study reduced the potential of being confounded by the Hawthorne Effect. A fourth strong point is that stroke severity was evaluated in our study [14] to a greater degree than in other studies [4].

Nevertheless, this study still has some limitations. First, acupoints are hard to define using the NHI database; moreover, different acupuncturists use different acupoints in different patients, depending on the symptoms and severity of stroke complications. However, some clinical studies have shown that even sham-acupuncture may have treatment effects in some diseases. Thus, there may be a positive effect even without considering the location of acupoints in different individuals in our study. Second, disability is an important predictor of PSD, but the severity of disabilities is hard to define using the NHI database. However, we controlled for stroke severity and comorbidities to minimize the effects of the severity of disability. Third, potential confounders, such as brain lesion of stroke [22], cognitive impairment after stroke, dysphagia [10], incontinence [10], anxiety, and social isolation [10], are not included in the NHI database, and so may confound our research results. Accordingly, future work is needed to further this understanding. Fourth, patients in the acupuncture group may have also received other complementary treatments such as massage, herbs, and aromatherapy, among others. Thus, we may overestimate the treatment effect of acupuncture. As such, the effects of the more specific acupuncture mechanisms or interactions deserves future investigation when data is available. Moreover, we conducted the exclusion criteria for depression within the first 3 months following their stroke for the purpose of minimizing survivorship bias. Further sensitivity analysis (table not shown) was conducted and was found to be similar to the present results, suggesting the possible role of acupuncture in preventing PSD development. Fifth, because the benefits of medicines and psychotherapy or pre-acupuncture depression screening in preventing PSD were not available in our dataset or relevant to acupuncture treatment, we did not control for these variables in our study. Sixth, we cannot know the total number of dropouts and the main reasons for dropping out because our study used NHIRD, and so the reasons that patients choose not to continue acupuncture were based on individual will. Accordingly, further research examining the choice to dropout or remain is therefore warranted.

5. Conclusions

In conclusion, controlling for potential confounders, stroke patients who receive acupuncture may have a lower risk of PSD than those who do not. Moreover, acupuncture after a stroke may have a protective effect on depression, thus stemming further deterioration. Further strictly designed randomized controlled trials are needed to better understand the specific mechanisms of acupuncture and its impact on psychological health outcomes.

Acknowledgments: This work was supported by the Office of Research and Development at National Cheng Kung University (P.I.: Ching-Ju Chiu, Ph.D. D100-35B19).

Author Contributions: Shuo-Ping Tseng, Yu-Ching Hsu reviewed the literature, analyzed the data, and wrote the draft of the manuscript. Ching-Ju Chiu guided the study design, had full access to all of the data in the study and takes responsibility for the integrity of the data and the accuracy of the discussion. Shang-Te Wu contributed to the discussion.

References

1. Hsieh, F.I.; Chiou, H.Y. Stroke-Morbidity, Risk Factors, and Care in Taiwan. *J. Stroke* **2014**, *16*, 59–64. [CrossRef] [PubMed]
2. Pohjasvaara, T.V.R.; Vataja, R.; Leppävuori, A.; Kaste, M.; Erkinjuntti, T. Cognitive functions and depression as predictors of poor outcome 15 months after stroke. *Cerebrovasc. Dis.* **2002**, *14*, 228–233. [CrossRef] [PubMed]
3. Hackett, M.L.; Anderson, C.S.; House, A.; Halteh, C. Interventions for preventing depression after stroke. *Cochrane Database Syst. Rev.* **2008**. [CrossRef]
4. Hou, W.H.; Liang, H.W.; Hsieh, C.L.; Hou, C.Y.; Wen, P.C.; Li, C.Y. Effects of stroke rehabilitation on incidence of poststroke depression: A population-based cohort study. *J. Clin. Psychiatry* **2013**, *74*, 859–866. [CrossRef] [PubMed]
5. Chang, C.C.; Lee, Y.C.; Lin, C.C.; Chang, C.H.; Chiu, C.D.; Chou, L.W.; Sun, M.F.; Yen, H.R. Characteristics of traditional Chinese medicine usage in patients with stroke in Taiwan: A nationwide population-based study. *J. Ethnopharmacol.* **2016**, *186*, 311–321. [CrossRef] [PubMed]
6. Andersen, G.; Vestergaard, K.; Ingemann-Nielsen, M.; Lauritzen, L. Risk factors for post-stroke depression. *Acta Psychiatrica Scand.* **1995**, *92*, 193–198. [CrossRef]
7. Hirata, S.; Ovbiagele, B.; Markovic, D.; Towfighi, A. Key factors associated with major depression in a national sample of stroke survivors. *J. Stroke Cerebrovasc. Dis.* **2016**, *25*, 1090–1095. [CrossRef] [PubMed]
8. De Ryck, A.; Brouns, R.; Geurden, M.; Elseviers, M.; De Deyn, P.P.; Engelborghs, S. Risk factors for poststroke depression identification of inconsistencies based on a systematic review. *J. Geriatr. Psychiatry Neurol.* **2014**, *27*, 147–158. [CrossRef] [PubMed]
9. Caeiro, L.; Ferro, J.M.; Santos, C.O.; Figueira, M.L. Depression in acute stroke. *J. Psychiatry Neurosci.* **2006**, *31*, 377–383. [PubMed]
10. Ayerbe, L.; Ayis, S.; Rudd, A.G.; Heuschmann, P.U.; Wolfe, C.D. Natural history, predictors, and associations of depression 5 years after stroke the South London Stroke Register. *Stroke* **2011**, *42*, 1907–1911. [CrossRef] [PubMed]
11. Chen, H.-F.; Lee, S.-P.; Li, C.-Y. Sex differences in the incidence of hemorrhagic and ischemic stroke among diabetics in Taiwan. *J. Women's Health* **2009**, *18*, 647–654.
12. American Psychiatric Association. *Diagnostic and Statistical Manual of Mental Disorders*; American Psychiatric Association: Washington, DC, USA, 2000.
13. Liu, C.-Y.; Hung, Y.T.; Chuang, Y.L.; Chen, Y.J.; Weng, W.S.; Liu, J.S.; Liang, K.Y. Incorporating development stratification of Taiwan townships into sampling design of large scale health interview survey. *J. Health Manag.* **2006**, *4*, 1–22.
14. Sung, S.F.; Hsieh, C.Y.; KaoYang, Y.H.; Lin, H.J.; Chen, C.H.; Chen, Y.W.; Hu, Y.H. Developing a stroke severity index based on administrative data was feasible using data mining techniques. *J. Clin. Epidemiol.* **2015**, *68*, 1292–1300. [CrossRef] [PubMed]
15. Post Stroke Depression. Available online: https://www.researchgate.net/publication/228850728_18_Post-Stroke_Depression (accessed on 13 March 2017).
16. Salom-Moreno, J.; Sánchez-Mila, Z.; Ortega-Santiago, R.; Palacios-Ceña, M.; Truyol-Domínguez, S.; Fernández-de-las-Peñas, C. Changes in Spasticity, Widespread Pressure Pain Sensitivity, and Baropodometry After the Application of Dry Needling in Patients Who Have Had a Stroke: A Randomized Controlled Trial. *J. Manip. Physiol. Ther.* **2014**, *37*, 569–579. [CrossRef] [PubMed]

17. Man, S.-C.; Hung, B.H.; Ng, R.M.; Yu, X.-C.; Cheung, H.; Fung, M.P.; Li, L.S.; Leung, K.-P.; Leung, K.-P.; Tsang, K.W.; et al. A pilot controlled trial of a combination of dense cranial electroacupuncture stimulation and body acupuncture for post-stroke depression. *BMC Complement. Altern. Med.* **2014**. [CrossRef] [PubMed]
18. Gosman-Hedström, G.; Claesson, L.; Klingenstierna, U.; Carlsson, J.; Olausson, B.; Frizell, M.; Fagerberg, B.; Blomstrand, C. Effects of acupuncture treatment on daily life activities and quality of life a controlled, prospective, and randomized study of acute stroke patients. *Stroke* **1998**, *29*, 2100–2108. [CrossRef] [PubMed]
19. Liu, F.; Li, Z.M.; Jiang, Y.J.; Chen, L.D. A Meta-Analysis of Acupuncture Use in the Treatment of Cognitive Impairment After Stroke. *J. Altern. Complement. Med.* **2014**, *20*, 535–544. [CrossRef]
20. Hsu, Y.-C.; Chiu, C.-J.; Wray, L.A.; Beverly, E.A.; Tseng, S.-P. Impact of traditional Chinese medicine on age trajectories of health: Evidence from the Taiwan longitudinal study on aging. *J. Am. Geriatr. Soc.* **2015**, *63*, 351–357. [CrossRef] [PubMed]
21. Salinas, J.; Beiser, A.; Himali, J.; Rosand, J.; Seshadri, S.; Dunn, E. Incidence and Predictors of Poststroke Depression: Results from the Framingham Heart Study (P5. 034). *Neurology* **2015**, *84* (Suppl. 14), 35–41.
22. Robinson, R.G.; Jorge, R.E.; Moser, D.J.; Acion, L.; Solodkin, A.; Small, S.L.; Fonzetti, P.; Hegel, M.; Arndt, S. Escitalopram and problem-solving therapy for prevention of poststroke depression: A randomized controlled trial. *Jama* **2008**, *299*, 2391–2400. [CrossRef] [PubMed]

13

The Pilot Study of Evaluating Fluctuation in the Blood Flow Volume of the Radial Artery, a Site for Traditional Pulse Diagnosis

Masashi Watanabe [1], Soichiro Kaneko [1,2], Shin Takayama [1,2,*], Yasuyuki Shiraishi [3], Takehiro Numata [1,2], Natsumi Saito [1], Takashi Seki [4], Norihiro Sugita [5], Satoshi Konno [3], Tomoyuki Yambe [3], Makoto Yoshizawa [6], Nobuo Yaegashi [7] and Tadashi Ishii [1]

1 Department of Education and Support for Regional Medicine, Department of Kampo Medicine, Tohoku University Hospital, 1-1 Seiryou-machi, Aoba-ku, Sendai, Miyagi 980-8574, Japan; egao.2008@wine.ocn.ne.jp (M.W.); souichi0134@gmail.com (S.K.); numatatakehiro@gmail.com (T.N.); natsu.beauty.summer@gmail.com (N.S.); t-ishi23@green.ocn.ne.jp (T.I.)
2 Comprehensive Education Center for Community Medicine, Graduate School of Medicine, Tohoku University, 2-1 Seiryou-machi, Aoba-ku, Sendai, Miyagi 980-8575, Japan
3 Institute of Development, Aging and Cancer, Tohoku University, 4-1 Seiryo-machi, Aoba-ku, Sendai, Miyagi 980-8575, Japan; shiraishi@idac.tohoku.ac.jp (Y.S.); konnos@idac.tohoku.ac.jp (S.K.); yambe@idac.tohoku.ac.jp (T.Y.)
4 Division of Cyclotron Nuclear Medicine, Cyclotron and Radioisotope Center, Tohoku University, 6-3 Aoba, Aramaki, Aoba-ku, Sendai, Miyagi 980-8578, Japan; tseki.tohoku@gmail.com
5 Department of Management Science and Technology, Graduate School of Engineering, Tohoku University, 6-6-05 Aramaki Aza Aoba, Aoba-ku, Sendai, Miyagi 980-8579, Japan; sugita@yoshizawa.ecei.tohoku.ac.jp
6 Research Division on Advanced Information Technology, Cyberscience Center, Tohoku University, 6-3 Aramaki Aza Aoba, Aoba-ku, Sendai, Miyagi 980-8578, Japan; yoshizawa@yoshizawa.ecei.tohoku.ac.jp
7 Department of Obstetrics and Gynecology, Graduate School of Medicine, Tohoku University, 1-1 Seiryou-machi, Aoba-ku, Sendai, Miyagi 980-8574, Japan; yaegashi@med.tohoku.ac.jp
* Correspondence: takayama@med.tohoku.ac.jp

Academic Editor: Gerhard Litscher

Abstract: Background: Radial artery (RA) pulse diagnosis has been used in traditional Asian medicine. Blood pressure (BP) and pulse rate related to heart rate variability (HRV) can be monitored via the RA. The fluctuation in these parameters has been assessed using fast Fourier transform (FFT) analytical methods that calculate power spectra. Methods: We measured blood flow volume (Volume) in the RA and evaluated its fluctuations. Normal participants (n = 34) were enrolled. We measured the hemodynamics of the right RA for approximately 50 s using ultrasonography. Results: The parameters showed the center frequency (CF) of the power spectrum at low frequency (LF) and high frequency (HF). More than one spectral component indicated that there were fluctuations. The CF at LF for Volume was significantly different from that for vessel diameter (VD); however, it was significantly correlated with blood flow velocity (Velocity). On the other hand, the CF at HF for Volume was significantly different from that for Velocity; however, it was significantly correlated with VD. Conclusion: It is suggested that fluctuation in the Volume at LF of RA is influenced by the fluctuation in Velocity; on the other hand, fluctuation in the Volume at HF is influenced by the fluctuation in VD.

Keywords: pulse diagnosis; radial artery; blood flow volume; fluctuation; ultrasonography

1. Introduction

Pulse diagnosis has been used in traditional medicine since ancient times (e.g., traditional Chinese medicine [1], Ayurveda [2], Unani medicine [3] and Tibetan medicine [4–7]). It is performed on the radial artery in the area around the radial styloid process, carotid artery and other arteries [8]. Traditional pulse diagnosis depends on experience, and quantification is very difficult. Therefore, it is difficult to carry out by education in Western medicine. Recently, a technique to measure a pulse wave was developed. Additionally, it is expected that various things become clear by evaluating the fluctuation included in the pulse wave [9].

Blood pressure (BP) and heart rate (HR) related to heart rate variability (HRV) can be monitored via the radial artery [10]. Fluctuations in the HR and BP have been assessed using fast Fourier transform (FFT) analytical methods that calculate power spectra [11–15]. Low frequency (LF) and high frequency (HF) components are observed in the spectrum of HRV [14,16,17]. The LF fluctuations in HRV are mediated by both the sympathetic and parasympathetic nervous systems, whereas the HF fluctuations are mediated solely by the parasympathetic system [14]. The blood flow volume is calculated using the vascular diameter (VD) and blood flow velocity (velocity). VD and velocity are evaluated using ultrasonic diagnostic equipment. VD is affected by the fluid content and through neurogenic control. The cell membranes of the smooth muscle cells in the vessels contain α- and β-adrenergic receptors that bind to neurotransmitters. Activation of α-adrenergic receptors promotes vasoconstriction, while the activation of β-adrenergic receptors mediates the relaxation of muscle cells, resulting in vasodilation. Normally, α-adrenergic receptors predominate in the smooth muscle of resistance vessels. Thus, vascular smooth muscle is ruled out of the sympathetic nerve-mediated tonicity. In addition, there are few reports about vasomotor fluctuation [18,19]. However, there are no studies yet that have measured the variability of the blood flow volume (Volume) in the radial artery. We measured the Volume in the radial artery and evaluated its fluctuations at the site of traditional pulse diagnosis using a high-resolution ultrasonography in the participants at rest.

The purpose of the pilot study was to measure the blood flow in the pulse diagnosis site and to explore its fluctuation related to the physiological parameters.

2. Experimental Section

2.1. Subjects

Thirty-three healthy volunteers (26 men and 7 women; mean age 34.2 ± 7.6 years) were enrolled in the study. All participants provided written informed consent before participation, and the study protocol was approved by the Ethics Committee of Tohoku University Graduate School of Medicine, Project identification code (2009-175) and approval date (27 July 2009) (Table 1).

Table 1. Participant's characteristics for this study.

Characteristic		Variable
Age (y)		34.2 ± 7.6
Sex (n)	Male	26
	Female	7
Body height (cm)		168.4 ± 6.7
Body weight (kg)		67.0 ± 13.0

2.2. Study Protocol

All investigations were performed under fasting conditions in a quiet air-conditioned room (constant temperature of 25–26 °C). Each participant was at rest in the supine position, and three electrocardiography electrodes (BP-608 Evolution II, Colin Healthcare Co. Ltd., Kyoto, Japan) were attached to the chest for monitoring. Radial artery hemodynamics were assessed using ultrasonography

(Prosound $\alpha10^{®}$; Hitachi-Aloka Medical, Ltd., Tokyo, Japan). This system had a high-resolution linear array transducer (13 MHz, Prosound $\alpha10^{®}$; Hitachi-Aloka Medical, Ltd., Tokyo, Japan) and computer-assisted analysis software (e-Tracking system®; Hitachi-Aloka Medical, Ltd., Tokyo, Japan) that could automatically detect a blood vessel edge and continuously measure the vessel diameter and Volume [20]. The right arm was fixed and the right radial artery was scanned longitudinally at 1–2 cm above the radial styloid process at a point where the vessel diameter and Doppler wave readings were stable. At a site where the clearest B-mode image of the anterior and posterior intimal interfaces between the lumen and vessel wall was obtained, the transducer was fixed in place using a special probe holder (MP-PH0001; Hitachi-Aloka Medical, Ltd., Tokyo, Japan). Compression of the artery was carefully avoided (Figure 1). When the tracking gate was placed on the intima, the radial artery diameter was monitored automatically, and a waveform representing the changes of vessel diameter during a cardiac cycle was displayed in real time using the e-Tracking system® (Figure 2). To obtain accurate measurements, a Doppler angle of $\leqslant$60 degrees was maintained [21,22]. Volume was calculated automatically as the Doppler flow velocity (corrected for the angle) multiplied by the vessel cross-sectional area [21–23]. We measured right radial artery hemodynamics for approximately 50 s after 10 min of rest in the supine position [24,25]. The hemodynamic parameters, including the radial artery diameter and Volume, and the HR were recorded continuously. To minimize the influence of respiration on the hemodynamic data, the participants were asked to breathe every 6 s during the test. Measured parameters were systolic vessel diameter (Sys-VD) per beat, diastolic vessel diameter (Dia-VD) per beat, Velocity per second, volume per beat and HR per minute.

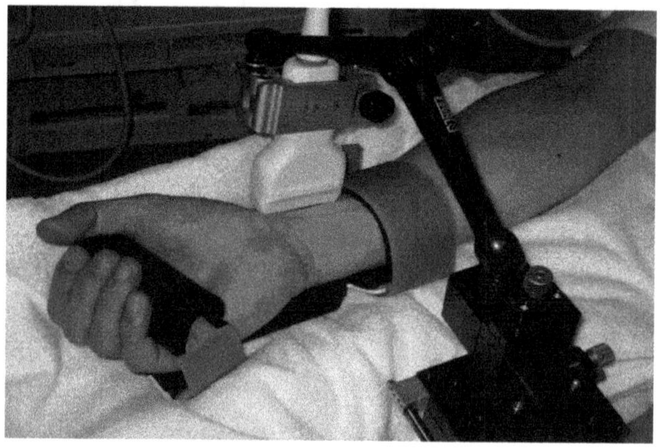

Figure 1. Ultrasonography measurement of radial artery using a special probe holder.

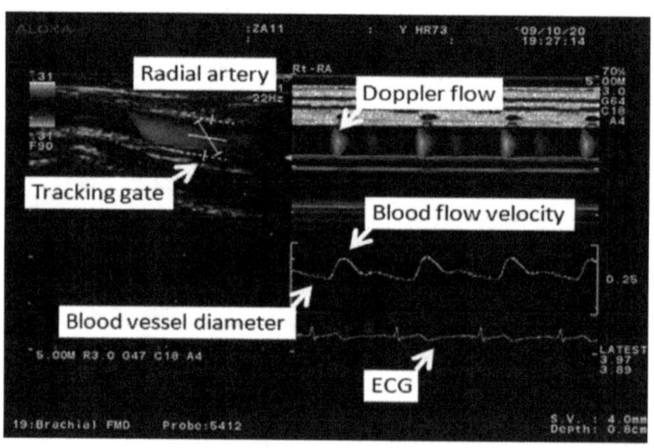

Figure 2. The image on the left shows the radial artery and the position of the tracking gate on the artery. The image on the right shows the changes in the vessel diameter, Doppler flow and flow velocity determined using an automated edge detection device and computer analysis software.

2.3. Analysis

In order to produce an evenly-sampled time series prior to FFT-based spectral estimation, linear spline interpolation and resampling of measured parameter data are usually employed [26,27]. After removal of linear trends included in the data, FFT analysis was applied using MATLAB software (Version 2007b; MathWorks, Natick, MA, USA) to obtain power spectra (periodogram) for Sys-VD, Dia-VD, HR, Velocity and Volume. In a low frequency component (LF; 0.04–0.15 Hz), we compared each of the center frequencies (CF) as follows: (1) Volume with Sys-VD; (2) Volume with Dia-VD; and (3) Volume with Velocity. In a high frequency component (HF; <0.15 Hz), we compared each of the CF as follows: (1) Volume with Sys-VD; (2) Volume with Dia-VD; and (3) Volume with Velocity.

2.4. Statistical Methods

Statistical analyses were performed using the PASW software (Version 17.0, SPSS Japan Inc., Tokyo, Japan). Comparisons between parameters were performed using ANOVA with Dunnett's *post hoc* tests and Pearson's product-moment correlation coefficient. Statistical significance was assumed at $p < 0.05$. Values are the mean ± standard deviation (SD).

3. Results

In all participants, the CF was seen in the LF and HF (Table 2). Comparisons of the CF of the LF and HF are shown in Figure 3a,b, respectively. There were significant differences in the CF between (1) the LF in Volume and the LF in HR ($p < 0.01$) and (2) the LF in Volume and the LF in Sys-VD ($p < 0.05$). There were significant correlate in the CF between (3) the LF in Volume and the LF in Velocity ($r = 0.64$, $p < 0.01$) and (4) the LF in Sys-VD and the LF in Dia-VD ($r = 0.57$, $p < 0.01$). On the other hand, there were significant differences in the CF between (5) the HF in Volume and the HF in Velocity ($p < 0.01$). There were significant correlate in the CF between (6) the HF in Volume and the HF in Sys-VD ($r = 0.39$, $p < 0.05$), (7) the HF in Sys-VD and the HF in Dia-VD ($r = 0.59$, $p < 0.01$) and (8) the HF in Dia-VD and the HF in HR ($r = 0.61$, $p < 0.01$).

Table 2. Center frequencies (Hz) and low frequency (LF)/high frequency (HF) ratio in the LF component and HF component of all subjects in blood flow volume (Volume), blood flow velocity (Velocity), systolic vessel diameter (Sys-VD), diastolic vessel diameter (Dia-VD) and heart rate (HR).

Participant	Volume		Velocity		Sys-VD		Dia-VD		HR	
No.	LF (Hz)	HF (Hz)	LF (Hz)	HF (Hz)	LF (Hz)	HF (Hz)	LF (Hz)	HF (Hz)	LF (Hz)	HF (Hz)
1	0.137	0.156	0.137	0.156	0.049	0.156	0.049	0.166	0.049	0.146
2	0.049	0.166	0.049	0.166	0.137	0.176	0.049	0.156	0.068	0.166
3	0.137	0.166	0.137	0.156	0.137	0.166	0.049	0.166	0.137	0.166
4	0.049	0.156	0.098	0.166	0.059	0.166	0.068	0.146	0.059	0.166
5	0.059	0.166	0.059	0.166	0.049	0.156	0.049	0.156	0.059	0.156
6	0.078	0.156	0.088	0.186	0.107	0.156	0.049	0.156	0.137	0.146
7	0.059	0.234	0.059	0.313	0.078	0.273	0.078	0.225	0.068	0.156
8	0.078	0.146	0.088	0.410	0.137	0.146	0.137	0.146	0.137	0.146
9	0.049	0.146	0.088	0.146	0.137	0.156	0.049	0.488	0.137	0.146
10	0.049	0.303	0.049	0.293	0.078	0.264	0.088	0.332	0.088	0.273
11	0.049	0.146	0.049	0.303	0.049	0.176	0.088	0.488	0.049	0.498
12	0.049	0.156	0.059	0.332	0.049	0.156	0.049	0.146	0.127	0.146
13	0.049	0.146	0.117	0.342	0.049	0.146	0.049	0.146	0.137	0.146
14	0.049	0.176	0.049	0.215	0.088	0.488	0.078	0.498	0.088	0.195
15	0.049	0.166	0.049	0.166	0.137	0.156	0.137	0.156	0.137	0.156
16	0.059	0.156	0.059	0.156	0.137	0.166	0.117	0.166	0.059	0.166
17	0.049	0.156	0.049	0.322	0.137	0.166	0.088	0.166	0.068	0.166
18	0.049	0.146	0.049	0.371	0.049	0.215	0.049	0.166	0.137	0.146
19	0.049	0.166	0.049	0.244	0.049	0.146	0.117	0.156	0.049	0.166
20	0.049	0.166	0.107	0.166	0.049	0.166	0.049	0.166	0.137	0.166
21	0.059	0.166	0.068	0.166	0.137	0.166	0.098	0.166	0.137	0.156
22	0.049	0.166	0.078	0.361	0.137	0.156	0.137	0.156	0.117	0.166
23	0.098	0.176	0.127	0.176	0.049	0.166	0.098	0.166	0.088	0.166

Table 2. *Cont.*

Participant	Volume		Velocity		Sys-VD		Dia-VD		HR	
No.	LF (Hz)	HF (Hz)	LF (Hz)	HF (Hz)	LF (Hz)	HF (Hz)	LF (Hz)	HF (Hz)	LF (Hz)	HF (Hz)
24	0.068	0.166	0.068	0.166	0.098	0.166	0.107	0.176	0.049	0.166
25	0.137	0.166	0.137	0.166	0.049	0.166	0.049	0.166	0.137	0.166
26	0.049	0.146	0.049	0.205	0.049	0.166	0.049	0.156	0.137	0.146
27	0.049	0.195	0.049	0.146	0.049	0.146	0.049	0.244	0.078	0.156
28	0.049	0.166	0.049	0.166	0.049	0.166	0.049	0.166	0.137	0.166
29	0.127	0.146	0.049	0.166	0.137	0.166	0.137	0.166	0.137	0.156
30	0.059	0.146	0.137	0.166	0.127	0.186	0.127	0.186	0.078	0.186
31	0.117	0.146	0.127	0.146	0.127	0.146	0.127	0.146	0.117	0.146
32	0.049	0.146	0.049	0.146	0.137	0.156	0.137	0.156	0.137	0.156
33	0.049	0.166	0.068	0.166	0.049	0.166	0.049	0.166	0.137	0.166
34	0.049	0.166	0.049	0.322	0.068	0.156	0.107	0.176	0.137	0.166
Mean ± SD	0.066 ± 0.030	0.166 ± 0.030	0.076 ± 0.033	0.219 ± 0.082	0.089 ± 0.040	0.179 ± 0.062	0.082 ± 0.035	0.200 ± 0.098	0.104 ± 0.036	0.173 ± 0.062
LF/HF Mean ± SD	2.1 ± 1.6		0.9 ± 0.5		0.8 ± 0.5		0.9 ± 0.5		0.8 ± 0.4	

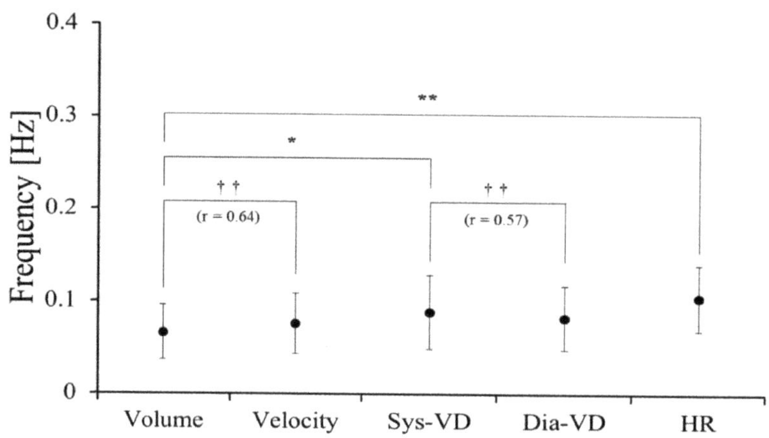

(a)

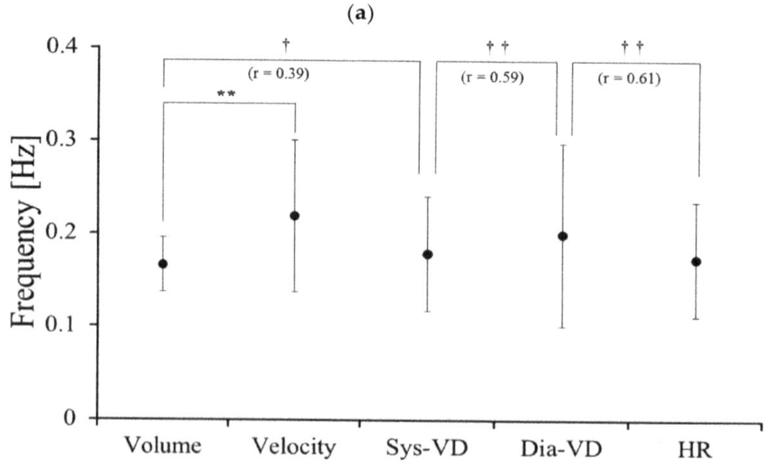

(b)

Figure 3. Comparison among the center frequency of blood flow volume (Volume), blood flow velocity (Velocity), systolic vessel diameter (Sys-VD), diastolic vessel diameter (Dia-VD) and heart rate (HR) in (**a**) the low-frequency component (LF) and (**b**) the high-frequency component (HF). Values represent the mean ± standard deviation (SD). Comparisons between parameters were performed using ANOVA with Dunnett's *post hoc* tests (* $p < 0.05$; ** $p < 0.01$) and Pearson's product-moment correlation coefficient (r: correlation coefficient, † $p < 0.05$; †† $p < 0.01$). Statistical significance was assumed at $p < 0.05$.

4. Discussion

A peak appears in the spectrum only due to the superposition of a number of waves from a time series comprising multiple waves [28]. HRV has different LF and HF that are observed in a spectrum for individual peaks [28]. In our analysis, we observed LF and HF in Sys-VD, Dia-VD, HR, Velocity and Volume in the radial artery while subjects were at rest. More than one spectral component indicated that there were fluctuations in each of these parameters. In a previous study on fluctuations in the circulatory system, only HRV and BP were studied [10,13,16,17,28–34], but there has been no report on Volume of the peripheral artery. In this study, to our knowledge, this is the first report of the investigation of the fluctuations in Volume of the radial artery. Frequencies of 0.085 and 0.09 Hz have been reported as the CF in the LF, and those of 0.21 and 0.24 Hz have been reported as the CF in the HF [17,31]. The LF appears to correspond to Mayer waves, while the HF is synchronous with respiration and has been considered as a quantitative evaluation of respiratory arrhythmia [17]. The HF varies in its CF with variations in the respiratory cycle [35]. In this study, the participants were asked to breathe every 6 s during the test, and this could have influenced the HF. The frequency during breathe control is 0.167 Hz, which was equivalent to that of the HF (0.166 Hz) in our results. It will be necessary to repeat the study without breath control. According to our results, in LF, there was a significant difference in the CF between Volume and HR/vessel diameter, while there was significant correlation between Volume and Velocity. In HF, there was a significant difference in the CF between Volume and Velocity, while there was significant correlation between Volume and vessel diameter. These results show that the CF of the Volume in LF is correlated with the CF of the Velocity in LF; on the other hand, the CF of the Volume in HF is correlated with the CF of the vessel diameter in HF.

In peripheral arteries, such as radial arteries, there are influences of local vasoconstrictor and vasodilator nerves, as well as the influence of the autonomic nerves on the heart. There are differences with regard to the LF. Some studies suggest that LF is a quantitative marker of sympathetic modulations, while other studies view LF as reflecting both sympathetic and vagal activities. Consequently, an LF/HF ratio is considered by some investigators to mirror a sympathovagal balance or to reflect sympathetic modulations [30]. In this study, the value of the LF/HF ratio for the Volume was 2.10. According to the previous reports, this value shows a rest state, but there is a difference by some reports [36–39].

Investigators from the Framingham Heart Study reported that HRV offers prognostic information independent of and beyond that provided by traditional risk factors [30]. The fluctuations of the LF/HF ratio in Volume of the radial artery could be a new index for the prognosis of cardiac vascular disease. The CF of the LF in Volume of the radial artery indicates a cycle of 7–25 s. This suggests that more than 25 s might be required for pulse diagnosis.

At the site of a pulse diagnosis using a radial artery, the blood vessel diameter is so small that the instrument used for measurement points can slip off due to slight movements by the participants. Therefore, in this study, it was difficult to make measurements for prolonged periods. For future investigations, an easier, more stable method of measurement must be established. The limitation of this study is also a lack of measurements of continuous BP and the sampling duration. To evaluate the relation among the HR, BP and blood flow, simultaneous measurements of these parameters are needed. We have conducted a further study that solves these problems and the evaluation introduced to investigate acupuncture effects. The duration of blood flow sampling used for analysis is a little shorter than ideal. Generally, the spectral analysis requires over 60 s of data. In the present study, the arms of the subjects were fixed to measure blood flow using ultrasonography; however, occasionally, the subjects moved their arms during long duration measurements. We have tried analyzing over 60 s of data for spectral analysis; unfortunately, error is introduced once the subjects move their arm. Therefore, we used data for a shorter period (50 s), which was free of errors. Thus, the sampling duration is one of the limitations of this study. The present study is a pilot study; therefore, we will conduct experiments using a revised protocol in the future. We also intend to increase the number of subjects and to perform these studies with considerations of gender, age and disease.

Further investigation will be needed for healthy subjects and patients with cardiovascular disease to show the clinical difference and meanings.

5. Conclusions

We measured the blood flow volume in the radial artery and evaluated its fluctuations at the site of traditional pulse diagnosis using ultrasonography in the participants at rest. We observed LF and HF in vessel diameter, HR, Velocity and Volume. More than one spectral component indicated that there were fluctuations in each of these parameters. This study showed that the CF of the Volume in LF was correlated with CF of the Velocity in LF, on the other hand, the CF of the Volume in HF was correlated with CF of the vessel diameter in HF.

Acknowledgments: We thank all of the participants who took part in this study. This work was supported by Special Coordination Funds for Promoting Science and Technology from the Japanese Ministry of Education, Culture, Sports, Science and Technology.

Author Contributions: Masashi Watanabe, Soichiro Kaneko, Shin Takayama, Yasuyuki Shiraishi, Takehiro Numata, Natsumi Saito, Takashi Seki, Norihiro Sugita, Satoshi Konno, Tomoyuki Yambe, Makoto Yoshizawa, Nobuo Yaegashi and Tadashi Ishii conceived and designed the experiments; Shin Takayama performed the experiments; Masashi Watanabe, Soichiro Kaneko, Yasuyuki Shiraishi, Natsumi Saito, Satoshi Konno, Tomoyuki Yambe, and Makoto Yoshizawa analyzed the data; all authors wrote the paper.

References

1. King, E.; Cobbin, D.; Ryan, D. The reliable measurement of radial pulse: Gender differences in pulse profiles. *Acupunct. Med.* **2002**, *20*, 160–167. [CrossRef] [PubMed]
2. Lad, V. *Secrets of the Pulse: The Ancient Art of Ayurvedic Pulse Diagnosis*, 2nd ed.; The Ayurvedic Press: Albuquerque, NM, USA, 2006.
3. Subbarayappa, B.V. The roots of ancient medicine: An historical outline. *J. Biosci.* **2001**, *26*, 135–143. [CrossRef] [PubMed]
4. Hsu, E. A hybrid body technique: Does the pulse diagnostic cun guan chi method have Chinese-Tibetan origins? *Gesnerus* **2008**, *65*, 5–29. [PubMed]
5. Steiner, R.P. Tibetan medicine: Part II: Pulse diagnosis in Tibetan medicine: Translated from the first chapter for the fourth tantra (rGyud-bzi). *Am. J. Chin. Med.* **1987**, *15*, 165–170. [CrossRef] [PubMed]
6. Steiner, R.P. Tibetan medicine. Part III: Pulse diagnosis in Tibetan medicine. Translated from the first chapter of the Fourth Tantra (rGyud-bzi). *Am. J. Chin. Med.* **1988**, *16*, 173–178. [CrossRef] [PubMed]
7. Steiner, R.P. Tibetan medicine Part IV: Pulse diagnosis in Tibetan medicine. *Am. J. Chin. Med.* **1989**, *17*, 79–84. [CrossRef] [PubMed]
8. Zhu, W. *Zhongyi Zhenduanxue (Study of the Chinese Medicine Diagnosis)*; Renmin Weisheng Chuban: Beijing, China, 1999.
9. Yambe, T.; Yoshizawa, M.; Taira, R.; Tanaka, A.; Iquchi, A.; Tabayashi, K.; Tobita, S.; Nitta, S. Fluctuations of Emax of the left ventricle: Effect of atrial natriuretic polypeptide. *Biomed. Pharmacother.* **2001**, *55* (Suppl. S1), 147s–152s. [CrossRef]
10. Sato, T.; Nishinaga, M.; Kawamoto, A.; Ozawa, T.; Takatsuji, H. Accuracy of a continuous blood pressure monitor based on arterial tonometry. *Hypertension* **1993**, *21*, 866–874. [CrossRef] [PubMed]
11. Castiglioni, J.; Frattola, A.; Parati, G.; Rieenzo, M. 1/f-modelling of blood pressure and heart rate spectra: Relations to aging. In Proceedings of the 1992 14th Annual International Conference of the IEEE Engineering in Medicine and Biology Society, Paris, France, 29 October–1 November 1992; pp. 465–466.
12. Kuusela, T.A.; Kaila, T.J.; Kahonen, M. Fine structure of the low-frequency spectra of heart rate and blood pressure. *BMC Physiol.* **2003**, *3*, 11. [CrossRef] [PubMed]
13. Marsh, D.J.; Osborn, J.L.; Cowley, A.W., Jr. 1/f fluctuations in arterial pressure and regulation of renal blood flow in dogs. *Am. J. Physiol.* **1990**, *258*, F1394–F1400. [PubMed]
14. Pomeranz, B.; Macaulay, R.J.; Caudill, M.A.; Kutz, L.; Adam, D.; Gordon, D.; Kilborn, K.M.; Barger, A.C.; Shannon, D.C.; Cohen, R.J.; *et al.* Assessment of autonomic function in humans by heart rate spectral analysis. *Am. J. Physiol.* **1985**, *248*, H151–H153. [PubMed]

15. Parati, G.; Saul, J.P.; di Rienzo, M.; Mancia, G. Spectral analysis of blood pressure and heart rate variability in evaluating cardiovascular regulation. A critical appraisal. *Hypertension* **1995**, *25*, 1276–1286. [CrossRef] [PubMed]
16. Akselrod, S.; Gordon, D.; Ubel, F.A.; Shannon, D.C.; Berger, A.C.; Cohen, R.J. Power spectrum analysis of heart rate fluctuation: A quantitative probe of beat-to-beat cardiovascular control. *Science* **1981**, *213*, 220–222. [CrossRef] [PubMed]
17. Pagani, M.; Lombardi, F.; Guzzetti, S.; Rimoldi, O.; Furlan, R.; Pizzinelli, P.; Sandrone, G.; Malfatto, G.; Dell'Orto, S.; Piccaluga, E.; *et al.* Power spectral analysis of heart rate and arterial pressure variabilities as a marker of sympatho-vagal interaction in man and conscious dog. *Circ. Res.* **1986**, *59*, 178–193. [CrossRef] [PubMed]
18. Hall, J.E. *Guyton and Hall, Textbook of Medical Physiology*; SAUNDERS ELSEVIE: Philaclclphia, PA, USA, 2011.
19. Griffith, T.M. Vasomotioin: The case for chaos. *J. Biorheol.* **2009**, *23*, 11–23. [CrossRef]
20. Soga, J.; Nishioka, K.; Nakamura, S.; Umemura, T.; Jitsuiki, D.; Hidaka, T.; Teragawa, H.; Takemoto, H.; Goto, C.; Yoshizumi, M.; *et al.* Measurement of flow-mediated vasodilation of the brachial artery: A comparison of measurements in the seated and supine positions. *Circ. J.* **2007**, *71*, 736–740. [CrossRef] [PubMed]
21. Burns, P.N.; Jaffe, C.C. Quantitative flow measurements with Doppler ultrasound: Techniques, accuracy, and limitations. *Radiol. Clin. N. Am.* **1986**, *23*, 641–657.
22. Taylor, K.J.; Holland, S. Doppler US. Part I. Basic principles, instrumentation, and pitfalls. *Radiology* **1990**, *174*, 297–307. [CrossRef] [PubMed]
23. Gill, R.W. Measurement of blood flow by ultrasound: Accuracy and sources of error. *Ultrasound. Med. Biol.* **1985**, *11*, 625–641. [CrossRef]
24. Corretti, M.C.; Anderson, T.J.; Benjamin, E.J.; Celermajer, D.; Charbonneau, F.; Creager, M.A.; Deanfield, J.; Drexler, H.; Gerhard-Herman, M.; Herrington, D.; *et al.* Guidelines for the ultrasound assessment of endothelial-dependent flow-mediated vasodilation of the brachial artery: A report of the International Brachial Artery Reactivity Task Force. *J. Am. Coll. Cardiol.* **2002**, *39*, 257–265. [CrossRef]
25. Deanfield, J.; Donald, A.; Ferri, C.; Giannattasio, C.; Halcox, J.; Halligan, S.; Lerman, A.; Mancia, G.; Oliver, J.J.; Pessina, A.C.; *et al.* Endothelial function and dysfunction. Part I: Methodological issues for assessment in the different vascular beds: A statement by the Working Group on Endothelin and Endothelial Factors of the European Society of Hypertension. *J. Hypertens.* **2005**, *23*, 7–17. [CrossRef] [PubMed]
26. Clifford, G.D.; Tarassenko, L. Quantifying errors in spectral estimates of HRV due to beat replacement and resampling. *IEEE Trans. Biomed. Eng.* **2005**, *52*, 630–638. [CrossRef] [PubMed]
27. Daskalov, I.; Christov, I. Improvement of resolution in measurement of electrocardiogram RR intervals by interpolation. *Med. Eng. Phys.* **1997**, *19*, 375–379. [CrossRef]
28. Hayano, J. *Therapeutic Research*; Life Science Publishing: Tokyo, Japan, 1996.
29. Berger, R.D.; Saul, J.P.; Cohen, R.J. Transfer function analysis of autonomic regulation. I. Canine atrial rate response. *Am. J. Physiol.* **1989**, *256*, H142–H152. [PubMed]
30. Malik, M. Heart rate bvariability: Standards of measurement, physiological interpretation, and clinical use. *Circulation* **1996**, *93*, 1043–1065.
31. Montano, N.; Ruscone, T.G.; Porta, A.; Lombardi, F.; Pagani, M.; Malliani, A. Power spectrum analysis of heart rate variability to assess the changes in sympathovagal balance during graded orthostatic tilt. *Circulation* **1994**, *90*, 1826–1831. [CrossRef] [PubMed]
32. Perini, R.; Veicsteinas, A. Heart rate variability and autonomic activity at rest and during exercise in various physiological conditions. *Eur. J. Appl. Physiol.* **2003**, *90*, 317–325. [CrossRef] [PubMed]
33. Persson, P.B. Spectrum analysis of cardiovascular time series. *Am. J. Physiol.* **1997**, *273*, R1201–R1210. [PubMed]
34. Kudaiberdieva, G.; Gorenek, B.; Timuralp, B. Heart rate variability as a predictor of sudden cardiac death. *Anadolu Kardiyol. Derg.* **2007**, *7* (Suppl. S1), 68–70. [PubMed]
35. Hirsch, J.A.; Bishop, B. Respiratory sinus arrhythmia in humans: How breathing pattern modulates heart rate. *Am. J. Physiol.* **1981**, *241*, H620–H629. [PubMed]
36. De Angelis, C.; Perelli, P.; Trezza, R.; Casagrande, M.; Biselli, R.; Pannitteri, G.; Marino, B.; Farrace, S. Modified autonomic balance in offsprings of diabeties detected by spectral analysis of heart rate variability. *Metab. Clin. Exp.* **2001**, *50*, 1270–1274. [CrossRef] [PubMed]

37. Mendonca, G.V.; Fernhall, B.; Heffernan, K.S.; Pereira, F.D. Spectral methods of heart rate variability analysis during dynamic exercise. *Clin. Auton. Res.* **2009**, *19*, 237–245. [CrossRef] [PubMed]
38. Pichon, A.; Roulaud, M.; Antoine-Jonville, S.; Bisschop, C.D.; Denjean, A. Spectral analysis of heart rate variability: Interchangeability between autoregressive analysis and fast Fourier transform. *J. Electrocardiol.* **2006**, *39*, 31–37. [CrossRef] [PubMed]
39. Takada, H.T.; Katayama, M.A. The significance of "LF-component and HF-component which resulted from frequency analysis of heart rate" and "the coefficient of the heart rate variability": Evaluation of autonomic nerve function by acceleration plethysmography. *Health Eval. Promot.* **2005**, *32*, 504–512. [CrossRef]

14

Individual Differences in Responsiveness to Acupuncture: An Exploratory Survey of Practitioner Opinion

David F. Mayor [1,*], Lara S. McClure [2] and J. Helgi Clayton McClure [2]

1 Department of Allied Health Professions and Midwifery, School of Health and Social Work, University of Hertfordshire, Hatfield AL10 9AB, UK
2 Northern College of Acupuncture, York YO1 6LJ, UK; LaraMcClure@chinese-medicine.co.uk (L.S.M.); helgi.claytonmcclure@oxon.org (J.H.C.M.)
* Correspondence: davidmayor@welwynacupuncture.co.uk

Abstract: Background: Previous research has considered the impact of personal and situational factors on treatment responses. This article documents the first phase of a four-stage project on patient characteristics that may influence responsiveness to acupuncture treatment, reporting results from an exploratory practitioner survey. **Methods:** Acupuncture practitioners from various medical professions were recruited through professional organisations to complete an online survey about their demographics and attitudes as well as 60 questions on specific factors that might influence treatment. They gave categorical ("Yes", "No", and "Don't know") and free-text responses. Quantitative and qualitative (thematic) analyses were then conducted. **Results:** There were more affirmative than negative or uncertain responses overall. Certain characteristics, including ability to relax, exercise and diet, were most often considered relevant. Younger and male practitioners were more likely to respond negatively. Limited support was found for groupings between characteristics. Qualitative data provide explanatory depth. Response fatigue was evident over the course of the survey. **Conclusions:** Targeting and reminders may benefit uptake when conducting survey research. Practitioner characteristics influence their appreciation of patient characteristics. Factors consistently viewed as important included ability to relax, exercise and diet. Acupuncture practitioners may benefit from additional training in certain areas. Surveys may produce more informative results if reduced in length and complexity.

Keywords: acupuncture; responsiveness; practitioner survey; patient characteristics; thematic analysis; Shannon entropy

---

1. Introduction

Outcomes from acupuncture treatment have been considered to depend on many interacting factors, including—among others—the condition treated, treatment parameters (acupuncture points and procedures used), setting, practitioner experience, characteristics and attitude, the patient–practitioner relationship, advice given, co-interventions, conditioning (e.g., from treatment repetition) and expectation [1–11].

What about the patient in the acupuncture scenario? The respected German-born British pioneering medical acupuncture practitioner Felix Mann (1931–2014) introduced the term "strong reactor" to describe a subset of patients who respond particularly strongly to acupuncture [12], with very rapid alleviation of their symptoms, although he was not able to define such patients otherwise than by observing that they seemed more likely to be artistic or inclined toward religious belief than less strong reactors. Similar to Mann, some British proponents of medical acupuncture such as Anthony Campbell and Peter Baldry have noted that strong reactors are also often "good responders" to acupuncture [1,13], with Campbell following a suggestion by Johnson et al. [14] concerning transcutaneous electrical nerve stimulation (TENS) that strong reactors could be people whose central nervous system, including the limbic system, is particularly sensitive to sensory stimulation [13]. Among the present authors, in D.F.M.'s experience over 36 years of clinical practice and in line with Campbell's findings [15], some patients have certainly seemed to respond well to acupuncture and benefit a great deal from receiving treatment, whereas others have appeared to respond less well, or even poorly, and benefit less from treatment—almost regardless of what that treatment is.

A central aim of this paper is to explore what practitioners consider as possible individual characteristics, attitudes and experiences that may contribute to someone being a "good" or "poor" responder. We make no claims about what actually are the factors that influence responsiveness, but contribute to a framework for assessing the impact of patient characteristics on treatment outcomes. This may ultimately assist in developing models of patient response tendencies, such as that of the "good responder" [1,13]. Further aims are to present some preliminary findings concerning such general questions as: "Are some patients more receptive to acupuncture in general, with a better, faster or more enduring response to treatment than others?", "Can acupuncture responders be consistently categorised as 'good', 'average' or 'poor', or does this vary?", or "Is placebo responsiveness considered materially to contribute to acupuncture responsiveness?"

Investigating such characteristics and questions is potentially important for any therapeutic intervention, and certainly not acupuncture alone, but they are rarely addressed in the literature except in a very limited way. In recent years, for example, genetic polymorphism (genotyping) has been investigated for its effects on treatment outcome in several fields—particularly in hepatology [16,17]—with a view to developing more personalised approaches to treatment or improving outcome prediction. Genomic correlates of the placebo response (the "placebome") have also been proposed [18,19], and such an approach has been used, if sparsely, in the field of acupuncture. Thus, response to acupuncture for smoking cessation was found in one Korean study to vary with genetic polymorphisms [20], and using serotonin transporter polymorphism techniques has been proposed as a method of guiding individualised treatment of irritable bowel syndrome in Chinese medicine [21]. More generally, genetic polymorphism has been shown to regulate the default mode network (DMN) in the brain, and so to regulate response to acupuncture stimulation [22]. In a very different approach, poor response to acupuncture used as an adjuvant treatment for In Vitro Fertilisation was found to be more likely in those with high peak levels of follicular stimulating hormone, longer histories of infertility and worse sperm morphology [23], but a quick PubMed search revealed no other studies that looked explicitly at the effects of such factors on treatment outcome.

Furthermore, genetic testing is highly technical and costly, and offers little insight to the clinician in daily practice. Similarly, although there are many studies on the endocrinology [24] and neurochemistry of acupuncture [25,26], again few are relevant in everyday practice. Therefore, a simpler, more accessible questionnaire-based research protocol was developed in an attempt to assess whether there might be any simple answers to the question "who responds well to acupuncture?" without recourse to complex and costly biomarkers (a similar approach, using psychometric data to evaluate the effects of patient personality on their response to placebo acupuncture, was explored by Kaptchuk and colleagues [27]). Such a protocol might seem not just simple but naïve and simplistic to those used to large-scale scientific research, but its feasibility and limited funding requirements recommended it for the current exploratory work. Development was by D.F.M. in association with a small focus group comprising six other experienced acupuncturists and researchers (one of whom previously published a paper about the effects of attachment style on response to acupuncture [28]), one neurofeedback practitioner and a retired medical doctor/government advisor.

To contextualise this paper, the protocol, still in development, is in four phases:

A A survey of UK acupuncture practitioners to find why members of the profession think some patients respond better to acupuncture than others.

B Use of self-report personality scales with around 100 participants who have taken part in acupuncture-related studies conducted at the University of Hertfordshire since 2011, to assess whether there are any meaningful associations between these traits and their electroencephalography (EEG), heart rate variability (HRV) and outcomes data already collected.

C A (blinded) retrospective survey of acupuncture teaching clinic patients who have responded either well or poorly to acupuncture, using a variety of short, established self-report personality questionnaires to determine whether any of the traits assessed have a bearing on outcome.

D A prospective study of patients using a smaller selection of self-report questionnaires (based on Phases A–C above), together with outcome measures such as the Measure Yourself Medical Outcome Profile (MYMOP) and perhaps a multiple measure of mood change similar to those developed and piloted by D.F.M. and other collaborators [29,30].

Phase A of the project is presented here. The survey process is described in Sections 2.1 and 2.2; a quantitative analysis of the categorical "Yes"/"No"/"Don't know" survey responses is undertaken in Section 3.2.3, with a nested qualitative analysis of the free-text responses in Section 3.3; the main conclusions are given in Section 5. The survey questions and the actual data gathered are provided in the Supplementary Materials (http://www.mdpi.com/2305-6320/5/3/85/s1).

Data for Phase B have now been collected and are currently in process of analysis. Phases C and D are still in the planning stage. In preparation, some small pilot studies have been undertaken to test the use of selected self-report questionnaires for the retrospective self-assessment of acupuncture's effectiveness and prospective assessment of mood changes in response to electroacupuncture in a teaching situation [30,31], with a further pilot study still in process.

2. Materials and Methods

Ethics approval was obtained from the University of Hertfordshire for Phases A and B of this project (Protocol HSK/SF/UH/02930, 3 August 2017).

Initially, the acupuncture literature as well as general literature on factors having an impact on health and wellbeing was reviewed to locate possible individual characteristics and experiences that might possibly affect treatment responsiveness and for which validated self-report questionnaires exist. Based on this review, the pilot studies mentioned above and prior experience of running acupuncture surveys [32,33], a survey was developed in consultation with the focus group, members of which were recruited informally from among those with an interest in the survey subject matter. The survey was then trialled by the group prior to launch. Several revisions were made at each stage of this process until the survey was finally considered ready for use.

2.1. The Survey

The final online version of the survey, hosted by Jisc (Bristol Online Surveys), was launched on 16 October 2017 and closed after 19 weeks on 28 February 2018. Before respondents could take the survey, they were informed about its purpose, origins and how long it was likely to take them to complete, and then asked for their consent to continue [34]. The 13-page survey included three initial questions about the respondents themselves, four about their acupuncture training, professional affiliation and practice, and one (Q9) asking whether—before becoming aware of the survey—they had ever considered that patient characteristics (such as temperament or personality traits) might affect treatment response.

Then followed the main part of the survey, consisting of 60 questions on particular patient characteristics, attitudes or experience that could contribute to how well (or poorly) they respond to acupuncture, derived from the literature on what can affect health (Q10.1 to Q12.18). Respondents were asked which of the listed suggestions they currently considered might have an important effect on treatment response ("What you THINK NOW"). They were also asked whether, in their own clinical practice, they thought at the time of giving a treatment or shortly afterwards that any of the listed suggestions had an impact on an individual patient's response to acupuncture ("What you THOUGHT THEN"). Answers could be "Yes", "No" or "Don't know" ("Yes", "No" and blank for the "THEN" responses). NOW and THEN questions were separately included deliberately to encompass responses based on both current knowledge (or opinion) and historical experience, which could relate to a single, specific past experience or on the practitioner's career experience as a whole. Explanations were provided for terms used in 10 of the questions which might be unfamiliar to those taking the survey. The survey also included 69 free-text boxes where respondents could choose to qualify their categorical answers with further comments.

In addition, respondents were asked further questions about their views on consistency of response to acupuncture treatment (Q13), short-term and long-term response to acupuncture treatment (Q14), three questions on their own response to acupuncture (Q15), two about their patients' response to acupuncture (Q16–17), and a final two about conditions they consider as responding particularly well or badly to acupuncture (Q18–19).

The survey questions and responses are summarised in the Supplementary Materials.

2.2. Recruitment

Information about the survey was sent to all the major (and some less established) UK professional acupuncture associations (Table 1), and also to selected training institutions whose graduates tended to become members of these associations. A template was provided for them to inform their members/graduates about the survey using various methods—newsletters (printed and/or electronic), emails, member forums and social media. No incentives were offered for completing the survey. Survey uptake was monitored by D.F.M.; reminders were sent to the associations, and by them to their members, some five weeks before the survey closed. Clearly, the reminder appears to have been effective (Figure 1); it also seems possible that members of the smaller associations (apart from the Chinese Medical Institute and Register (CMIR)) were more likely to take the survey; although the correlation between membership numbers and percentages of these that took the survey was not significant ($r_s = -0.464$, $p = 0.294$), the trendline of a scatterplot for the two remaining sets of six numbers—without the CMIR data—shows a tantalisingly clear power distribution, so that overall numbers were low (median percentage of membership 1.43%, interquartile range 0.43–1.94%).

Table 1. Acupuncture Associations and training institutions informed about the survey, showing percentage of association members who completed the survey.

Association/Institution	Membership *M*	Respondents *R*	*R*/*M* (%)
Acupuncture Association of Chartered Physiotherapists (AACP)	6000	5	0.08%
Acupuncture Society (AS)	1000	20	2.0%
Association of Traditional Chinese Medicine (ATCM)	700	10	1.43%
British Academy of Western Medical Acupuncture (BAWMA)	150	12	8.00%
British Acupuncture Council (BAcC)	3000	56	1.87%
British Medical Acupuncture Society (BMAS)	2300	10	0.43%
Chinese Medical Institute and Register (CMIR)	240	1	0.42%
College of Chinese Medicine (CCM)		unknown	n/a
College of Integrated Chinese Medicine (CICM)		unknown	n/a
Northern College of Acupuncture (NCA)		unknown	n/a

Notes: Some membership numbers are taken from Mayor and Bovey 2016 [33], so percentage figures are indicative; 13 respondents stated they were members of "Other" associations, and 12 were concurrently members of two associations.

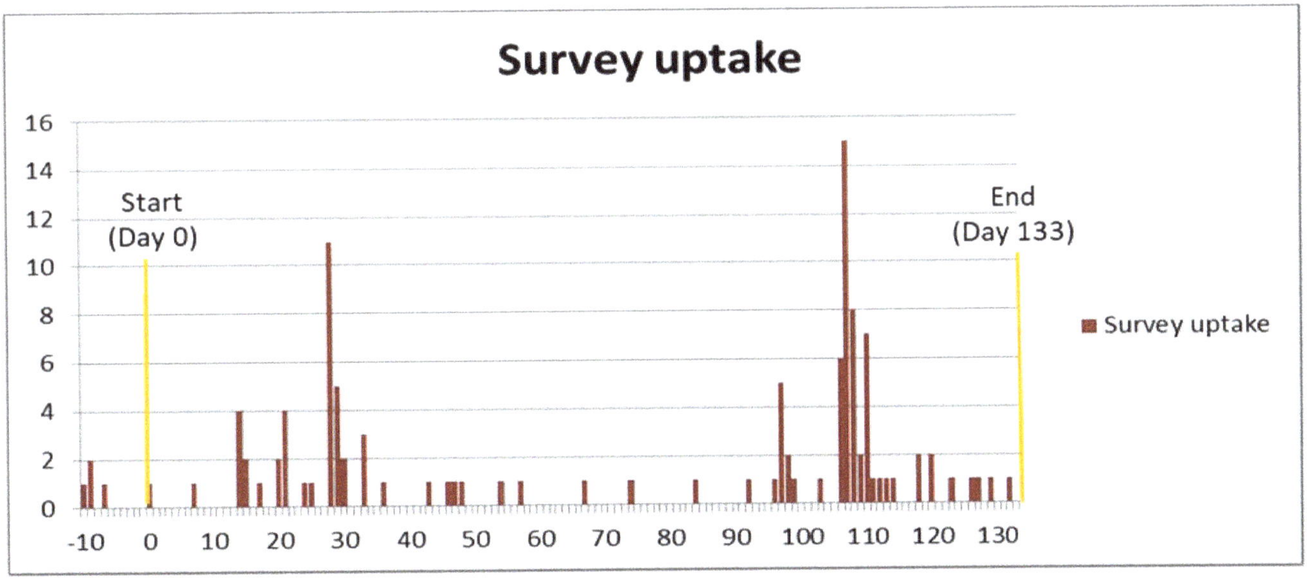

Figure 1. Survey uptake over time, showing the effects of the reminder sent five weeks before closure.

2.3. *Analysis*

For the most part, data were not normally distributed when tested using the Shapiro–Wilk test and for skewness and kurtosis. Analysis was therefore conducted using non-parametric methods in SPSS (v23) and Excel (2010). Randolph's free-marginal multi-rater *kappa* was calculated using the online calculator (at http://justusrandolph.net/kappa/), and Shannon entropy using the simple Excel-based method described in a previous study [30].

3. Results

3.1. *The Respondents*

In total, 114 people completed the survey, including four members of the focus group before the official survey start date (the results for these four are not included in the Supplementary Materials). One of these was not an acupuncture practitioner, one other respondent was also not an acupuncturist (although trained), and one completed the survey prior to training.

There were 79 female and 35 male respondents, the median age for both genders being 52 (interquartile ranges, IQR, being 42–57 and 48–64, respectively).

Most respondents (83) considered themselves primarily as acupuncturists or practitioners of traditional Chinese medicine (TCM), as against only seven as medical doctors, six as physiotherapists or nurses (including midwives) and two as chiropractors. There were more male than female medical doctors and chiropractors among the respondents, although not significantly.

Median ages for the acupuncturists/TCM practitioners, chiropractors and other professionals who completed the survey were very similar (52, IQR 46–58). However, those for medical doctors were much greater (63, IQR 59.5–69.5), and those for physiotherapists much less (35.5, IQR 30.5–48).

There was a strong correlation between respondents' age and how long they had used acupuncture in clinical practice (Spearman's rank correlation coefficient *rho* or $r_s = 0.535$, $p < 0.0001$); this was more marked for men ($r_s = 0.712$) than for women ($r_s = 0.438$).

Respondents had used acupuncture for a median of ten years (IQR 5–19), with medical doctors using it for longest (20 years, IQR 13.5–35) and "other" practitioners for the shortest time (3 years, IQR 1.5–10).

Different styles of acupuncture treatment were used, which could be categorised as more "traditional" (e.g., TCM, Five-Element, Japanese or "Tung's style"), used by 88 respondents, and more "modern" or "Western" (e.g., Western medical, Trigger point or "Formula"), used by 23. Those using more Western styles tended to be older (median age 56, IQR 47–63) than the traditionalists (median age 52, IQR 42.25–57), although not significantly. There was also a higher proportion of males among those using Western styles (72.7%) than those using more traditional methods (65.2%), but again this difference was not significant.

Of those who classed themselves as good responders to acupuncture (Q15), 34 were older than the median age for the sample, and 26 younger, whereas this was reversed for those who considered themselves only as average responders (20 being younger and 15 older than the median age). Those who considered themselves good responders were also more likely than those who thought of themselves as average responders to assess their own patients as good responders (Q16): 65.6% of the former described 80% or 100% of their patients as good responders, as against only 43.2% of the latter (with good responder practitioners correspondingly less likely to describe their patients as poor responders (Q17)). However, none of these differences were significant.

3.2. *The Questions*

3.2.1. Questions Requiring "Yes" or "No" Responses—An Overview

In total, 124 questions required a "Yes" or "No" response. The 60 questions on particular patient characteristics, attitudes or experience could be answered as "What you THINK NOW" and "What you THOUGHT THEN", with "Yes", "No" or "Don't know" responses, and a further four more general questions could be answered simply with "Yes" or "No". A full list of responses for these questions is given in Appendix A.

The 60 specific questions were generally answered in the affirmative, both when considered by respondent and by question (Table 2). This is consistent with the fact that 96 respondents (84.2%) stated that they had previously considered that patient characteristics (such as their temperament or personality traits) might affect their response to treatment (Q9), and that 70 respondents (61.4%) stated their believe that that some patients respond consistently well or poorly to acupuncture, almost regardless of other factors such as the condition treated or their state of health at the time (Q13).

Table 2. Medians and IQRs of "Yes", "No" and "Don't know" (DK) answers to the 60 main survey questions, as percentages of total possible counts (60 by respondent, 114 by question).

"Now" or "Then"	How counted	"Yes" responses	"No" responses	"DK" responses
NOW	By respondent	53.3 (35.4–66.7)	25.0 (8.3–38.3)	15.0 (6.7–29.6)
	By question	53.1 (40.6–62.3)	25.4 (19.5–31.8)	16.2 (12.8–26.5)
THEN	By respondent	42.5 (18.8–63.3)	21.7 (5.0–44.2)	13.3 (1.7–47.9)
	By question	43.9 (35.3–49.8)	25.4 (20.8–33.1)	28.9 (23.7–34.2)

Note: "DK" responses THEN calculated as 60—("Yes" + "No" counts).

There were strong correlations between "Yes" (NOW) and "Yes" (THEN) responses ($r_S = 0.655$, $p < 0.0001$), between "No" (NOW) and "No" (THEN) responses ($r_S = 0.609$, $p < 0.0001$), and between "Yes" and "No" (NOW) responses ($r_S = -0.685$, $p < 0.0001$). There was also a slightly weaker correlation between "Don't know" (NOW) and "Don't know" (THEN) responses ($r_S = 0.487$, $p < 0.0001$), but none between "Yes" and "No" (THEN) responses ($r_S = 0.001$, $p = 0.989$).

3.2.2. On Specific Questions Requiring "Yes" or "No" Responses

Of the 60 questions in the main part of the survey, those in the upper and lower deciles for numbers of "Yes" and "No" scores are shown in Table 3 (with numbers of responses in each case).

Table 3. "Yes", "No" and "Don't know" (DK) responses in the upper and lower deciles for the 60 main survey questions (numbers of responses in brackets). Items shown in bold red type appear in the same deciles both NOW and THEN; those underlined appear in Most "Yes" responses and Least "No" responses (NOW or THEN), or vice versa.

	NOW		THEN	
	Most responses	Fewest responses	Most responses	Fewest responses
Yes	**Willing to follow advice** (101) **Able to relax** (93) **Self-motivated** (90) **Exercise** (89) **Diet** (85) **General health** (85) Openness (85)	**Gender issues** (17) **Ethnicity** (21) **Alexithymia** (21) Education (28) Relnship status (30) (and 4 **others**, [a] tied 31)	**Willing to follow advice** (84) **Exercise** (74) **Able to relax** (73) **General health** (73) **Self-motivated** (72) **Diet** (71)	**Ethnicity** (13) **Alexithymia** (15) **Gender issues** (16) **Character when young** (22) Birth/prenatal (23) **Child poverty** (26)
No	**Gender** (75) **Ethnicity** (74) **Education** (69) **Relnship status** (60) **Age** (59) Sceptical (57)	**Willing to follow advice** (9) Central sensitisn (13) Able to relax (14) Alexithymia (15) Psychotic (15) **Self-motivated** (15)	**Ethnicity** (73) **Gender** (68) **Education** (56) **Relnship status** (53) Gender issues (50) **Age** (47)	**Willing to follow advice** (7) Commitment (14) General health (14) Openness (16) **Self-motivated** (16) Exercise (17)
DK	Alexithymia (78) Gender issues (52) Central sensitsn (51) TCM pattern (47) Child poverty (45) Character when young (44)	Willing to follow advice (5) Able to relax (6) Age (6) Negativity (7) Gender (7) Self-motivated (8)		

[a] *gender, character when young, childhood poverty* and *extraverted/introverted*. Two of these also appear under "Fewest responses (THEN)".

A graphical representation of salient findings for "Yes" and "No" responses is given in Figure 2.

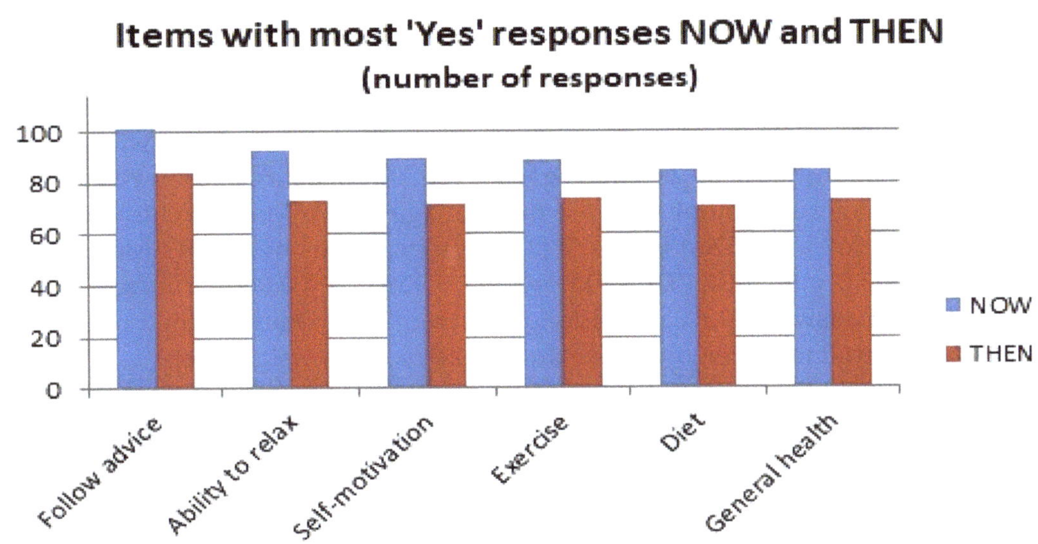

(a)

Figure 2. *Cont.*

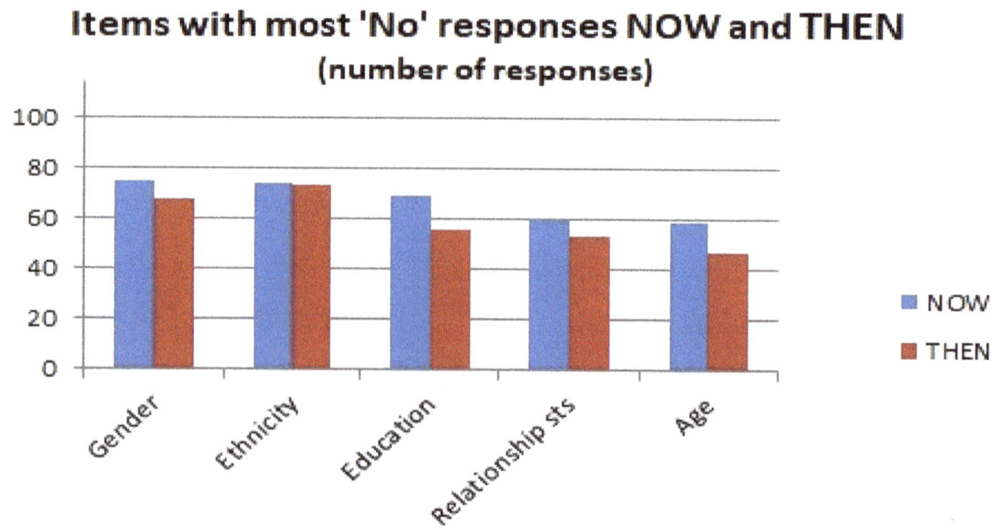

(b)

Figure 2. Salient findings for the "Yes" and "No" responses in Table 3. (**a**): Items with most "Yes" responses; (**b**): Items with most "No" responses.

As for the "Yes" and "No" responses in general, there is thus considerable agreement between the patient characteristics perceived to affect treatment outcome in past clinical practice and at the time of responding.

Attributes most consistently considered to affect response are *willingness to follow advice*, *self-motivation*, *general health status*, *ability to relax*, *exercise* and *diet*. Those most consistently considered *not* to affect response are *patient age*, *gender*, *ethnicity*, *education* and *relationship status* ("Relnship status" in Table 3).

Respondents were least likely to hazard a guess for the somewhat abstract characteristics of *alexithymia* and *central sensitisation* ("Central sensitisn" in Table 3), as well as *gender issues*, *child poverty*, *character when young* and *TCM pattern*.

3.2.3. Respondent Characteristics and Yes/No Responses

Age and Years in Practice

Other than a small negative correlation between respondent age and the number of "No" (THEN) answers given ($r_s = -0.215$, $p = 0.022$), there were no particular correlations between numbers of "Yes" or "No" responses and either respondents' ages or years in practice. However, if the sample was divided into those younger and older than the median age (52), a Mann–Whitney test showed significant differences of "No" and "Don't know" (THEN) responses between older and younger respondents ("No": $U = 903.0$, $p = 0.004$; "Don't know": $U = 928.5$, $p = 0.006$). Younger respondents (THEN) were more likely to answer "No", and older to answer "Don't know" (the same was true for the NOW responses considered together, but these differences were nonsignificant).

These patterns in age differences were significant for responses to ten of the 60 questions (three NOW and seven THEN), with a Kruskal–Wallis test indicating p values < 0.01 for three of them: Birth and prenatal experience (NOW) ($p = 0.008$, $\chi^2 = 9.57$), Housing situation (THEN) ($p = 0.002$, $\chi^2 = 12.19$) and Work situation (NOW) ($p = 0.005$, $\chi^2 = 10.54$).

There were also eight significant differences among responses to specific questions with years in practice (p values < 0.05), those in practice for longer being more likely to consider central sensitisation (both NOW and THEN) a relevant factor, for example, but also less likely to consider optimism (both NOW and THEN) as having an impact on treatment outcome.

Gender

Table 4 illustrates differences in response frequencies by respondent gender.

Table 4. Median numbers of "Yes", "No" and "Don't know" responses for female and male respondents.

	NOW			THEN		
Gender	**Yes**	**No**	**DK**	**Yes**	**No**	**DK**
Female	33 (22–42)	15 (4–21)	10 (4–17)	31 * (15–40)	16 (3–27)	6 * (1–21)
Male	27 (20–36)	15 (6–30)	8 (3–21)	20 * (0–34)	8 (0–27)	19 * (2–59)

Note: "DK" responses THEN calculated as 60—("Yes" + "No" counts); significant differences indicated with (*).

A Mann–Whitney test indicated that significantly more women than men gave "Yes" (THEN) responses (two-tailed significance, $U = 941.5$, $p = 0.007$), but this difference was not significant for the "Yes" (NOW) responses ($p = 0.071$). Conversely, men provided significantly more "Don't know" (THEN) responses (i.e., did not answer these questions) than women ($U = 1000.0$, $p = 0.018$).

One particular question exemplifies this difference between female and male respondents, as shown in Figure 3: most women considered NOW that childhood health could impact treatment response, whereas men generally did not (Pearson's $\chi^2 = 7.30$, $p = 0.026$).

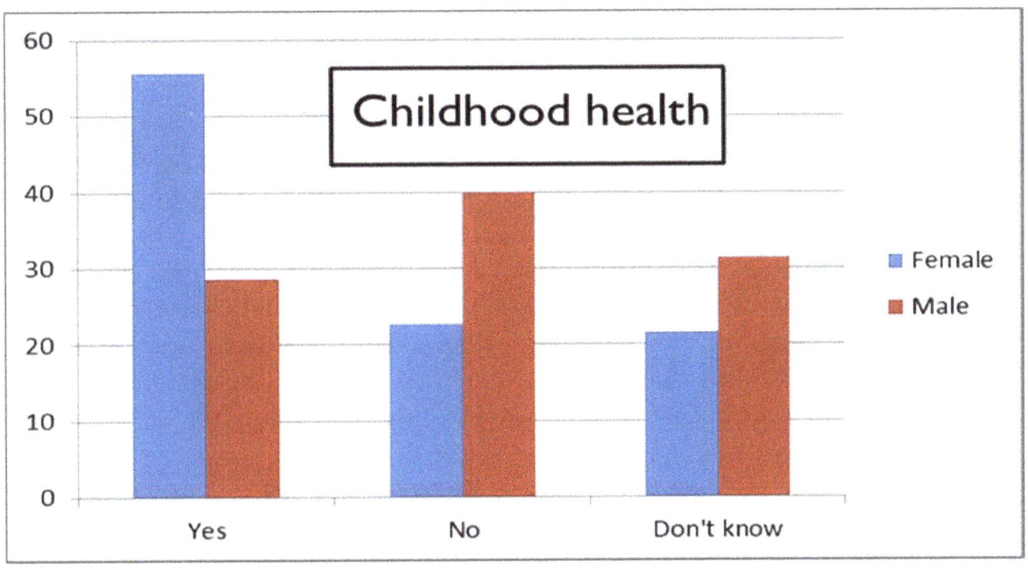

Figure 3. Percentages of female and male respondents giving "Yes", "No", and "Don't know" responses regarding the item on *childhood health* (NOW responses).

A very similar result was found for *family health in the patient's childhood* (Pearson's $\chi^2 = 7.26$, $p = 0.027$). In all there were 11 questions (three NOW, seven THEN) for which female and male responses differed significantly. As in Table 4 for the 60 questions considered together, more males than females replied "Don't know" to these individual questions.

Main Profession

The medical doctors (who were mostly male) gave fewer "Yes" responses than the remainder of the respondents, although a Kruskal–Wallis test showed these difference not to be significant. When ratios of numbers of "Yes" to "No" scores are considered, acupuncturists appear least likely to consider that individual patient characteristics may affect outcome. In contrast, physiotherapists and nurses (including midwives) showed the highest ratio of numbers of "Yes" to "No" scores (both NOW and THEN) (Table 5).

Table 5. Yes-to-No count ratios NOW and THEN, by profession, showing medians and IQRs.

Profession	Yes-To-No Count Ratios NOW	Yes-To-No Count Ratios THEN
Acupuncturists	1.7 (0.9–5.1)	1.4 (0.6–4.9)
Medical doctors	2.3 (2–2.7)	2.4 (1.3–2.5)
Physiotherapists	6.2 (1.8–17.6)	2.9 (1.7–4.1)
Nurses (and midwives)	4.8 (1.3–12.5)	3.5 (2.5–5.1)
Others	2.4 (1.5–2.9)	2.1 (1.0–3.1)

Note: Cases with no "No" responses are omitted, and as this only left one chiropractor, this category was removed from analysis.

Taking only those professions showing the most extreme NOW ratios from the table above (acupuncturists and physiotherapists), responses for the individual questions were examined. Mostly Yes-to-No count ratios were of a similar order and in the same direction for both professions; they were only significantly different and definitively in the opposite direction for one question: religious beliefs or practices ($p = 0.005$, $\chi^2 = 10.41$). All the physiotherapists considered this might be a factor in treatment response, whereas only 33.8% of the acupuncturists did.

Professional Association Membership

BAcC and ATCM members, although all acupuncturists, responded in different ways to this survey. The median ages of those belonging to the two associations were comparable, but, whereas there were equal numbers of female and male ATCM respondents, there were many more female than male BAcC respondents (47 versus 9). The former recorded the most "No" (THEN) responses of any association members (median per member 18.5, IQR 4–28), and the latter the least (median 4.5, IQR 0.8–9.3), a significant difference (p values of between 0.014 and 0.043 using the Mann–Whitney test, depending on analysis of multiple-affiliated respondents). Correspondingly, median Yes-to-No count ratios THEN were highest for ATCM members (although ratios NOW were highest for AACP members). Otherwise, association membership did not appear to have a significant effect on the total number of "Yes", "No" or "Don't know" responses (NOW or THEN). Lowest Yes-to-No count ratios (whether NOW or THEN) were for those stating they belonged to another association than those listed.

Analysing only the THEN responses for ATCM and BAcC members using the same procedure as for acupuncturists and physiotherapists in the previous section, again Yes-to-No count ratios were mostly of a similar order and in the same direction for both groups.

Style of Practice

There were no significant differences in numbers of "Yes" or "No" responses (either NOW or THEN) with style of practice—more "traditional" or more "Western"—although the former tended to respond more definitively (whether with "Yes" or "No") and the latter more with "Don't know" (both NOW and THEN).

Prior Opinion That Patient Characteristics Might Affect Treatment Response

In total, 113 respondents answered the question on whether in the past they had considered that patient characteristics might affect treatment response, 97 of them in the affirmative.

Those who held the prior opinion that patient characteristics might affect their response to treatment were more likely to respond "Yes" to both NOW ($U = 366.0$, $p = 0.001$) and THEN ($U = 480.0$, $p = 0.015$) questions than those who did not, and were correspondingly less likely to give "No" responses.

3.2.4. Associations between the 60 Main Questions in the Survey

There is no unique or perfectly precise way of classifying the 60 questions on individual characteristics that might affect treatment outcome, and the list itself is not exhaustive. An initial attempt was made to group them under 14 different headings, such as early life, social/financial, behavioural attitudes, and so forth. A confirmatory cluster analysis was then undertaken on the basis of these groupings, but did not yield useful results. Therefore, an alternative approach was used, assessing associations among "Yes", "No" and "Don't know" responses for the different questions using χ^2 tests.

These showed strong associations (low p values) between "Yes", "No" and "Don't know" responses for some measures within the anticipated groupings. However, not all of these supported the groupings initially proposed, so that these were adjusted in an attempt to maximise significance of the associations, resulting in the final groupings shown in Appendix A. Even so, some groupings have more explanatory value than others.

The limited convergence of the χ^2 (or phi or Cramer's V) measures of association and the results of the hierarchical cluster analysis for NOW (only 19 of 100 tested associations appearing at the first stage of the agglomeration process) led to the decision not to investigate such a relationship for the THEN questions.

Some of the χ^2 groupings appeared as consecutive questions in the original survey, so this may have swayed respondents to answer similarly. To test this, associations between eight consecutive but unrelated questions were also explored (see Appendix A). The results of this test indicate that just because questions follow each other consecutively, they are not necessarily answered in the same manner.

As for internal consistency, Cronbach's alpha was 0.930 for the NOW responses, and 0.981 for the THEN responses. Removal of individual items did not greatly affect these values—for NOW, alpha ranged from 0.928 to 0.931, and, for THEN, from 0.981 to 0.982.

3.2.5. Agreement between Respondents, Variability and Variance of Responses

Three methods were used to assess the consistency of responses across respondents. Firstly, Randolph's free-marginal multi-rater *kappa* [35,36] was calculated for both NOW and THEN questions and used to derive a measure of "overall agreement" between participants on each question. The questions for which *kappa* exceeded 0.4 (considered at least a moderate level of agreement [37]) are tabulated in Appendix A. Secondly, Shannon Entropy (SE) values were calculated for each question, both NOW and THEN. SE is a measure of the inherent "informativity" (uncertainty or randomness of information) in a given string of data, where higher values indicate more uncertainty or informativity [38]; we have used this approach in previous pilot studies [30,31]. Randolph's *kappa* and SE are corollaries, since they respectively measure agreement and variability in a data sample. This was reflected by extremely strong negative correlations between *kappa* (or overall agreement) and SE across all questions in both NOW and THEN responses ($r_s \leq -0.998$, $p < 0.0001$). This pattern is shown graphically in Appendix A. A third measure, a non-parametric version of coefficient of variance (CV), defined as inter-quartile range divided by the median and multiplied by 100, produced significant correlations in the variance of both "Yes" and "No" responses between NOW and THEN ($r_s = 0.870$ and 0.632, $p < 0.0001$ and $p = 0.006$), but was omitted from further analysis due to its lack of convergence with *kappa* or SE (correlations ns).

When individual questions were considered, there was considerable overlap with the previous analysis of "Yes", "No" and "Don't know" response frequencies outlined in Table 3 (Section 3.2.2). Only two questions with lowest inter-rater agreement (or greatest SE) appear in that table, both under "DK" responses. Thus, our analysis of respondent agreement (or variability) tallies with our previous analysis of consistency of response by question.

3.2.6. Patterns in Survey Completion Assessed from Numbers of "Yes", "No" and "Don't know" Answers

There are clear trends in the numbers of "Yes" and "No" responses to the 60 main questions over the course of the survey, with considerable agreement between the NOW and THEN responses, but rather less pronounced trends in the numbers of "Don't know" responses (Figure 4).

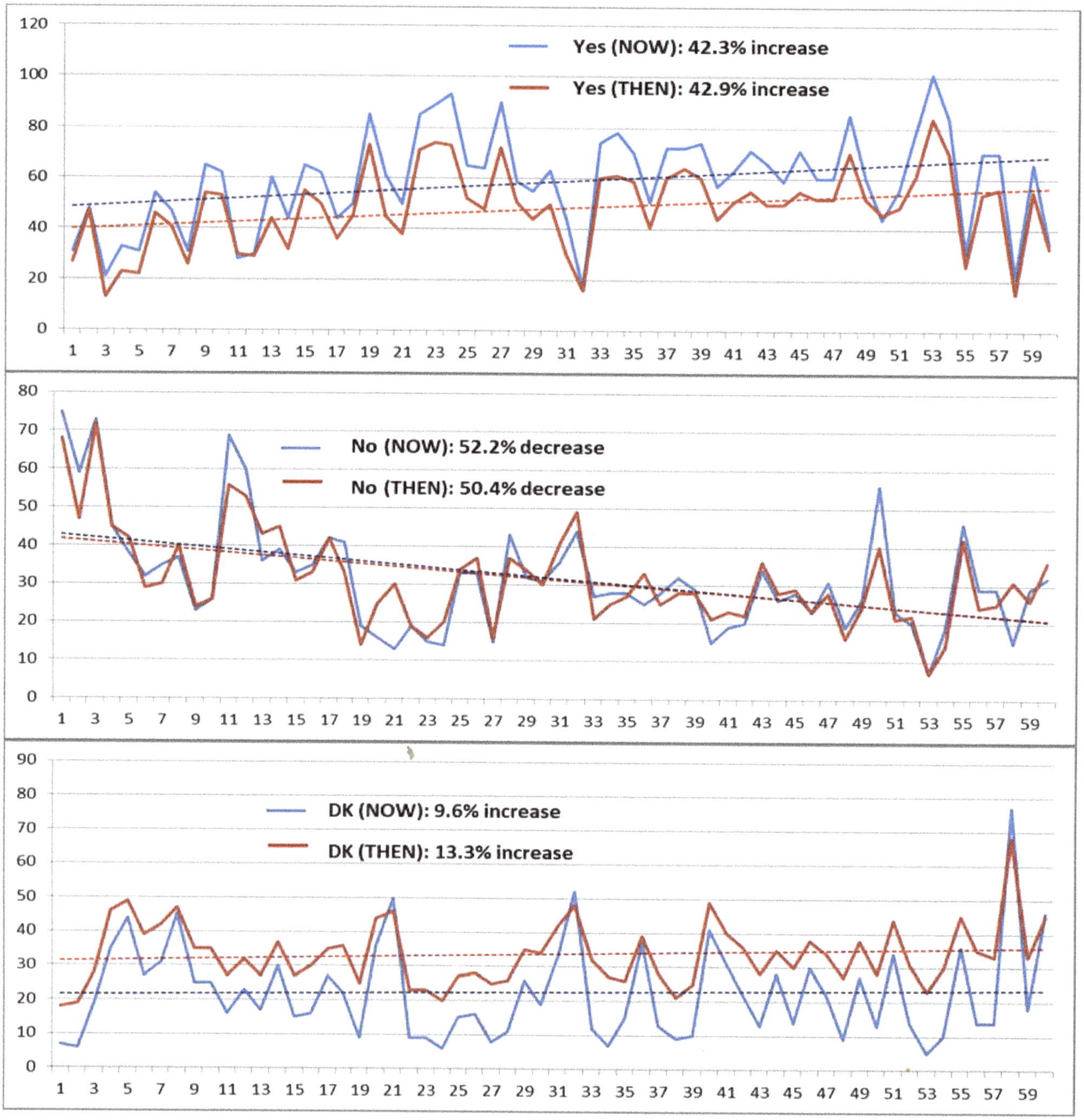

Figure 4. Changes in numbers of "Yes", "No" and "Don't know" responses to the 60 main questions over the course of the survey completing them.

When variability values were computed for four consecutive quarters of the main questions (1–15, 16–30, etc.), a similar pattern was observed, with 95.3% and 80.0% overall increases in the *kappa* values for NOW and THEN questions between the first and last quarter, but generally smaller corresponding changes in SE and non-parametric CV (npCV).

3.3. Thematic Analysis of Free-Text Responses

Respondents providing qualitative responses are self-selecting participants; by first ticking a box to indicate understanding of a question's underlying premise ("Yes", "No", "Don't know"), and then deciding at each free-text prompt whether to provide further information, respondents declare buy-in at two levels. Simple counts of the number of responses made to each question (Figure 5) show where this second level of buy-in is strongest.

The maximum number of free-text responses to any survey item was 106, and the minimum 1 (median 10, IQR 7–13). The maximum number of free-text responses for any respondent was 65, and the minimum 0 (median 5, IQR 4–10), as shown in Figure 5. In what follows, respondents are identified by number (from 1 to 114), and the questions to which they respond by their alphanumeric code (from 9.a to 20); thus, "11.4.c/63" refers to Respondent 63's answer to question 11.4.c.

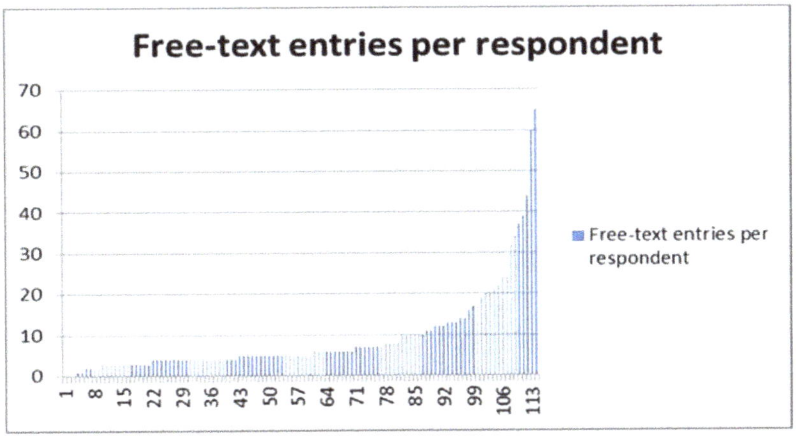

Figure 5. Free-text entries across all parts of the survey, shown in ascending order by respondent.

Questions that elicited the most free-text responses were the general questions (9, 15, 18 and 19), with fewest in the areas of *resilience* (3 responses), *self-regulation* (3), *suggestibility* (3) and *extraversion–introversion* (1).

It is perhaps unsurprising that Question 9, the first and most fundamental question—"Before you knew about this survey, did you ever consider that patient characteristics (such as their temperament or personality traits) might affect their response to treatment?"—elicited the largest number of responses (94/114), indicating a perceived need for qualification of the key issue at the outset. Some respondents pick out a single characteristic to highlight here—for example, "calm" patients (9.a/68) are deemed more responsive, "anxious or hostile" (9.a/66) or "depressed and negative" patients (9.a/71) less so. Variation in response intensity is allowed, with some patients identified as "super responders" (9.a/100).

This questionnaire deliberately uses the distinction between the general and the particular, asking respondents to both consider their general opinion at the time of responding, and give deliberately separate consideration to their opinion of a specific patient interaction in the past. A response of "Don't know" is only possible in the "NOW" answers, demanding concrete judgment of the evoked historical event.

Some characteristics are in themselves symptoms or medical conditions and could be the reason for treatment being sought—e.g., anxiety, depression. One respondent highlights this with a repeat response—"depends if this is a symptom/being treated" (verbatim at 11.4.c/63, 11.5.c/63, 11.19.c/63).

Respondents' comments about patient response are predicated on their own understanding of what "response" means in this context. Notions of "response" are unpacked in the introductory matter for the survey, with a range of meanings suggested encompassing improvement in symptoms and changes in wellbeing and quality of life. However, no formal definition of a "good" or "poor" response or responder was provided.

Texts were extracted from the optional free-text fields to a spreadsheet for thematic analysis. Whilst these texts are researcher-instigated data, they have been generated independently by respondents without the researcher present and so remain subjective, "re-presentations of reality rather than simply true or false" [39] (p. 275). These occupy a middle ground within the continuum of qualitative data between the "gold standard" interview and "naturally occurring" texts such as transcribed conversations and fieldnotes [40] (pp. 669–670). We allow that unique statements have as much potential importance as frequently-found words [41].

A relatively informal approach to analysis was appropriate, as "the qualitative text analysis is not at the core of the research but instead is in a subsidiary or complementary role" [40] (p. 670). Immersion in the data led to emergence of themes, illustrated below by means of in vivo quotes. Mason's tripartite levels of analysis were used to arrange the themes at literal, interpretive, and reflexive levels [42] (p. 180) to gain understanding of what acupuncturists think about their patients' identity as "responders" to acupuncture. These themes apply axially across the different question areas [43].

3.3.1. Literal Analysis

Literal analysis assigns literal meaning to statements. Many emergent literal themes (indicated here in italics) in the present data directly stem from specific topic areas established in the survey.

Questions about the impact of *gender* and *age* on response elicit high levels of response (23 responses to each, the second-highest count amongst all the free-text responses). There is broad consensus that women are better responders than men, and younger patients better than older (for multiple examples, see the data repository at http://www.mdpi.com/2305-6320/5/3/85/s1). Respondent 99 is a lone voice opining that neither gender nor age affects response (10.1.c/99 and 10.2.c/99).

By contrast, there is no consensus on the effect of *ethnicity* on response, and only 11 responses are made, perhaps indicating that responder fatigue is already in play by this point in the survey [44].

Of the 15 free-text responses offered in relation to *work*, seven mention *stress*.

Childhood aspects are important for a small set of respondents, but as the factors listed multiply, answers become less specific, with certain respondents opting for generic "Ibid"-type responses (see, for example, 10.6.c/45 and 10.6.c/70, and Respondent 5's generic approach to all answers). Others rephrase ideas already expressed in connection with the age question, perhaps indicating some theoretical saturation and respondent fatigue as well as consistency of views. Some respondents may not have been able to make subtle distinctions between overlapping categories such as *self-motivation* and *optimism*, *self-efficacy* and *resilience*—in some cases declaredly so, despite the provision of glossary information in the survey itself.

An important outcome of the present survey is an update to the acupuncture profession's perceived *scope of expertise* as represented by the list of conditions that these practitioners find respond well to acupuncture. There is strong consensus around certain conditions, including musculoskeletal problems, anxiety, depression, irritable bowel syndrome (IBS), headaches and chronic pain conditions (see data repository for full details). There is clear overlap between this list and the "effectiveness gaps" identified in UK GP care over a decade ago [45], and also with those conditions identified as having the strongest published evidence for the effectiveness of acupuncture [46].

3.3.2. Interpretive Analysis

Interpretive analysis assigns contextualised meaning to statements. Emergent themes are again indicated here in italics.

Paired polarised positions of *belief* and *scepticism* are given as baseline patient characteristics for some respondents, with general consensus that belief improves response, although the premise is also contested—"Belief is irrelevant" (9.a/11), "non believers can get the same benefit as well!" (9.a/21). Belief finds 69 direct mentions in the data and can also be discerned in "softened" forms such as expectation of positive outcome (9.a/5) and willingness to engage (9.a/34). Scepticism (24 mentions) is depicted as an undesirable starting-point characteristic which acupuncture treatment can shift—"attitude changes with improvement in their condition" (9.a/114). A reinforcing cycle of improved outcomes with increased buy-in to the system responsible is perceived, and acupuncture's capacity to potentiate *positive change* and enhance *self-efficacy* is acknowledged as it is in current literature [47]. Respondent 43 (amongst others) is repeatedly concerned with acupuncture's impact on individuals' *ability to cope*, emphasising that this is a more important factor than changes to symptoms, in particular pain levels (see, for e.g., 10.12.c/43 and 10.13.c/43).

Placebo finds frequent mention both as a pejorative and as a self-evident absolute—"Positivity helps the placebo response" (9.a/40). Individual respondents' understanding of and political attitude towards the term influences response. Debate on the elusive nature of a plausible inert placebo for use in clinical trials of acupuncture is not new [48]. Superficial needling or the application of non-penetrative devices to acupuncture points is recognised to stimulate these points in a manner equitable to a lower dose of the same treatment [49,50] and subsequent research in this area has led to the development of pragmatic trial models which assess the effectiveness of acupuncture treatment against active comparators in ecologically valid settings [51,52]. Awareness of this context is discernible in many responses here.

Appearing in relation to hypochondria (now more formally known as "illness anxiety disorder"), and elsewhere, the notion of *sick role* is important to several respondents, with reference to patients who "may not want to get well" (11.20.c/37), "have an identity with being ill" (11.20.c/109) or even "a victim complex" (9.a/77). Notions of belief are again in play—"some people are clearly stuck in the 'sick role' mindset and therefore physically get better but don't believe they are" (9.a/30).

The experience of appropriately-placed experts is being deliberately sought by this survey, so evocation of the *theoretical knowledge base* particular to the profession is perhaps inevitable: "more metal types can be more resistant" (9.a/29). *Specialisms* appear too, with Respondent 74 focusing on pregnancy and Respondent 43 on chronic pain. Information being elicited is to some degree held as *self-evident*—"anyone qualified would know this as part of their studies if not common sense" (9.a/27), "pretty obvious" (10.8.c/45).

Individual patient diagnosis emerges as a priority with regard to response/non-response, with consensus found across many areas and specifically with regard to depression (see, for example, 11.18.c/4 and 11.18.c/18) that the innate and unique characteristics of each individual patient are the deciding factor with regard to response level. There are repeated pleas for the diagnostic specificity of the medicine (such as Respondent 63's answers above) and acknowledgement of the non-specific treatment effects known to accompany it [47,53,54].

3.3.3. Reflexive Analysis

Reflexive analysis assigns reflexive meaning to statements. In this context, this analysis considers the data in relation to the acupuncture profession as a whole. Emergent themes are again indicated here in italics.

Belief reappears in the form of witness-type statements when respondents are asked about themselves as responders, with 18 counts of "I believe" as well as mentions of "faith". Pseudo-religious language may stem from the acupuncture profession's self-identification as distinct, special and "other". This question also prompts *ego*-driven statements: "since I started practising I've become quite adept at predicting who will respond well based on the initial consultation" (9.a/82).

Consideration of *Belief* and *scepticism* may have roots in the dichotomy-driven nature of Traditional Chinese Medicine theory. Thirty-two responses detail specific TCM/5-element diagnostic patterns, again indicating recourse to the *theoretical knowledge base* of the profession. Evocation of the particulars of a medicine system about which respondents are passionate indicates a desire to establish professional *credibility* and *expertise*. This is in places wielded with discernible *defensiveness* against the survey instrument, the questions, and the non-responsive *sick role* patient, who is "never satisfied" (11.20.c/30) and "not quite engaged into getting well" (9.a/39). Focus on *scepticism* may indicate a defensiveness on behalf of a medicine seen as contested—"there is always an element of you having to prove yourself continually" (9.a/49): "Some patients seem to be self sabotaging and come convinced that acupuncture does not work" (9.a/54). *Judgmental language* permeates the discourse of certain individuals (e.g., Respondent 43).

The response trajectory of specific individual *respondent personalities* can be traced through the data set. Respondent 45, a 69 year old male, gives 65 free-text answers, the maximum number of free-text responses by any respondent (minimum = 1, median = 5). Respondent 45 establishes a distinctive "voice" early on, taking issue with the fundamental premise of the endeavour—"characteristics such as temperament or personality traits seem a little fuzzy to me" (9.a/45), and succumbing to petulant exasperation later on—"I repeat: a patient with a healthy, balanced qi will respond better to acupuncture treatment and vice versa" (10.8.c/45). Respondent 45's desire to return to a repeated universal answer reiterates his perception of the universality of the medicine he practises. When asked about factors like housing and work, he consistently holds that these things have relevance only insofar as they "affect the state of the person's qi" (verbatim at 10.14.c/45 and 10.15.c/45).

45 personifies the survey instrument, adopting a tone of debate with the researcher, who is assigned an assumed medicopolitical stance—"all actions (external, internal, emotional, etc.) that affect the state of our qi, blood, jing, shen, etc. will have an effect on how we function, both in the language of CM or that of biomedical science, which you seem to favour" (11.1.c/45).

4. Discussion

This study resulted in several unexpected and useful findings. The first of these (Figure 1) is that it may clearly be useful, when survey uptake is flagging, to remind potential respondents of its existence. Another finding on recruitment (Table 1) is that members of the smaller professional associations were more likely to take the survey, suggesting that personal contact with association staff may be an important factor in increasing uptake. Even so, only 114 people completed the survey out of more than 12,000 potential respondents, an uptake of less than one percent. However, in this age of internet marketing, low response rates are not uncommon. As another organiser of acupuncture surveys has stated, "The number of acupuncture practitioners who respond to electronic surveys tends to be disappointing, but reasons are unclear why this is so" [55]. Personal contact may always be useful, but equally may bias responses.

Considerably more women than men took the survey (Section 3.1), as in our previous survey on electroacupuncture usage, where this was particularly true for UK respondents [33]. Again, as in the earlier survey, male respondents outnumbered females among medical doctors and chiropractors (osteopaths in the earlier survey), although numbers were too small for this to reach significance. Medical doctors tended to be older, and physiotherapists younger, than the majority of survey respondents. It is possible that those doctors that did respond had an interest in the subject matter of the survey because of early contact or training with the doyens of medical acupuncture who first proposed the notions of "strong reactor" and "good responder". Acupuncturists often enter the profession as a second career, but for physiotherapists acupuncture is usually an add-on to their first main career, so it makes sense that physiotherapists would be the youngest group.

A high proportion (84.2%) of respondents stated that in the past (before they knew about this survey) they had considered that patient characteristics might affect their response to treatment (Section 3.2.1). Correspondingly, the vast majority of individual THEN and NOW questions were given "Yes" answers. This suggests that responses to the main body of the survey were generally made in a manner congruent with existing practitioner attitudes, rather than being arbitrary. The qualitative evidence indicating clear conceptual understanding of relevant patient characteristics supports this, also suggesting that the respondents answered with reference to theoretical frameworks central to their practice (Section 3.3). The fact that respondents generally did not make suggestions for additional attributes that ought to be included suggests that the "long-list" of 60 questions was quite comprehensive in terms of the factors readily encountered in a treatment context.

The overall positive correlation between "NOW" and "THEN" responses may be driven by various factors, including a simple tendency to tick the same box twice while completing the survey (response perseveration). Although it is of course possible that previous clinical experience heavily shapes later attitudes (i.e., a true similarity between what they thought THEN and NOW), it is difficult to conclude this from the current data alone, since the clinical context(s) on the basis of which practitioners made their THEN judgments were not controlled. More recently qualified practitioners (50 of 114 within the last 10 years) may have made these judgments in a very different manner from those who have had both greater subsequent experience and longer to forget!

The specific questions that elicited most and fewest responses (Section 3.2.2) merit particular attention. Those characteristics/behaviours which were most often considered to impact on treatment outcome (Table 3) included what acupuncture author Bob Flaws once called "the three frees"—relaxation, diet and exercise—but also *self-motivation*, *willingness to follow advice* given, *general state of health* and *openness* to new experiences. In the HRV literature on acupuncture, parasympathetic activation or an improvement in sympathovagal balance is often found to result from acupuncture treatment [56–58], so a pre-existing ability to relax could facilitate this. The remaining items are all quite straightforward and easy to interpret in the context of acupuncture, where for instance patients less open to new experiences are presumably less likely to procure treatment in the first place.

The items judged least often to impact outcome included age and gender. Statements are often found in the paediatric acupuncture literature [59,60] to the effect that children tend to respond particularly well, but at the other end of the age spectrum there appears to be little information available on whether elderly patients respond better or worse than those in their middle years, despite the existence of many studies on the use of acupuncture for conditions of old age. This is in sharp contrast with the qualitative findings, where many of the free-text comments regarding patient age and gender emphasised their general significance for treatment response—with younger and female patients perceived as likely to respond better to acupuncture. It is important to qualify this apparently contradictory result by noting that, although both were relatively popular items for free-text commentary, only 23 qualitative responses were given regarding patient age and gender across 114 respondents.

There was considerable agreement that relationship status per se does not have much effect on responsiveness to acupuncture, although arguments could be made that a lack of close satisfactory relationship(s) is likely to affect general health as well as the practitioner-patient relationship [28]. Other general characteristics such as level of education and ethnicity were also thought to have little effect on treatment outcome. It is certainly of interest that 50% of respondents were of the opinion that scepticism does not affect outcome—implying a lack of consensus from a quantitative perspective. The qualitative data help to clarify this by showing distinct schools of thought about the impact of *belief* in the treatment technique, with some mentioning a positive impact, while most respondents acknowledged that patients show different levels of scepticism—whether it is influential on treatment outcomes.

Items about which respondents were least certain included *alexithymia* and *central sensitisation* (which may be unfamiliar or difficult to grasp), *gender issues* (which have only become salient *zeitgeist* issues fairly recently), and *TCM* or *Five-element* pattern. It was unexpected that this last item should appear here, as both models differentiate diagnostic categories by their expected response to treatment: dampness and phlegm are considered relatively difficult to treat in TCM, for instance [61]. Theoretical constructs such as the three major blocks to treatment, namely "possession", "husband/wife imbalance" and "aggressive energy" [62], further imply that choice of theoretical framework may have an impact on how patient characteristics are expected to influence treatment response.

All in all, only around 20 items appear in Table 3; there was no clear convergence of opinion among respondents about the remaining two-thirds of the questions. The groupings for which the lowest proportions of items were included in the table are shown in Table A20 in Appendix A. Those groupings which produced least consensus (from which fewest items are therefore included in Table 3) were

4 (Trauma), 6 (Beliefs/attitudes), 5 (Social/financial) and particularly 12 (Psychological attitudes 1), whereas those producing the clearest consensus were 1 (Demographic 1), 2 (Demographic 2), 7 (Lifestyle) and 15 (Behavioural attitudes).

It may well be the case that groupings where respondents did not show clear consensus include items which really do have little impact on treatment outcome, and those where they concurred, items which do have an impact. However, it is also possible that acupuncture practitioners in general may not be trained to have sufficient awareness of the impacts on health and recovery of such things as social and financial situations [63] and psychological attitude [64,65]. This gap in knowledge may be pertinent for those who design acupuncture training courses (especially those for continuing professional education).

There was some variation in response patterns between groups of practitioners (Section 3.2.3). For example, younger respondents (i.e., those earlier in their acupuncture careers) were more likely than their elders to discount particular patient characteristics as having a possible impact on treatment outcome, whereas older respondents (those likely to have had more experience of actual practice) were less decided (Age and Years in Practice). This may in part be due to changes in acupuncture education over the years, with younger/more recently trained practitioners placing more emphasis on core protocols and theory; older practitioners, on the other hand, may have had less information-rich instruction and so more of a desire to explore for themselves. However, such an interpretation is conjectural, and would need to be confirmed with further investigation. Furthermore, male respondents appeared slightly less inclined than female respondents to consider particular patient characteristics as having a possible impact on treatment outcome. This gender difference was significant for several specific questions (Gender). Medical doctors (who were mostly male) gave fewer "Yes" responses than the remainder of the respondents, physiotherapists and nurses more; physiotherapists were unanimous in their view that *religious beliefs or practices* might be a factor in treatment response, as against only a third of the acupuncturists (Main Profession); however, this could be a chance finding, the result of small sample size and asking a large number of questions, and should certainly not be taken to imply that physiotherapists have a fundamentally more positive view on the influence of religious beliefs.

The differences in survey responses between BAcC and ATCM members are intriguing (Professional Association Membership). In addition to the observed difference in gender profile in the two groups of respondents, it is worth noting that ATCM members are mostly TCM doctors trained in China. As already discussed, (Western) medical doctors tended to give fewer affirmative responses than non-doctors, but there is perhaps a greater tendency to conformity among Chinese than Western practitioners, which may have influenced their responses [66]. Style of practice (Style of Practice) and prior opinion that patient characteristics might affect treatment response (Prior Opinion That Patient Characteristics Might Affect Treatment Response) did not appear to affect survey responses in any striking or unexpected ways.

Different methods of grouping the questions were attempted (Section 3.2.4), from prima facie to cluster analysis to χ^2 tests. A compromise set of 17 groupings, using three methods, was arrived at, and performed well (using χ^2 tests) against a set of unrelated but consecutive questions in the survey, indicating that the groupings were not simply the result of perseveration of responses over strings of questions (Appendix A). When numbers of "Yes", "No" and "Don't know" responses for the groupings were calculated, as a generalisation, respondents appear to have considered Lifestyle, Stress/relaxation and Behavioural attitudes as having more of an impact on treatment outcomes than Early life, Attitudes to religion or nature, basic Demographics and some of the more complex (less behavioural) issues such as *attachment* or *central sensitisation*, which clearly did not strike a chord with many respondents.

This again perhaps suggests a lack of awareness of some less behavioural psychological perspectives on health among acupuncture practitioners.

Three measures of consistency of response were explored (Section 3.2.5), namely Randolph's free-marginal multi-rater *kappa*, Shannon entropy (SE) and a novel non-parametric equivalent of the coefficient of variation (npCV). As expected from their complementary mathematical basis, *kappa* and SE values showed strong negative correlations.

Surprisingly, given its origin in information theory, SE has rarely been used in the analysis of questionnaire responses, with only two relevant citations found in PubMed [67,68], although the long-term dynamics of questionnaire mood responses have been studied using a similar measure, *approximate entropy* [69]. To our knowledge, this is the first time that an explicit association between SE and *kappa* has been reported, although given that the former is a measure of response variability and the latter of agreement, the negative correlation between them would be expected. Indeed, SE-based measures of consensus and dissention for Likert scale data have been suggested before [70,71], although they do not appear to have been used except by their originators. For both datasets (NOW and THEN), a *kappa* value of 0.4 corresponds to SE of 1.02; thus, an intermediate or better value of *kappa*, using Fleiss's definitions, corresponds to a SE of 1.02 or less. Conversely, an SE of 1 corresponds to a *kappa* value of 0.41–0.42. This suggests a useful rule of thumb for interrogating questionnaire SE data, and further avenues for exploring relationships between other measures of inter-rater agreement and measures of entropy.

In contrast to the very strong inverse association between *kappa* and SE, correlations between npCV and *kappa* or SE were not significant. Thus, npCV measures a different construct from the other two methods. Further research will be needed to determine if it is useful in the context of analysing questionnaire or survey responses.

Survey fatigue is suggested by the trending of "Yes" and "No" responses over the course of the survey (Section 3.2.6), although numbers of "Don't know" responses did not increase markedly, as can sometimes occur when respondents experience fatigue [72]. Increases in *kappa*, as well as decreases in SE and (for the most part) npCV, also suggest that participants were fatigued by the end of the survey, perhaps tending to fall into a pattern of repeating responses without giving each question due attention.

This was indeed a long survey for people to take, and it is not known how many of those targeted started but did not complete it, or did not even contemplate taking the survey because the topic did not interest them. Many of the questions may have seemed irrelevant, strange or even bewildering to some acupuncture practitioners unfamiliar with the vast literature on other therapeutic approaches or the sociology of health. It may indeed be "a waste of time" (as one respondent put it) to try to determine whether individual characteristics or attributes can affect response to acupuncture in general, but results from our other pilot studies are encouraging, and the results of this survey, together with those from Phase B of this project, will be useful in designing Phase C before, we hope, moving on to a prospective study to investigate the question of whether good and poor responders to acupuncture can be predicted in advance from their psychometric or other data.

Looking at the qualitative arm alone, the existence of "good responders" appears confirmed by this survey of opinion—with some areas of consensus as to the nature of that "good response" and an understanding that it can vary in intensity.

The acupuncturists who responded to this survey appear to have clear concepts of the characteristics that contribute to their patients' response to acupuncture treatment—although probably for a variety of reasons—and found a range of ways to link these characteristics to the core theoretical base of their medicine. Individual variation is a priority. Acupuncture treatment is characterised by these respondents as a collaborative endeavour which builds self-efficacy in a cycle of reinforcement and has an important preventative aspect. The agendas of both individuals and the whole of the profession they represent can be discerned in these texts [40] (p. 686).

5. Conclusions

The main conclusions from this study are:

1 If appropriate, reminders sent out a few weeks before a survey is closed could well increase uptake. Authors of acupuncture surveys should not expect enthusiastic uptake unless their survey is of particular relevance to their pool of potential respondents. In addition, members of smaller professional organisations may be more likely to respond than those of larger acupuncture associations.

2 Practitioner age and gender influence how they view the importance of patient characteristics, as do the practitioner's main profession and potentially their own ethnicity.

3 Attributes most consistently reported to affect treatment outcome were diet, exercise and the ability to relax (Bob Flaws' "Three frees"), together with general health, self-motivation and a willingness to follow advice.

4 However, a lack of awareness of more complex or difficult psychological and social issues may have skewed the current findings, obscuring the potential importance of some less obvious attributes.

5 Attempts to group characteristics according to item response patterns met with limited success, perhaps relating to the aforementioned skewing.

6 Survey fatigue was observed in terms of numbers of "Yes" and "No" responses, as well as changes in response variability, over the course of completing the survey.

7 Qualitative data may support different and subtler conclusions regarding acupuncturists' appreciation of factors influencing their practice. A key example here is the varying views on belief and scepticism, which "fall through the net" of the quantitative arm of the study.

Limitations

This is a relatively small survey with a relatively large number of questions. It is also not known to what extent responses represent those of the population of UK acupuncture practitioners as a whole, or, of course, whether the results of the survey are transferrable to other populations (e.g., chiropractors, or acupuncture practitioners in other countries). Furthermore, respondents were asked about some individual characteristics and attributes about which they may have had little prior knowledge. Results should therefore be interpreted with caution. In addition, qualitative responses were optional and in many cases not given—whereas the picture provided by the quantitative data appears more comprehensive.

A serious problem with the survey—as with any survey—is that the outcomes reflect the respondents' own characteristics, attributes, and bias. The results should therefore be considered as representing trends in practitioner opinion—a first step towards further confirmatory research, and not necessarily as truly representative of patient characteristics and attributes that may underlie their responsiveness to acupuncture. Nonetheless, we hope that the results of this survey will help practitioners gain insight into their patients' responses in the clinical setting.

It is also important to note that this paper does not establish true impacts on responsiveness to acupuncture, but it does not intend to; in fact, it is preliminary to other studies which will actually investigate the effects of a subset of the characteristics currently explored.

Author Contributions: D.F.M. drafted the survey wording, organised recruitment for the survey, carried out much of the quantitative analysis and prepared the first draft of this paper. L.S.M. conducted the qualitative analysis of free-text responses. J.H.C.M. carried out additional analysis, and edited and rewrote the article.

Acknowledgments: The very helpful staff at the acupuncture associations and training institutions involved in recruiting their members for this project and for good-humouredly sending out reminders to them when asked, and of course all the respondents themselves for taking the time to answer quite a lengthy online survey; The eFocus Group who assisted with survey design, wording and piloting (Ashley Bennett, Mark Bovey, Karen

Charlesworth, Amy Din, Diana Ernaelsteen, Roz Gibbs, Bea Masters and Tony Steffert); Amanda Apponyi, for sharing her recollections of Felix Mann; Justus Randolph, for assistance in calculating his free-marginal multi-rater *kappa*, and for an enlightening discussion on the relationship between this measure and Shannon entropy (Personal communication, 11 June 2018); Neil Spencer for his view of this relationship (Personal communication, 22 June 2018); Nicola Robinson for her comment about acupuncture surveys; and the anonymous reviewers (and Mark Bovey) who judiciously helped to reshape this article; and of course our families for continuing to support us in our never-ending research projects are gratefully acknowledged.

Appendix A

Groupings of the 60 main questions in the survey.

Seventeen groupings were selected based on strong χ^2 associations (low p values) among "Yes", "No" and "Don't know" responses for the measures within them. However, despite adjustments to maximise p values, some questions remain uneasy bedfellows, such as the items in the "Trauma" grouping (Table A4), whereas others could be included in several different groupings (see, for example, the Note to Table A14, "Psychological characteristics"). The corresponding agglomeration stage for each NOW association was assessed from a dendrogram of a nine-stage confirmatory cluster analysis (using the hierarchical method, Ward's method and squared Euclidean distances), and is indicated in each of Tables A1–A17 by an asterisk and the stage number for each association.

Table A1. Demographic 1.

NOW	Gender	Ethnicity	Education
Gender		<0.0001 [*1]	<0.0001 [*2]
Ethnicity			<0.0001 [*2]
Education			
THEN	**Gender**	**Ethnicity**	**Education**
Gender		<0.0001	<0.0001
Ethnicity			<0.0001
Education			

[*1]: Agglomeration stage 1; [*2]: Agglomeration stage 2.

Table A2. Demographic 2.

NOW	Age	General Health
Age		0.001 [*3]
General health		
THEN	**Age**	**General Health**
Age		<0.0001
General health		

[*3]: Agglomeration stage 3.

Table A3. Early life.

NOW	Birth/Prenatal	Characteristics	Health	Family Health	Poverty
Birth/prenatal		<0.0001 [*3]	<0.0001 [*2]	<0.0001 [*2]	<0.0001 [*1]
Characteristics			<0.0001 [*3]	<0.0001 [*3]	<0.0001 [*3]
Health				<0.0001 [*1]	<0.0001 [*2]
Family health					<0.0001 [*2]
Poverty					
THEN	**Birth/Prenatal**	**Characteristics**	**Health**	**Family Health**	**Poverty**
Birth/prenatal		<0.0001	<0.0001	<0.0001	<0.0001
Characteristics			<0.0001	<0.0001	<0.0001
Health				<0.0001	<0.0001
Family health					<0.0001
Poverty					

[*1]: Agglomeration stage 1; [*2]: Agglomeration stage 2; [*3]: Agglomeration stage 3.

Table A4. Trauma.

NOW	Early Trauma	Later Trauma	Past Invasive Med
Early trauma		<0.0001 *[1]	0.023 *[4]
Later trauma			0.045 *[4]
Past invasive med			
THEN	**Early Trauma**	**Later Trauma**	**Past Invasive Med**
Early trauma		<0.0001	<0.0001
Later trauma			<0.0001
Past invasive med			

*[1]: Agglomeration stage 1; *[4]: Agglomeration stage 4.

Table A5. Social/financial.

NOW	Relationship	Soc Support	Housing	Work	Finances
Relationship		<0.0001 *[4]	<0.0001 *[4]	<0.0001 *[4]	<0.0001 *[4]
Soc support			<0.0001 *[2]	<0.0001 *[2]	<0.0001 *[2]
Housing				<0.0001 *[2]	<0.0001 *[2]
Work					<0.0001 *[1]
Finances					
THEN	**Relationship**	**Soc Support**	**Housing**	**Work**	**Finances**
Relationship		<0.0001	<0.0001	<0.0001	<0.0001
Soc support			<0.0001	<0.0001	<0.0001
Housing				<0.0001	<0.0001
Work					<0.0001
Finances					

*[1]: Agglomeration stage 1; *[2]: Agglomeration stage 2; *[4]: Agglomeration stage 4.

Table A6. Beliefs/attitudes.

NOW	Religion	Nature/Technology
Religion		<0.0001 *[2]
Nature/technology		
THEN	**Religion**	**Nature/Technology**
Religion		<0.0001
Nature/technology		

*[2]: Agglomeration stage 2.

Table A7. Lifestyle.

NOW	Nutrition	Exercise
Nutrition		<0.0001 *[1]
Exercise		
THEN	**Nutrition**	**Exercise**
Nutrition		<0.0001
Exercise		

*[1]: Agglomeration stage 1.

Table A8. Hypothalamic–pituitary–adrenal axis 1: Stress and relaxation.

NOW	SensStress	Anxiety	RelaxAbil
SensStress		<0.0001 *1	0.002 *4
Anxiety			<0.0001 *4
RelaxAbil			
THEN	**SensStress**	**Anxiety**	**RelaxAbil**
SensStress		<0.0001	<0.0001
Anxiety			<0.0001
RelaxAbil			

*1: Agglomeration stage 1; *4: Agglomeration stage 4.

Table A9. Hypothalamic–pituitary–adrenal axis 2: "Central sensitisation" and biochemistry.

NOW	CentrSens	Neuroch
CentrSens		<0.0001 *1
Neuroch		
THEN	**CentrSens**	**Neuroch**
CentrSens		<0.0001
Neuroch		

*1: Agglomeration stage 1.

Table A10. Somatisation (MUS), catastrophising, hypochondria and psychosis.

NOW	MUS	Catastr	Hypoch	Psychosis [a]
MUS		<0.0001 *4	0.001 *4	0.002 *4
Catastr			<0.0001 *1	<0.0001 *2
Hypoch				<0.0001 *2
Psychosis				
THEN	**MUS**	**Catastr**	**Hypoch**	**Psychosis**
MUS		<0.0001	<0.0001	<0.0001
Catastr			<0.0001	<0.0001
Hypoch				<0.0001
Psychosis				

[a] This may not appear the most likely grouping to include Psychosis, but, although it fits naturally in "Psychological characteristics" (#14 below), p is high at 0.010 for its association with Extravert/introvert (p is low, <0.0001, for the associations of Extravert/introvert with Depressive and Emotionally unstable). *1: Agglomeration stage 1; *2: Agglomeration stage 2; *4: Agglomeration stage 4.

Table A11. Attachment, addiction and identity.

NOW	Attachment	Addiction	Doctor Shopping	Gender Issues
Attachment		0.007 *3	<0.0001 *3	<0.0001 *5
Addiction			0.007 *1	0.001 *5
Doctor shopping				0.007 *5
Gender issues				
THEN	**Attachment**	**Addiction**	**Doctor shopping**	**Gender issues**
Attachment		<0.0001	<0.0001	<0.0001
Addiction			<0.0001	<0.0001
Doctor shopping				<0.0001
Gender issues				

*1: Agglomeration stage 1; *3: Agglomeration stage 3; *5: Agglomeration stage 5.

Table A12. Psychological attitudes 1.

NOW	LifeSatis	Incontrol	S/Esteem	S/Efficacy	Resilience	Optim	Valency	S/Regul
LifeSatis		<0.0001 *1	<0.0001 *1	<0.0001 *5	<0.0001 *2	<0.0001 *4	<0.0001 *4	<0.0001 *5
InControl			<0.0001 *1	<0.0001 *5	<0.0001 *2	<0.0001 *4	<0.0001 *4	<0.0001 *5
S/Esteem				<0.0001 *5	<0.0001 *2	<0.0001 *4	<0.0001 *4	<0.0001 *5
S/Efficacy					<0.0001 *5	<0.0001 *5	<0.0001 *5	<0.0001 *1
Resilience						<0.0001 *4	<0.0001 *4	<0.0001 *5
Optim							<0.0001 *1	<0.0001 *5
Valency								<0.0001 *5
S/Regul								
THEN	**LifeSatis**	**InControl**	**S/ESteem**	**S/Efficacy**	**Resilience**	**Optim**	**Valency**	**S/Regul**
LifeSatis		<0.0001	<0.0001	<0.0001	<0.0001	<0.0001	<0.0001	<0.0001
InControl			<0.0001	<0.0001	<0.0001	<0.0001	<0.0001	<0.0001
S/ESteem				<0.0001	<0.0001	<0.0001	<0.0001	<0.0001
S/Efficacy					<0.0001	<0.0001	<0.0001	<0.0001
Resilience						<0.0001	<0.0001	<0.0001
Optim							<0.0001	<0.0001
Valency								<0.0001
S/Regul								

*1: Agglomeration stage 1; *2: Agglomeration stage 2; *4: Agglomeration stage 4; *5: Agglomeration stage 5.

Table A13. Psychological attitudes 2, including placebo responsiveness.

NOW	Defensive	Open	Suggestible	Sceptical	Trusting	Placebo
Defensive		<0.0001 *5	<0.0001 *1	<0.0001 *6	<0.0001 *4	0.001 *2
Open			<0.0001 *5	0.005 *5	<0.0001 *3	0.003 *5
Suggestible				<0.0001 *6	<0.0001 *4	<0.0001 *4
Sceptical					<0.001 *4	<0.001 *5
Trusting						0.001 *4
Placebo						
THEN	**Defensive**	**Open**	**Suggestible**	**Sceptical**	**Trusting**	**Placebo**
Defensive		<0.0001	<0.0001	<0.0001	<0.0001	<0.0001
Open			<0.0001	<0.0001	<0.0001	<0.0001
Suggestible				<0.0001	<0.0001	<0.0001
Sceptical					<0.0001	<0.0001
Trusting						<0.0001
Placebo						

*1: Agglomeration stage 1; *2: Agglomeration stage 2; *3: Agglomeration stage 3; *4: Agglomeration stage 4; *5: Agglomeration stage 5; *6: Agglomeration stage 6.

Table A14. Psychological characteristics.

NOW	Depressive	Unstable	Extrav/Introv
Depressive		<0.0001 *2	<0.0001 *5
Unstable			<0.0001 *5
Extrav/Introv [a]			
THEN	**Depressive**	**Unstable**	**Extrav/Introv**
Depressive		<0.0001	<0.0001
Unstable			<0.0001
Extrav/Introv [a]			

a. Extravert/Introvert also demonstrated *p*-values < 0.0001 for groupings #11 and #13, for example. *2: Agglomeration stage 2; *5: Agglomeration stage 5.

Table A15. Behavioural attitudes.

NOW	Self-Motivated	Follows Advice	Commitment
Self-motivated		<0.0001 *[1]	<0.001 *[3]
Follows advice			<0.0001 *[3]
Commitment			
THEN	**Self-Motivated**	**Follows Advice**	**Commitment**
Self-motivated		<0.0001	<0.0001
Follows advice			<0.0001
Commitment			

*[1]: Agglomeration stage 1; *[3]: Agglomeration stage 3.

Table A16. Self-awareness.

NOW	Bodily Aware	Emotionally Aware	Alexithymic
Bodily aware		<0.0001 *[1]	<0.0001 *[5]
Emotionally aware			<0.0001 *[5]
Alexithymic			
THEN	**Bodily Aware**	**Emotionally Aware**	**Alexithymic**
Bodily aware		<0.0001	<0.0001
Emotionally aware			<0.0001
Alexithymic			

*[1]: Agglomeration stage 1; *[5]: Agglomeration stage 5.

Table A17. TCM.

NOW	*Qi* Strong/Weak	TCM/5E Diagnosis
Qi strong/weak		<0.0001
TCM/5E diagnosis		

Some of the χ^2 groupings appeared as consecutive questions in the original survey, so this may have swayed respondents to answer similarly. To test this, associations between eight consecutive but unrelated questions were also explored (Table A18).

Table A18. Associations between consecutive survey questions from different groupings. Shown in **bold** are the χ^2 associations from Table A17.

NOW	Religion	Nature/Tech	Health	Neurochem	Central Sens	Nutrition	Exercise	Ability to Relax
Religion		**<0.0001**	<0.0001	0.005	0.006	n.s.	n.s.	n.s.
Nature/Tech			<0.001	0.006	<0.001	0.034	n.s.	0.010
Health				<0.001	0.042	**<0.0001**	**<0.0001**	n.s.
Neurochem					**<0.0001**	n.s.	n.s.	n.s.
Central Sens						n.s.	n.s.	0.039
Nutrition							**<0.0001**	0.001
Exercise								0.014
Ability to Relax								

n.s.: not significant.

Thus, the χ^2 associations between closely *consecutive* items does not necessarily imply that they are answered in the same manner.

Table A19 shows values of *kappa*, median SE and npCV for the 17 groupings. Table A20 shows the numbers of items from each grouping included and not included in Table 3.

Table A19. Values of *kappa*, median SE and npCV for the 17 groupings.

Grouping	NOW				THEN			
	Kappa	Median SE	npCV Yes	npCV No	*Kappa*	Median SE	npCV Yes	npCV No
1	0.22	1.29	18.97	4.05	0.14	1.36	32.14	12.50
2	0.29	1.13	27.41	51.28	0.14	1.37	21.31	54.10
3	0.01	1.57	45.45	7.89	0.02	1.54	69.23	29.27
4	0.13	1.40	3.03	23.08	0.04	1.52	4.72	23.08
5	0.09	1.43	40.38	24.00	0.02	1.55	41.45	15.91
6	0.03	1.54	6.38	2.38	0.00	1.58	11.11	13.16
7	0.43	1.00	1.71	8.57	0.21	1.30	1.37	5.56
8	0.33	1.22	14.38	32.14	0.14	1.41	13.11	16.00
9	0.11	1.40	9.91	10.34	0.01	1.55	8.43	9.09
10	0.15	1.37	14.18	21.79	0.04	1.51	10.85	38.64
11	0.06	1.46	42.38	41.94	0.03	1.52	59.15	47.83
12	0.14	1.38	14.45	14.29	0.03	1.54	12.87	19.40
13	0.17	1.43	28.75	32.35	0.07	1.51	4.85	25.00
14	0.15	1.31	30.28	31.03	0.06	1.47	28.33	26.79
15	0.52	0.91	8.79	36.67	0.26	1.29	9.59	32.14
16	0.22	1.30	35.71	25.86	0.09	1.50	37.27	14.00
17	0.07	1.48	30.69	4.92	0.02	1.54	25.00	16.13

Table A20. Numbers of items from each grouping included and not included in Table 3.

Grouping	Included	Not Included	% Included
1	3	0	100
2	2	0	100
3	3	2	60
4	0	3	0
5	1	4	20
6	0	2	0
7	2	0	100
8	1	2	33
9	1	1	50
10	1	3	25
11	1	3	25
12	1	7	12.5
13	2	4	33
14	1	2	33
15	3	0	100
16	1	2	33
17	1	1	50

Table A21 shows the individual questions in the upper and lower deciles for SE and *kappa* scores. Note that *all* questions for which *kappa* $\geq$ 0.4 are included in this table, and that *kappa* for none of the THEN questions reached 0.4.

Comparing Table A21 and Table 3, there is considerable agreement between questions for which there was greatest inter-rater agreement (or lowest SE) and those for which most responses were "Yes" (either NOW or THEN), as well as for Ethnicity, for which most responses were "No", and also for Commitment, for which the fewest responses were "No". Only two questions with lowest inter-rater agreement (or greatest SE) appeared in Table 3, both under "DK" responses.

Values of Randolph's free-marginal multi-rater *kappa* can range from −1.0 (complete disagreement, below chance) to 1.0 (complete agreement, above chance), with 0.0 indicating agreement equal to chance. Values of *kappa* less than 0.40 are considered poor, values from 0.40 to 0.75 intermediate to good, and values above 0.75 excellent [37]. "Overall agreement", a slightly more sensitive measure derived from *kappa*, can range from around 33% (equivalent to *kappa* = 0) to 100% (for *kappa* = 1).

Table A21. Survey questions in the upper and lower deciles for SE and *kappa* scores. As in Table 3, items shown in bold red type appear in the same deciles both NOW and THEN.

	Shannon Entropy (SE)			Free-Marginal *Kappa*	
	NOW	THEN		NOW	THEN
SE Q3	**Birth/prenatal** **Char when young [a]** **Child poverty [a]** **Housing** **Attachment style** Extravert/introvert	**Religious beliefs** **Attitude to nature/t** **Self-efficacy** Attachment style **Self-regulation** **TCM diagnosis**	*κ* Q1	**Birth/prenatal** **Character when young [a]** **Child poverty [a]** **Housing** **Attachment style** TCM diagnosis	Family health young **Religious beliefs** **Attitude to nature/t** **Self-efficacy** **Self-regulation** **TCM diagnosis**
SE Q1	General health [b,d] **Diet [b,d]** **Exercise [b,d]** **Ability to relax [b,d]** **Self-motived [b,d]** **Will follow advice [b,d]**	**Ethnicity [c]** **General health [b]** **Exercise [b]** Ability to relax [b] **Self-motivated [b]** **Will follow advice [b]**	*κ* Q3	**Diet [b,d]** **Exercise [b,d]** **Ability to relax [b,d]** **Self-motivated [b,d]** Openness [b,d] **Will follow advice [b,d]**	**Ethnicity [c]** **General health [b]** **Exercise [b]** **Self-motivated [b]** **Will follow advice [b]** Commitment [c]

Notes: [a] "DK" in Table 3; [b] "Yes" in Table 3; [c] "No" in Table 3; [d] $kappa \geq 0.4$.

Values of SE can range from 0 (no variability or informativity), through 1 (which would result from repeated tosses using an unbiased coin [73]) to > 2.6 for some questionnaires (Body Awareness Questionnaire, data in course of analysis).

For the 60 main survey questions here, SE varies between 0.62 and 1.57, *kappa* between 0 and 0.7. When SE was plotted against *kappa* and overall agreement for each of the 60 question responses, very strong correlations were found between them (Figure A1).

These correlations are seemingly quite dramatic, but may in fact be trivial. They will be explored in a future paper.

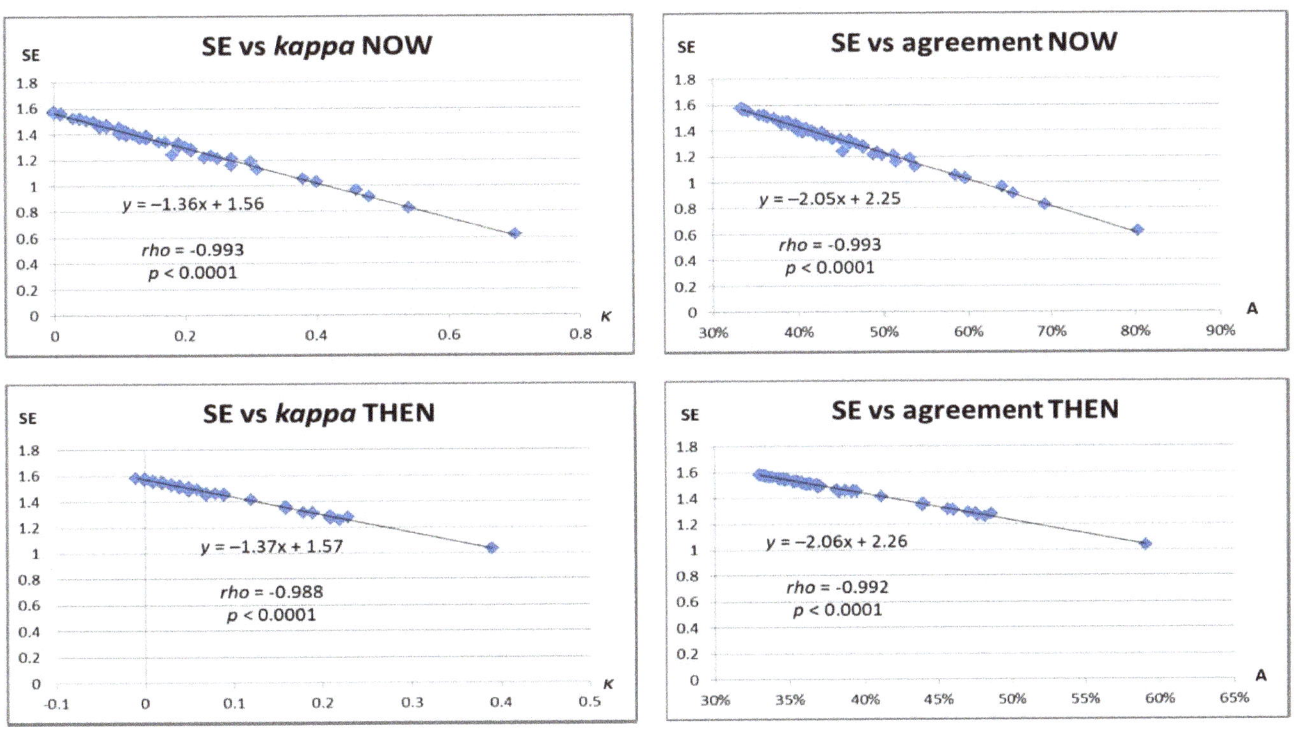

Figure A1. Scatter plots of Shannon entropy (SE) vs. free-marginal *kappa* and overall agreement for the 60 main survey questions.

References

1. Baldry, P. Superficial versus deep dry needling. *Acupunct. Med.* **2002**, *20*, 78–81. [CrossRef] [PubMed]
2. Grant, S.; Colaiaco, B.; Motala, A.; Shanman, R.M.; Sorbero, M.E.; Hempel, S. *Needle Acupuncture for Posttraumatic Stress Disorder (PTSD): A Systematic Review*; RAND Corporation: Santa Monica, CA, USA, 2017.
3. Paterson, C.; Britten, N. The patient's experience of holistic care: Insights from acupuncture research. *Chronic Illn.* **2008**, *4*, 264–277. [CrossRef] [PubMed]
4. McPhail, P.; Sandhu, H.; Dale, J.; Stewart-Brown, S. Acupuncture in hospice settings: A qualitative exploration of patients' experiences. *Eur. J. Cancer Care* **2018**, *27*. [CrossRef] [PubMed]
5. White, P.; Bishop, F.L.; Prescott, P.; Scott, C.; Little, P.; Lewith, G. Practice, practitioner, or placebo? A multifactorial, mixed-methods randomized controlled trial of acupuncture. *Pain* **2012**, *153*, 455–462. [CrossRef] [PubMed]
6. Powell, J.; Wojnarowska, F. Acupuncture for vulvodynia. *J. R. Soc. Med.* **1999**, *92*, 579–581. [CrossRef] [PubMed]
7. Ko, S.J.; Park, J.W.; Leem, J.; Kaptchuk, T.J.; Napadow, V.; Kuo, B.; Gerber, J.; Dimisko, L.; Yeo, I.; Lee, J.; et al. Influence of the patient-practitioner interaction context on acupuncture outcomes in functional dyspepsia: Study protocol for a multicenter randomized controlled trial. *BMC Complement. Altern. Med.* **2017**, *17*. [CrossRef] [PubMed]
8. MacPherson, H.; Elliot, B.; Hopton, A.; Lansdown, H.; Birch, S.; Hewitt, C. Lifestyle advice and self-care integral to acupuncture treatment for patients with chronic neck pain: Secondary analysis of outcomes within a randomized controlled trial. *J. Altern. Complement. Med.* **2017**, *23*, 180–187. [CrossRef] [PubMed]
9. Karst, M.; Schneidewind, D.; Scheinichen, D.; Juettner, B.; Bernateck, M.; Molsberger, A.; Parlesak, A.; Passie, T.; Hoy, L.; Fink, M. Acupuncture induces a pro-inflammatory immune response intensified by a conditioning-expectation effect. *Forsch. Komplementmed.* **2010**, *17*, 21–27. [CrossRef] [PubMed]
10. Kong, J.; Wang, Z.; Leiser, J.; Minicucci, D.; Edwards, R.; Kirsch, I.; Wasan, A.D.; Lang, C.; Gerber, J.; Yu, S.; et al. Enhancing treatment of osteoarthritis knee pain by boosting expectancy: A functional neuroimaging study. *Neuroimage Clin.* **2018**, *18*, 325–334. [CrossRef] [PubMed]
11. Mayor, D.F.; McClure, L.S.; McClure, J.H.C. Nonspecific feelings expected and experienced during or immediately after electroacupuncture: A pilot study in a teaching situation. *Medicines* **2017**, *8*. [CrossRef] [PubMed]
12. Mann, F. *Reinventing Acupuncture: A New Concept of Ancient Medicine*, 2nd ed.; Butterworth-Heinemann: Oxford, UK, 2000; ISBN 9780702038280.
13. Campbell, A. The limbic system and emotion in relation to acupuncture. *Acupunct. Med.* **1999**, *17*, 124–130. [CrossRef]
14. Johnson, M.I.; Ashton, C.H.; Thompson, J.W. The consistency of pulse frequencies and pulse patterns of transcutaneous nerve stimulation (TENS) used by chronic pain patients. *Pain* **1991**, *44*, 231–234. [CrossRef]
15. Campbell, A. Acupuncture: Where to place the needles and for how long. *Acupunct. Med.* **1999**, *17*, 113–117. [CrossRef]
16. Alborzi, A.; Hashempour, T.; Moayedi, J.; Musavi, Z.; Pouladfar, G.; Merat, S. Role of serum level and genetic variation of IL-28B in interferon responsiveness and advanced liver disease in chronic hepatitis C patients. *Med. Microbiol. Immunol.* **2017**, *206*, 165–174. [CrossRef] [PubMed]
17. Yan, Z.; Wang, Y. Viral and host factors associated with outcomes of hepatitis C virus infection (Review). *Mol. Med. Rep.* **2017**, *15*, 2909–2924. [CrossRef] [PubMed]
18. Hall, K.T.; Loscalzo, J.; Kaptchuk, T.J. Genetics and the placebo effect: The placebome. *Trends Mol. Med.* **2015**, *21*, 285–294. [CrossRef] [PubMed]
19. Wang, R.S.; Hall, K.T.; Giulianini, F.; Passow, D.; Kaptchuk, T.J.; Loscalzo, J. Network analysis of the genomic basis of the placebo effect. *JCI Insight* **2017**, *2*. [CrossRef] [PubMed]
20. Park, H.J.; Kim, S.T.; Yoon, D.H.; Jin, S.H.; Lee, S.J.; Lee, H.J.; Lim, S. The association between the DRD2 TaqI A polymorphism and smoking cessation in response to acupuncture in Koreans. *J. Altern. Complement. Med.* **2005**, *11*, 401–405. [CrossRef] [PubMed]
21. Wu, X.L.; Sun, J.H.; Liu, L.Y.; Fu, H.Y.; Jiao, D.Y.; Shu, Y.Y.; Chen, D.; Liu, C.Y.; Zhan, D.W.; Zhang, W. A feasibility analysis on individualized acupuncture treatment of irritable bowel syndrome under help of genetic polymorphism technique. *Zhen Ci Yan Jiu* **2014**, *39*, 252–255. [PubMed]

22. Yang, X.; Gong, J.; Jin, L.; Liu, L.; Sun, J.; Qin, W. Effect of catechol-O-methyltransferase Val158Met polymorphism on resting-state brain default mode network after acupuncture stimulation. *Brain Imaging Behav.* **2017**, *12*, 798–805. [CrossRef] [PubMed]
23. Magarelli, P.; Cridennda, D. Acupuncture & IVF poor responders: A cure? *Fertil. Steril.* **2004**, *81*. [CrossRef]
24. Jo, J.; Lee, Y.J.; Lee, H. Acupuncture for polycystic ovarian syndrome: A systematic review and meta-analysis. *Medicine* **2017**, *96*. [CrossRef] [PubMed]
25. Han, J.S. *The Neurochemical Basis of Pain Relief by Acupuncture. A Collection of Papers 1973–1987*; Beijing Medical University: Beijing, China, 1987.
26. Han, J.S. *The Neurochemical Basis of Pain Relief by Acupuncture*; Hubei Science and Technology Press: Xianning, China, 1998; Volume 2, ISBN 9787535221995.
27. Kelley, J.M.; Lembo, A.J.; Ablon, J.S.; Villanueva, J.J.; Conboy, L.A.; Levy, R.; Marci, C.D.; Kerr, C.E.; Kirsch, I.; Jacobson, E.E.; et al. Patient and practitioner influences on the placebo effect in irritable bowel syndrome. *Psychosom. Med.* **2009**, *71*, 789–797. [CrossRef] [PubMed]
28. Sochos, A.; Bennett, A. Psychological distress, physical symptoms, and the role of attachment Style in acupuncture. *Altern. Ther. Health Med.* **2016**, *22*, 8–16. [PubMed]
29. Mayor, D.; Steffert, T. Measuring mood—Relative sensitivity of numerical rating and Likert scales in the context of teaching electroacupuncture. Initial findings and the influence of response style on results. In Proceedings of the 18th ARRC International Acupuncture Research Symposium, London, UK, 19 March 2016. [CrossRef]
30. Mayor, D.; Steffert, T. Personality and treatment response to electroacupuncture. A new measure of mood change and further analysis of questionnaire response styles. In Proceedings of the 20th ARRC International Acupuncture Research Symposium, London, UK, 17 March 2018. [CrossRef]
31. Steffert, T.; Mayor, D. Mood changes in response to electroacupuncturetreatment in a classroom situation. Personality type, emotional intelligence and prior acupuncture experience, with an exploration of Shannon entropy, response style and graphology variables. In Proceedings of the 19th ARRC International Acupuncture Research Symposium, London, UK, 25 March 2017. [CrossRef]
32. Mayor, D.F. The teaching of electroacupuncture in North America: An informal survey. *Clin. Acupunt. Orient. Med.* **2001**, *2*, 116–128. [CrossRef]
33. Mayor, D.; Bovey, M. An international survey on the current use of electroacupuncture. *Acupunct. Med.* **2017**, *35*, 30–37. [CrossRef] [PubMed]
34. Eysenbach, G. Improving the quality of Web surveys: The Checklist for Reporting Results of Internet E-Surveys (CHERRIES). *J. Med. Internet Res.* **2004**, *6*. [CrossRef] [PubMed]
35. Randolph, J.J. Free-Marginal Multi-Rater *kappa*: An Alternative to Fleiss' Fixed-Marginal Multi-Rater *Kappa*. Ph.D. Thesis, University of Joensuu, Joensuu, Finland, 2005.
36. Randolph, J.J. Online *Kappa* Calculator. Available online: http://justus.randolph.name/kappa (accessed on 10 May 2018).
37. Fleiss, J.L.; Levin, B.; Paik, M.C. *Statistical Methods for Rates and Proportions*, 3rd ed.; John Wiley & Sons: Hoboken, NJ, USA, 2004; ISBN 9780471526292.
38. Shannon, C.E.; Weaver, W. *The Mathematical Theory of Communication*; University of Illinois Press: Chicago, IL, USA, 1949; ISBN 9780252725487.
39. Silverman, D. *Interpreting Qualitative Data*, 5th ed.; Sage: London, UK, 2015; ISBN 9781446295434.
40. Peräkylä, A.; Ruusuvuori, J. Analyzing talk and text. In *The Sage Handbook of Qualitative Research*, 5th ed.; Denzin, N.K., Lincoln, Y.S., Eds.; Sage: London, UK, 2017; pp. 669–690. ISBN 9781483349800.
41. Croke, S. *The Need for Novel Methodologies and Introduction to Theatricality*; Research Council for Complementary Medicine (CAMSTRAND): Manchester, UK, Unpublished Conference Paper, 2018.
42. Mason, J. *Qualitative Researching*, 3rd ed.; Sage: London, UK, 2018; ISBN 9781473912182.
43. Saldaña, J. *The Coding Manual for Qualitative Researchers*, 3rd ed.; Sage: London, UK, 2015; ISBN 9781473902497.
44. O'Reilly-Shah, V.N. Factors influencing healthcare provider respondent fatigue answering a globally-administered in-app survey. *PeerJ* **2017**, *5*. [CrossRef] [PubMed]
45. Fisher, P.; Van Haselen, R.; Hardy, K.; Berkovitz, S.; McCarney, R. Effectiveness gaps: A new concept for evaluating health service and research needs applied to complementary and alternative medicine. *J. Altern. Complement. Med.* **2004**, *10*, 627–632. [CrossRef] [PubMed]

46. McDonald, J.; Janz, S. The Acupuncture Evidence Project: A Comparative Literature Review, rev ed.; Brisbane: Australian Acupuncture and Chinese Medicine Association: Brisbane, Australia, 2017. Available online: https://www.acupuncture.org.au/wp-content/uploads/2017/11/28-NOV-The-Acupuncture-Evidence-Project_Mcdonald-and-Janz_-REISSUED_28_Nov.pdf (accessed on 2 July 2018).
47. Wenham, A.; Atkin, K.; Woodman, J.; Ballard, K.; MacPherson, H. Self-efficacy and embodiment associated with Alexander Technique lessons or with acupuncture sessions: A longitudinal qualitative sub-study within the ATLAS trial. *Complement. Ther. Clin. Pract.* **2018**, *31*, 308–314. [CrossRef] [PubMed]
48. Campbell, A. Hunting the Snark: The quest for the perfect acupuncture placebo. *Acupunct. Med.* **1991**, *9*, 83–84. [CrossRef]
49. Birch, S. A review and analysis of placebo treatments, placebo effects, and placebo controls in trials of medical procedures when sham is not inert. *J. Altern. Complement. Med.* **2006**, *12*, 303–310. [CrossRef] [PubMed]
50. Itoh, K.; Kitakoji, H. Acupuncture for chronic pain in Japan: A review. *Evid. Based Complement. Alternat. Med.* **2007**, *4*, 431–438. [CrossRef] [PubMed]
51. MacPherson, H.; Tilbrook, H.; Bland, J.M.; Bloor, K.; Brabyn, S.; Cox, H.; Kang'ombe, A.R.; Man, M.-S.; Stuardi, T.; Torgerson, D.; et al. Acupuncture for irritable bowel syndrome: Primary care based pragmatic randomised controlled trial. *BMC Gastroenterol.* **2012**, *12*. [CrossRef] [PubMed]
52. MacPherson, H.; Richmond, S.; Bland, M.; Brealey, S.; Gabe, R.; Hopton, A.; Keding, A.; Lansdown, H.; Perren, S.; Sculpher, M.; et al. Acupuncture and counselling for depression in primary care: A randomised controlled trial. *PLoS Med.* **2013**, *10*. [CrossRef] [PubMed]
53. Paterson, C.; Britten, N. Acupuncture as a complex intervention: A holistic model. *J. Altern. Complement. Med.* **2004**, *10*, 791–801. [CrossRef] [PubMed]
54. Linde, K.; Niemann, K.; Schneider, A.; Meissner, K. How large are the nonspecific effects of acupuncture? A meta-analysis of randomised controlled trials. *BMC Med.* **2010**, *8*, 1–14. [CrossRef] [PubMed]
55. Robinson, N.; London South Bank University. Personal communication, 2018.
56. Longhurst, J. Acupuncture's cardiovascular actions: A mechanistic perspective. *Med. Acupunct.* **2013**, *25*, 101–113. [CrossRef]
57. Villas-Boas, J.D.; Dias, D.P.; Trigo, P.I.; Almeida, N.A.; de Almeida, F.Q.; de Medeiros, M.A. Acupuncture affects autonomic and endocrine but not behavioural responses induced by startle in horses. *Evid. Based Complement. Alternat. Med.* **2015**, *2015*. [CrossRef] [PubMed]
58. Uchida, C.; Waki, H.; Minakawa, Y.; Tamai, H.; Hisajima, T.; Imai, K. Evaluation of autonomic nervous system function using heart rate variability analysis during transient heart rate reduction caused by acupuncture. *Med. Acupunct.* **2018**, *30*, 89–95. [CrossRef] [PubMed]
59. Scott, J.; Barlow, T. *Acupuncture in the Treatment of Children*, 3rd ed.; Eastland Press: Seattle, WA, USA, 1999; ISBN 9780939616305.
60. Loo, M. *Pediatric Acupuncture*; Churchill Livingstone: Edinburgh, UK, 2002; ISBN 9780443070327.
61. Maciocia, G. *The Foundations of Chinese Medicine. A comprehensive Test for Acupuncturists and Herbalists*; Churchill Livingstone: Edinburgh, UK, 1989; ISBN 9780443039805.
62. Franglen, N. *The Handbook of Five Element Practice*, rev ed.; Singing Dragon: London, UK, 2014; ISBN 9781848191884.
63. Marmot, M. *Status Syndrome: How Your Place on the Social Gradient Directly Affects Your Health*; Bloomsbury: London, UK, 2015; ISBN 9781408872680.
64. Náfrádi, L.; Nakamoto, K.; Schulz, P.J. Is patient empowerment the key to promote adherence? A systematic review of the relationship between self-efficacy, health locus of control and medication adherence. *PLoS ONE* **2017**, *12*. [CrossRef] [PubMed]
65. Pashang, S.; Khanlou, N.; Clarke, J. *Today's Youth and Mental Health: Hope, Power, and Resilience*; Springer: Cham, Switzerland, 2018; ISBN 9783319648361.
66. Meade, R.D.; Barnard, W.A. Conformity and Anticonformity among Americans and Chinese. *J. Soc. Psychol.* **2010**, *89*, 15–24. [CrossRef]
67. Glynn, L.M.; Howland, M.A.; Sandman, C.A.; Davis, E.P.; Phelan, M.; Baram, T.Z.; Stern, H.S. Prenatal maternal mood patterns predict child temperament and adolescent mental health. *J. Affect. Disord.* **2018**, *228*, 83–90. [CrossRef] [PubMed]

68. Handayani, P.W.; Hidayanto, A.N.; Pinem, A.A.; Sandhyaduhita, P.I.; Budi, I. Hospital nformation system user acceptance factors: User group perspectives. *Inform. Health Soc. Care* **2018**, *43*, 84–107. [CrossRef] [PubMed]
69. Pincus, S.M.; Schmidt, P.J.; Palladino-Negro, P.; Rubinow, D.R. Differentiation of women with premenstrual dysphoric disorder, recurrent brief depression, and healthy controls by daily mood rating dynamics. *J. Psychiatr. Res.* **2008**, *42*, 337–347. [CrossRef] [PubMed]
70. Tastle, W.J.; Wierman, M.J. An information theoretic measure for the evaluation of ordinal scale data. *Behav. Res. Methods* **2006**, *38*, 487–494. [CrossRef] [PubMed]
71. Tastle, W.J.; Wierman, M.J. Consensus and dissention: A measure of ordinal dispersion. *Int. J. Approx. Reason.* **2007**, *45*, 531–545. [CrossRef]
72. Lavrakas, P.J. *Encyclopedia of Survey Research Methods*; Sage: Thousand Oaks, CA, USA, 2008; ISBN 9781412918084.
73. Lesne, A. Shannon entropy: A rigorous notion at the crossroads between probability, information theory, dynamical systems and statistical physics. *Math. Struct. Comput. Sci.* **2014**, *24*. [CrossRef]

15

Acupuncture and Neural Mechanism in the Management of Low Back Pain

Tiaw-Kee Lim [1], Yan Ma [1,2], Frederic Berger [3] and Gerhard Litscher [1,4,*]

1 University Postgraduate Education of Principles and Practice of Traditional Chinese Medicine, Medical University of Vienna, 1090 Vienna, Austria; jalimee@gmail.com (T.-K.L.); yan.ma@meduniwien.ac.at (Y.M.)
2 Institute of Pathophysiology and Allergy Research, Center for Pathophysiology, Infectiology and Immunology, Medical University of Vienna, 1090 Vienna, Austria
3 Gregor Mendel Institute of Molecular Plant Biology GmbH, Austrian Academy of Sciences, 1030 Vienna, Austria; frederic.berger@gmi.oeaw.ac.at
4 Research Unit of Biomedical Engineering in Anesthesia and Intensive Care Medicine, Research Unit for Complementary and Integrative Laser Medicine, and TCM Research Center Graz, Medical University of Graz, 8036 Graz, Austria
* Correspondence: gerhard.litscher@medunigraz.at

Abstract: Within the last 10 years, the percentage of low back pain (LBP) prevalence increased by 18%. The management and high cost of LBP put a tremendous burden on the healthcare system. Many risk factors have been identified, such as lifestyle, trauma, degeneration, postural impairment, and occupational related factors; however, as high as 95% of the cases of LBP are non-specific. Currently, LBP is treated pharmacologically. Approximately 25 to 30% of the patients develop serious side effects, such as drowsiness and drug addiction. Spinal surgery often does not result in a massive improvement of pain relief. Therefore, complementary approaches are being integrated into the rehabilitation programs. These include chiropractic therapy, physiotherapy, massage, exercise, herbal medicine and acupuncture. Acupuncture for LBP is one of the most commonly used non-pharmacological pain-relieving techniques. This is due to its low adverse effects and cost-effectiveness. Currently, many randomized controlled trials and clinical research studies have produced promising results. In this article, the causes and incidence of LBP on global health care are reviewed. The importance of treatment by acupuncture is considered. The efforts to reveal the link between acupuncture points and anatomical features and the neurological mechanisms that lead to acupuncture-induced analgesic effect are reviewed.

Keywords: low back pain (LBP); acupuncture; mechanism of acupuncture; anti-nociceptive; purinergic receptors; adenosine triphosphate (ATP); adenosine

---

1. Introduction

Low back pain (LBP) is one of the most frequently encountered musculoskeletal disorders in today's society. LBP is defined as pain and discomfort, located in between the costal margin and the inferior gluteal folds, with or without referred leg pain [1–4]. LBP is categorised according to duration as acute (less than 6 weeks), sub-acute (between 6 and 12 weeks), or chronic (more than 12 weeks) [4–6].

LBP interferes with activities of daily living [7], work performance [8,9], and is a major reason for people to seek medical consultation [10,11]. This disorder contributes to a substantial burden on individuals, employers, the healthcare system and society in general. According to a report published by the World Health Organization (WHO) in 2013, back pain, together with neck pain, was the second highest cause amongst the 20 leading non-fatal health outcomes from the year 2000 to 2011 [12].

The survey, The Global Burden of Disease Study 2016 (GBD 2016), published in the Lancet in 2017 [13,14], highlights the extent of health loss due to diseases, injuries, risk factors, prevalence and mortality rate by age, sex, and geography at specific points in time. In the GBD 2016, LBP was the number one cause for the most years lived with disability (YLDs) in the world [13].

The disability-adjusted life years (DALYs) are calculated as the combination of years of life lost (YLLs) due to premature mortality and years lived with disability (YLDs) [14,15]. Because LBP does not cause mortality, therefore YLDs are the same as disability-adjusted life years (DALYs). DALYs for LBP, together with neck pain, was on the 4th position out of the 30 leading global DALYs in the GBD 2016 [14]. This was much higher than the average DALYs related to road injuries, HIV/AIDS, diabetes, chronic obstructive pulmonary disease (COPD) and lung cancer [14]. The overall estimation of DALYs for LBP in 2016 was 57.6 million, which represents more than 40% of the total number of 140 million DALYs of all the musculoskeletal disorders combined. In Austria, the GBD 2015 for YLDs and DALYs due to LBP and neck pain are ranked at No. 1 and No. 2, respectively [16].

The estimated global prevalence of the population affected by LBP was 9.2% according to WHO in 2010 [12]. Hoy et al. estimated that the ranges of prevalence of LBP at a point, 1-month, 1-year and over a lifetime were 18.3%, 30.8%, 38.0% and 38.9%, respectively [17]. In the GBD 2016, it was estimated that the prevalence of LBP for the year 2016 was more than 511 million of the world's population, an increase of 18.0%, as compared to 2006 [7]. LBP results in high costs to society due to increased demands on the healthcare system and work absence. In the USA alone, it has been estimated that LBP costed between US $100–200 billion yearly [1]. This amount has more than doubled from 1991 to 2016 [18].

In this scientific article, causes of LBP are surveyed and the links between anatomical features and acupuncture points are outlined. This is followed by a review of randomized controlled trials (RCTs) and of mechanisms potentially targeted by acupuncture treatments.

2. Causes and Risk Factors of Lower Back Pain

LBP is very common, and yet is a very complex multifactorial disorder with much possible etiology. These originate from injuries, trauma or fractures to the anatomical structure [19–21]; lumbar spine degeneration [22,23]; and disc herniation or nerve entrapment [24–26]. Other causes associated with an increased risk of LBP, include infections, autoimmune diseases, orthopedic diseases or tumours [27–33]. LBP results also from occupational ergonomic factors related to heavy physical work, repetitive actions due to occupational requirements [1,2,34–39]; as well as sports activities or sports-related injuries [40,41]; sedentary lifestyle, prolonged sitting or inactivity and lack of exercises [42–44]; post operation or surgery-induced [45,46]; secondary from other medical conditions [47–49]; lifestyle factors [50]; poor trunk control and postural impairment [51]; psychosocial and behavior-related factors from smoking, alcohol abuse, obesity, depression and stress [1,6,14,52–57]; socio-economic factors [58]; and ageing [59,60]. However, it is often difficult to identify the origin of LBP [1,5,6,61–65] and 85–95% of the total cases of back problems [1,63–65] are not associated with a specific patho-anatomical origin, or attributed to any recognizable pathology patterns.

2.1. *Age and Gender*

The age group 40–69 is affected with the highest incidence of LBP [17], and women have higher LPB prevalence than men [17,50,57,66–69].

Großschädl et al. studied the LBP prevalence of the Austrian population in 1983, 1991, 1999, and 2006/7. During this period, they found a marked increase in the rate of LBP for both sexes, especially more so in women over recent years [69]. This increasing trend of the rate of LBP is recorded worldwide and might be related to women's involvement in the workforce, while their house chores do not diminish [69,70]. LBP's risk factors specific to women comprise exposure to musculoskeletal loads due to pregnancy [71–73]; menstruation [74,75]; menopausal [66,76,77]; hormone [66,78]; osteoporosis [68,79]; low bone mineral density [80,81]; and conditions associated with ageing [59,82]. In contrast, certain studies show that men have a higher rate of LBP [1,2], especially those involved in heavy physical work and repetitive movements [1,2,6,38,39].

2.2. Obesity and Smoking

Schneider et al. reported that the prevalence of LBP is significantly higher for women affected by overweight, low level of social support, a sedentary lifestyle, smoking and lower income groups [67]. The association between obesity and LBP remains controversial. Few studies on the relation between obesity and LBP have been published so far. Obesity is considered as one of the elements that contributes to the increasing rate of LBP [56,57,67–69,83,84]. Heuch et al. estimated that the rate of LBP increases in parallel with the rate of body mass index (BMI) [83]. As stated by a guideline by WHO, an adult is viewed as overweight when the BMI is greater or equal to 25, and one is considered obese when the BMI has reached 30 or more [85]. In addition, increased BMI also affects the incidence of neck pain and arthritis [86]. A group of studies led to speculation of connections between smoking and obesity that may result in LBP [67,87]. Yet, such a conclusion was challenged by another study, which did not find such link between LBP, smoking and obesity [88].

3. Theories of Pain

For many centuries, people have been seeking the origin of pain and ways to alleviate it. Despite a marked progress in our understanding of pain, many aspects of the mechanisms involved remain unclear. Pain is a very subjective issue, as it is interpreted differently by each patient. Some people have a very high pain threshold, which allows them to tolerate pain extremely well. For others, even a slight trigger of stimulation might cause them to suffer in agony. Because of this huge difference in perception of pain magnitude, it is difficult to understand the degree of suffering by a patient. The visual analogue scale (VAS), which was created in 1921 by Hayes and Patterson [89], is a simple tool to judge a patient's perspective of pain, to translate a subjective level of pain into an objective measurement.

Pain is classified as a nociceptive pain (caused by excitation of nociceptors by external stimuli), inflammatory pain (intervened by inflammatory mediators released by an inflamed organ), or neuropathic pain (induced by lesions of the central or peripheral nervous system) [90]. According to Merskey and Bogduk, "pain is an unpleasant sensory and emotional experience associated with actual or potential tissue damage or described in terms of such damage" [91].

The discovery of nociceptor by Charles Sherrington in 1906, has changed forever the way we consider the concept of the central nervous system (CNS) [92]. This gave rise to many modern studies about pain management, such as nerve blocking and analgesic effect by acupuncture. The Gate Control Theory of Pain, which was proposed in 1965 by Melzack and Wall, suggested that the brain has a "gate" mechanism either blocking or allowing pain messages to reach the brain [93]. Although their theory was later proven to be flawed, it did provide a useful overall concept of how pain is experienced and many researchers engaged in this field of study. One of them resulted in the invention of transcutaneous electric nerve stimulation (TENS) for the management of LBP [94].

In 1973, Pert and Synder discovered the opiate receptor, the cellular binding site for endorphins in the brain [95]. Two years later, a group of British scientists led by Hughes and Kosterlitz, found the breakthrough in the field of molecular receptor studies, the discovery of enkephalin [96]. This was followed by studies that led to our current knowledge of endorphins, the body's very own natural mechanism of painkiller [97–100].

To be able to ease the pain experienced by patients, first we need to understand the root cause of pain and the mechanism that triggered the transmission of pain. Having a better understanding of the nervous system's own mechanism of analgesia, such as that triggered by the stimulation of needles by acupuncture, pain management of LBP by acupuncture is no longer a placebo or a contextual effect, but rather, an evidence-based scientific proof of an ancient practice. These topics are addressed in more detail below.

4. Pain Mechanism

The mechanism of pain is a very complex process, due to the involvement of multiple layers of the neural circuit, from the stimulation of the receptors to the chemical reaction in the CNS. The perception of pain is called nociception, and it is initiated by nociceptors present at free nerve endings [101]. The nociceptors, part of the architecture of neural circuits, are spread all over the body, from the superficial layers of skin to the deeper tissues and internal organs.

Tissue injury by noxious stimuli is detected by the nociceptors. This information is transmitted as electrical nerve impulses, or action potentials, via the nerve fibres, called the primary afferent neurons to the dorsal root ganglia (DRG). DRG are linked to dorsal root in the spinal cord through the dorsal root. The electrical signal synapses with the second afferent neuron at the dorsal horn of the grey matter. From here, the signal crosses over to the opposite side of the spinal cord, and connects to the ventral white matter and further links to the spinothalamic tract. The signal is now traveling upward from the spinal cord to the thalamus in the brain where pain is generated. In the thalamus, a third synapse occurs and the nerve impulse is transmitted via the thalamocortical tract to the cerebral cortex. This process tells us the exact location of the pain. Nociceptors enable humans to recognise pain stimuli and therefore to respond accordingly, such as pulling away our hand from a fire or sharp object [102–109].

4.1. Nerve Fibres

There are two types of nerve fibres, afferent and efferent. Afferent means ascending, and qualifies sensory fibres sending signals to the brain. While efferent signifies descending, and defines motor fibres, which relay messages away from the CNS. The afferent nerve fibres convey signals concerning potential damage or injury from outside and inside the body.

The afferent nerve fibres in the human's body are further divided into four major types of primary sensory neurons, which can be differentiated morphologically and functionally into A-alpha (Aα), A-beta (Aβ), A-delta (Aδ) and C fibre [110]. Aα fibres represent motor fibres connected to voluntary muscles and include certain sensory fibres that transmit position sensation from skeletal muscles. Aβ fibres carry non-noxious stimuli and convey the sensations of touch, vibration and pressure from the skin [111]. There are only two types of nerve fibres involved in the transmission of painful impulses. The Aδ fibre is myelinated, enables fast transmission of impulses and produces sharp and well localised pain. The second type, the unmyelinated C fibre, is slow in transmission and produces dull or burning pain, the exact location of which is diffused and poorly localised [105–107,109]. Kagitani et al. demonstrated that acupuncture stimulation enables production of various autonomic functions on both Aδ and C fibres [110]. While Zhao suggested that stimulation by manual acupuncture (MA) and electroacupuncture (EA) activates Aδ and C fibres to produce an analgesic effect [112].

4.2. Inflammatory Soup

Tissue damage causes release of a variety of chemical substances into the extracellular space around the receptor terminals. These chemical substances comprise bradykinin, histamine, serotonin, prostaglandins, nerve growth factor (NGF), substance P, adenosine triphosphate (ATP), calcitonin gene-related peptide (CGRP), protons (H^+) and other purines and indolamines. Altogether, they form the "inflammatory soup" and are able to interact and activate the nociceptive fibres that cause localised pain and inflammation [102–109].

5. Treatment of LBP by Acupuncture

The goal of LBP treatment is to control or reduce pain, to improve structure impairment of the spine and to return to the normal life activities as soon as possible. Most current international guidelines recommend pharmacological management for pain relief of LBP, including paracetamol, non-steroidal anti-inflammatory drugs (NSAIDs), muscle relaxant, opioid analgesics, epidural steroid, anticonvulsants, antidepressants, and corticosteroids, among others [1,5,61,65,113–116]. However, most of these pharmacological treatments produce limited pain relief and are accompanied by serious side effects, such as drowsiness, dizziness, addiction, allergic responses, reversible reduction of liver function, and negative impacts on gastrointestinal functions [1,5,61,113,114,116,117]. At least one of these side effects is experienced in approximately 25 to 30% of patients treated with opioids [118]. The major problem with this approach is that pain may be temporarily relieved but the source of LBP is not identified and alternative treatments of LBP are required. These include multidisciplinary rehabilitations based on physiotherapy, spinal manipulation, exercise therapy, massage therapy, cognitive-behaviour therapy, yoga, tai-chi, and acupuncture [5,61,65,113,115]. Here, the focus is on a critical assessment of the benefits of acupuncture in LBP treatment.

5.1. Acupuncture

Acupuncture is part of the healing system of Traditional Chinese Medicine (TCM). It consists of insertion of thin needles into the muscle, on specific acupuncture points placed along meridians to treat a variety of conditions. Apart from the traditional manual acupuncture (MA), there are other methods to stimulate acupuncture points for therapeutic purposes, such as electroacupuncture (EA), acupressure, laser acupuncture and moxibustion.

The practice of acupuncture as pain relief is widely used in many of the countries throughout the world [119]. Despite a lack of well-designed clinical studies supporting its efficacy, and skeptical opinions from many, it is nevertheless well accepted by many patients globally. Acupuncture is legally recognised by many countries in Asia, Australia, America, Canada, and some parts of Europe and Latin America [120].

World Health Organization (WHO) estimated that one-third of the world's population has no regular access to modern medicines, especially in many parts of Africa, Asia and Latin America. Fortunately, complementary and alternative medicine (CAM) such as herbal and traditional medicine and acupuncture are available and accessible [120].

In the USA alone, the number of acupuncture users increased by 50% between 2002 and 2012 [121]. As of December 2010, there were approximately 305,000 registered Complementary & Alternative Medicine (CAM) providers across Europe, including 96,380 acupuncturists. Eighty-thousand were medical and 16,380 were non-medical practitioners [122]. In Austria, there were 3531 doctors qualified with the diploma of acupuncture from the Austrian Medical Association (Diplom für Akupunktur der Österreichischen Ärztekammer) in 2011 [123]. According to the Law of Health Services Austria (Bundesgesetz über die Gesundheit Österreich), acupuncture is a scientifically recognized treatment that can be provided in hospitals [124]. In contrast with increasing interest and practice of acupuncture, there is a persistent lack of infrastructure and funding dedicated to research and teaching in this field [125].

5.2. Brief History of Acupuncture

The root of Traditional Chinese Medicine (TCM) can be traced back over 3000 years ago in China. While acupuncture is the best known modality of TCM in the West, TCM has a long history of great use of herbal remedies. Apart from acupuncture and herbal medicine, TCM also comprises of Qigong, Taichi and Tuina. The first written medical text on acupuncture was mentioned in the Huang Di Nei Jing (The Yellow Emperor's Internal Classic). It comprised of two volumes: The first one is Su Wen (Basic Questions), which covers the diagnostic methods and theoretical foundation of TCM [126]. The second part is called Ling Shu (The Spiritual Pivot) and explains acupuncture therapy such as the description of meridians, functions of the acupuncture points, needling techniques, types of Qi and the location of 160 points [127]. Two other classic texts which mention acupuncture in depth are Nan Jing (The Classic of Difficult Issues) [128] and Zhen Jiu Jia Yi Jing (The Systematic Classic of Acupuncture and Moxibustion). The latter was written by Huangfu Mi, who added another 189 acupuncture points to reach a total of 349 [129]. The precise history of these four books is unclear as they were edited, annotated and reinterpreted several times. Another obstacle of learning and understanding the teaching of TCM is the difficulty in translating these ancient Chinese texts [130].

Unlike western medicine, which has a clear distinct path that can be traced back to Hippocrates [131], there is undocumented evidence to when and where the origin of acupuncture came from due to the loss of many of the valuable ancient texts. The archaeological discovery of "bian shi" (a kind of flattened and sharpened stone) from the era of the New Stone Age in China (8000–2000 BC), was believed to represent the ancient acupuncture needle for treating illnesses by pricking certain parts of the body. During the Warring States (475–221 BC), metal needles were developed to substitute the stone needles [132].

In the 6th century, acupuncture together with the teaching of TCM spread to Korea and Japan. Later in the 10th century, acupuncture arrived in Vietnam through the commercial routes. The practice of acupuncture was brought back to France by the Jesuit missionaries in the 16th century [133]. The very first acupuncture description that appeared in the West was written by Wilhelm Ten Rhyne in 1683, a physician employed by the Dutch East India Company, who was based in Japan [134].

In the USA, acupuncture has gained sudden attention and popularity thanks to the New York Times writer James Reston's article in 1971, entitled "Now, About My Operation in Peking" [135]. He described his first-hand experience of acupuncture with an emergency appendectomy and post-operative care while on his assignment to China prior to President Nixon's visit. This has prompted many doctors visiting China to observe and study the effectiveness and benefits of acupuncture, with a specific interest in its use for surgical analgesia [136–140].

5.3. Theory of Traditional Chinese Medicine

Traditional Chinese Medicine (TCM), one of the most important components of Chinese culture, has a long-established history and consists of a wealth of experience and a profound source of knowledge. It has made a great contribution to the overall welfare of its people. At present, TCM is also becoming well known globally, playing a unique role in the development of public healthcare [141].

In contrast to the anatomical and scientific perspective, the theories of the mechanism of action in TCM on LBP differ significantly from those of modern pharmacology. TCM states that pain is caused by internal disharmony between Yin and Yang, imbalance between Qi and Blood, and disparity within the Five Elements [142]. Qi, the essence of life, is believed to circulate within special conduits in the body termed meridians and collaterals that connect all parts of the body, including connecting the organ systems with each other and their related sense organs. When there is insufficiency of Qi, or when the meridians are blocked, this causes an imbalance between Yin and Yang, perturbs the meridians, hinders the smooth flowing of Qi and results in stagnation of Qi and blood, leading to pain and illness [143–146].

6. Acupuncture Principles

Acupuncture is based on the theory of channels, simply referred to as meridians and collaterals, which are the branches of the meridians. There are 14 main meridians, and each consists of an internal pathway that runs inside the body and links to an external pathway where acupuncture points are located. Qi flows through these pathways of meridians interconnecting with each other, and is linked to specific internal organs, which are also called Zangfu organs [146]. Stimulation on the acupuncture points by acupuncture needle enables unblocking of the meridians, hence promoting a smooth flow of Qi [147].

6.1. The Anatomical Structure of Acupuncture Points and Meridians

Detailed lists and definition of acupuncture points are provided in several textbooks [148–151]. Deadman et al., in their book, A Manual of Acupuncture [151], mentioned that "centuries of observation of the existence of tender spots on the body during the course of disease, and the alleviation of symptoms when they were stimulated by massage or heat, led to the gradual discovery of the acupuncture points". This sheds a bit of light on the origin of acupuncture. The meridians and the acupuncture points can be compared with airline travel routes: They exist on a map but cannot be "seen".

Many studies have been carried out to obtain concrete evidence supporting the existence of acupuncture points and the Qi flowing meridians. Back in 1963, the North Korean scientist, Kim Bong Han, discovered the Kyungrak System (it means acupuncture meridians and collaterals in Korean), better known as the primo vascular system (PVS). PVS is a threadlike structure defining a circulatory system entirely different from the vascular, nervous, and lymphatic systems. Kim established that the PVS represents anatomical structures linked to acupuncture points and meridians. He proposed that the PVS has the ability of hematopoietic functions as well as to regenerate injured tissues and heal wounds [152]. Many scientists tried to reproduce his result but failed. That was because Kim did not mention what kind of staining blue dye was used in his studies [153]. In 2002, Shin et al. confirmed the existence of PVS [154].

Stefanov et al. proposed that the PVS is the communication system between living organisms and the environment. They believed that this system is involved in channeling the flow of energy and information relayed by biophotons (electromagnetic waves of light) and is closely related to DNA [155]. Independent experiments involved injection of radioactive tracers at acupuncture points to attempt to map out and visualize the routes of meridians [156–158]. An alternative study by Langevin and Yandow led to the hypothesis that networks of interstitial connective tissue constitute the link between acupuncture points and meridians tissue [159]. Ultrasound imaging reveals a visible connective tissue forming an intramuscular cleavage plane at acupuncture points but not at control points [159]. Another anatomical distinctive feature of acupuncture points is high densities of nerve endings [160,161].

Other studies have explored the possibility of physiological differences between acupuncture points and surrounding tissues. Several reports conclude that the skin electrical impedance along meridians is lower than in their surroundings [162–164]. However, Stux and Pomeranz were quite skeptical about these kinds of electrical properties [165] and Kramer et al. concluded that skin electrical resistance at acupuncture points can either be lower or higher compared to the surrounding area [166]. In 2010, Litscher et al. developed a miniaturized 48-channel skin impedance measurement system for needle and laser acupuncture [164]. This system was further improved and a new multi-channel skin resistance measuring system, called GEDIS (Graz ElectroDermal Impedance measurement System) was used to differentiate the electrical skin resistance measurement between an acupuncture point and a placebo point. The system performs "electrodermal mapping", and shows that the skin resistance at the acupuncture point has lower impedance values as compared to the non-acupuncture point [167].

Other studies suggested that there are more mast cells distributed at acupuncture points [168–170]. Marcelli, Peuker and Cummings, and Cheng, have made some studies of the morphological characteristics between the meridians and the anatomical structure [171–174]. Shaw and McLennan did an anatomical dissection study based on investigation of cadaveric specimens. They concluded that acupuncture points and meridians are purposefully named to reflect the observable physical form, e.g., heart meridian, lung meridian, etc. [175]. Anatomical dissections in ancient China are mentioned in chapter 12 of the Huang Di Nei Jing Ling Shu. Here, the imperial physician Qi Bo explains the fundamental structures of the human organism to the emperor Huang Di. The physician says: "After someone has died his body can be anatomically dissected and be examined (for medical investigation)" [127]. As another source of evidence to prove that acupuncture points are anatomically correct, the chapter 42 of Nanjing describes the length, diameter, weight and capacity of the internal organs [120]. In chapter 7 of Book 3 from Mi Huang-Fu's Jia Yi Jing, the measurement of bones and intestines, and the volume of the stomach and intestines were clearly explained [129]. That is why the names for the internal organs used today are the same as the name of TCM organs defined more than 2000 years ago from Huang Di Nei Jing Ling Shu [127].

Acupuncture points are thus positioned at precise anatomical structures. For example, in TCM theory, the lung (LU) meridian is paired with the large intestine (LI) meridian [146]. LU 7 Lieque

(Broken Sequence) is also the Luo-Connecting Point of the Lung meridian. From LU 7, the meridian branches out and links to the large intestine meridian, at LI 4 Hegu (Joining Valley), also known as Yuan-Source Point [151]. From an anatomical point of view, both points are located at the branch from the main cephalic vein, which is supplied by the radial nerve [176]. This evidence supports that acupuncture points and meridians correspond to anatomically defined positions in the human body. Pushing this idea further at the molecular level, Zhang et al. studied the connection between the heart and stomach meridians to cardiovascular diseases (CVDs) and gastrointestinal disorders (GIDs) and found that both CVDs and GIDs express sets of genes which are functionally related [177].

According to Thomas Myers, the author of Anatomy Trains, the whole body is a unique linkage of myofascial and locomotor anatomy in which the muscles are connected to the fascial net. The fascia, with an appearance akin to a spider's web, is a continuous sheath of tissue, covering and interpenetrating every muscle, bone, nerve, artery, vein and lymph vessel, as well as, all internal organs, brain and spinal cord [178]. The fascial anatomy has a striking anatomical correlation to acupuncture points and meridians. Finando and Finando suggest that all fundamental characteristics of acupuncture treatment are consistent with stimulation of the fascia [179].

6.2. Acupuncture Points, Ashi Points, Myofascial Trigger Points (mTrPs) and Referral Pain

Interestingly, acupuncture points were rediscovered by researchers in western medicine. A study done by Kellgren in 1938 reported that intramuscular injection of sterile saline caused pain at locations away from the injection site [180]. Inspired by this study, Travell et al. realized that pressure applied to specific points (later defined as trigger points) relieved pain from shoulder and arm pain [181]. Later, Travell together with Simons, through their collaboration published their texts Myofascial Pain and Dysfunction, the Trigger Point Manual in 1983 [182,183]. Trigger points were described as locally tender points associated with focal areas of muscle shortening termed "taut bands". When palpated, trigger points can feel like small nodules within the muscle and may refer pain distally [182,183]. Dorsher, did a study based on Travell and Simons' texts, and found that 93.3% of the common myofascial trigger points (238 out of 255) correspond to the classical acupuncture points [184].

Translated into Chinese medicine terms, the above statement means that a trigger point is an area of Qi stagnation in the muscles. It also means that emotional stress may be the aetiological factor causing Qi stagnation in the muscles [144]. Ashi points, are very comparable to trigger points and were first mentioned in Bei Ji Qian Jin Yao Fang (Important Formulas Worth a Thousand Gold Pieces for Emergency) compiled by Sun Simiao in the Tang dynasty [185]. Chapter 13 of Huang Di Nei Jing Ling Shu, describes a treatment method, referring to Ashi points as "tenderness was taken as needling point" [127]. Ashi points are also used in other methods of treatment, such as Japanese shiatsu, Thai massage and Swedish deep tissue massage [186].

It is interesting to note that the route of referred pain from the heart, such as myocardial ischemia, is identical to the pathway of the heart meridian [187,188]. This kind of referred pain occurs due to the sharing of information between visceral and somatic afferent nerve fibres within overlapping spinal cord segments. The confusion about the origin of pain results from the density of sensory nerves higher in the skin than the heart [189].

Rong and Zhu suggested a common biological connection between the cardiac sympathetic nerve and the heart meridian (HM) [190]. Their findings provide a possible morphological and physiological explanation for the relation between referred cardiac pain and HM [190]. It is thus not surprising that traditionally, HM is being used to treat cardiac related illness, such as palpitation or cardiac arrhythmia, coronary heart disease, angina pectoris, myocardial infarction, ischaemic heart disease, cardiovascular disease and hypercholesterolemia [144,148,150,151,191–194].

7. Qi and Energy Fields

In the theory of TCM, Qi is thought to be a form of balancing energy that flows through the body. Qi keeps the body in harmony with the internal and the external environment that brings together the overall wellbeing of a person [126,129,142–144,150].

Chapter 18 of Huang Di Nei Jing Ling Shu [127], and Maciocia [192], give a detailed explanation about Qi formation. The production of Qi comes from the combination of food that we take and air that we breathe. Food is digested by the stomach and the nutrition is absorbed by the spleen and sent to the lung to form gathering Qi. The gathering Qi assists the lung in controlling Qi and breathing, and enhances the heart's function of governing blood and blood vessels. It combines with original Qi that originates from the kidney and can be compared to the dynamic motive force that activates and moves the functional activity of all the organs, to form true Qi. True Qi is the final stage in the process of refinement and transformation of Qi. True Qi is further divided into nutritive Qi and defensive Qi. The main function of nutritive Qi is to nourish the internal organs. Nutritive Qi is also related to blood, and flows in the channels and blood vessels. Nutritive Qi is activated whenever a needle is inserted in an acupuncture point. As the name implies, defensive Qi means to defend or to protect the body. Unlike nutritive Qi, it flows outside of the channels [192].

7.1. How to Relate Qi to Molecular Knowledge of Modern Medicine?

In modern medicine, energy is the product of metabolic degradation of food and nutrients. The process of energy formation involves a complex series of various types of chemicals, molecules and cellular reactions. The process of metabolism is a collection of chemical catabolic reactions that break down the food we eat, from protein into amino acids, fats into fatty acids, and carbohydrates into glucose by the enzymes of the digestive system. In a nutshell, the nutrients from food are converted into adenosine triphosphate (ATP), which provides the basic unit of energy required for all functions in the body. A molecule of ATP consists of adenine, ribose, and three phosphate groups. Energy together with adenosine diphosphate (ADP) and a phosphate group (symbolized as Ⓟ) are released when the terminal phosphate group is split off ATP. About 40% of the energy released in metabolism is used for cellular functions. The rest is converted to heat, some of which helps with maintaining the body temperature [188]. ATP is also involved in the process of muscle contraction and relaxation [188], inflammation [102] and the analgesic effect of acupuncture [195–201], as explained below.

7.2. Energy and Information

Albert Szent-Györgyi, was a Hungarian biochemist who discovered vitamin C (deficiency of vitamin C from malnutrition is the main cause of scurvy [131]) and won the Nobel Prize in Physiology or Medicine in 1937. He quoted "In every culture and in every medical tradition before ours, healing was accomplished by moving energy" [202]. The word "energy", for Szent-Györgyi, meant a cloud of electrons held together by nuclei [203]. He published a trilogy [202,204,205], based on his observation in the presence of energy in the living organisms during his study on cancer research. His study of energy in biology was linked to the role of purines and ATP as extracellular signaling molecules [206]. Later, this would have a great impact on the research of acupuncture. James Oschman, author of Energy Medicine, described the involvement of energy in the healing processes. The body is capable to take in, store, release, conduct, and utilise various kinds of energy and information [207].

Energy and information are also involved in the process of intercellular communication. This is done through action potential, an electrical signal conduction transporting information from one neuron to the next [102]. For example, action potential takes place by sending electrical impulses to the brain through afferent nerve fibres, such as in the event of pain or injury. To carry the information from one neuron to the next, neurotransmitters require energy in the form of ATP [208]. An action potential is also triggered by the stimulation of acupuncture needle insertion, which in turn affects the activities in the brain neuronal network [209].

Robert Becker, in his book, The Body Electric [210], hypothesizes that the acupuncture meridians are electrical conductors that send injury signals to the brain, which responds with the appropriate level of direct current to stimulate healing in the injured area. He also believed that the conductivity of the skin is much higher at acupuncture points.

Björn Nordenström, a Swedish radiologist and surgeon, and the author of Biologically Closed Electric Circuits [211], believed that Qi is equivalent to or perhaps the same as the electromagnetic energy found in biologically closed electrical circuits (BCEC). Its Yin and Yang components may be compared to the positive and negative electrical charges of closed circuit ionic flow. If the acupuncture needle is inserted through the normal muscle into the injured muscle, it thus acts as a short circuit to enable the flow of ions. This facilitates healing of the injured tissue. Both Becker [210] and Nordenström [211] believed that the process of healing might work electrically.

In 1980, Cohen et al. measured the magnetic fields produced by the human body with the sensitive magnetic detector called the Superconducting Quantum Interference Device (SQUID) [212]. The body's fluctuating magnetic fields, such as those from the heart are 100 times stronger than the field generated by the brain and can be detected up to a meter away from the body, in all directions, using SQUID-based magnetometers [213]. Both the magnetic fields produced by the heart and brain, can be measured via electrocardiogram (ECG) and electroencephalogram (EEG), respectively. Russek et al. proposed that the heart plays the major role in generating as well as integrating the flow of energy in the body [214].

Probably one of the best possible ways to explain the nature of Qi in a scientific manner is to relate it to the theory of extracellular and intracellular signaling. Qi can be considered to derive from signaling processes in the body, which include phosphorylation/dephosphorylation cascades, and guanine nucleotide-binding proteins (G protein) signaling involving cyclic adenosine monophosphate (cAMP) production and degradation, or calcium release and sequestration [215]. The balance between Yin and Yang that constitutes Qi could reflect cellular activities, which balance the actions of endogenous agonists and antagonists, and the sympathetic and parasympathetic nervous systems [216].

8. Is Acupuncture a Placebo Intervention?

Blinded controlled studies have addressed the following question. Do contextual effect and/or placebo acupuncture needle have the same therapeutic outcome as real acupuncture? The results from many randomized controlled trials (RCTs) have both proved and disproved the benefit of acupuncture. As compared to other types of pharmacological RCTs, the study of acupuncture is very complex due to the involvement of many issues, such as inadequate sample size, randomization, sham interventions, and blinding. The tendency that potential bias might arise from both the sham interventions and blinding procedures is another great challenge in such studies. Patients' expectation may also influence the final outcomes of the trials [217]. Table 1 summarized some of the RCTs of LBP treated with acupuncture. There was no special search strategy used to select the publications for Tables 1 and 2 and therefore it is rather an overview than evidence based on a systematic search method. Most articles can be found in the database Pubmed.

Table 1. Results of randomized control trials for acupuncture treatment of lower back pain.

Authors	Diagnosis	Intervention Group	Control Group	Outcome Measure	Result
Pach et al. (2013) [218]	CLBP	n = 73, standardized manual acupuncture; n = 66, individualized manual acupuncture	NA	VAS	Both intervention groups showed improvement in pain scale but there were no relevant difference between them
Molsberger et al. (2002) [219]	LBP	n = 65, manual acupuncture + conventional orthopaedic therapy	n = 61, sham acupuncture + conventional orthopaedic therapy; n = 60, conventional orthopaedic therapy	VAS	Acupuncture + conventional orthopaedic therapy were better than sham and conventional orthopaedic therapy alone
Weiß et al. (2013) [220]	CLBP	n = 74, manual acupuncture + inpatient rehabilitation program	n = 69, inpatient rehabilitation program	SF-36	Intervention group showed better results judging from SF-36 questionnaires
Inoue et al. (2006) [221]	LBP	n = 15, manual acupuncture	n = 16, sham acupuncture	VAS, Schober test	Both groups showed reduction in pain but intervention group showed better result than control group
Giles et al. (2003) [222]	CSP	n = 36, manual acupuncture; n = 36, spinal manipulation	n = 40, medication	ODI, NDI, SF-36, VAS	Manipulation achieved the best overall results, however, on the VAS for neck pain, acupuncture showed a better result than manipulation (50% vs. 42%)
Haake et al. (2007) [223]	CLBP	n = 387, manual acupuncture	n = 387, sham acupuncture; n = 388, conventional therapy (physiotherapy, exercise)	CPGS, HFAQ	Effectiveness of acupuncture, both verum and sham, was almost twice that of conventional therapy
Brinkhaus et a (2006) [224]	CLBP	n = 146, manual acupuncture; n = 73, minimal manual acupuncture	n = 79, waiting list	SF-36, VAS	Acupuncture was better than no acupuncture, but no significant differences between acupuncture and minimal acupuncture
Cho et al. (2013) [225]	CLBP	n = 57, manual acupuncture	n = 59, sham acupuncture	VAS	Acupuncture was better than sham acupuncture
Cherkin et al. (2001) [226]	CLBP	n = 94, manual acupuncture	n = 78, massage; n = 90, self-care	SBS, RDS	Massage was better than acupuncture and self-care
Cherkin et al. (2009) [227]	CLBP	n = 158, standardized manual acupuncture; n = 157, individualized manual acupuncture; n = 162, simulated acupuncture (using toothpick)	n = 161, usual care (medications, physiotherap)	RMDQ	All intervention groups showed better outcome than usual care, but no significant differences among the acupuncture groups

Table 1. *Cont.*

Authors	Diagnosis	Intervention Group	Control Group	Outcome Measure	Result
Yun et al. (2012) [228]	CLBP	n = 82, standardized manual acupuncture; n = 80, individualized manual acupuncture	n = 74, usual care (massage, physiotherapy, medications)	RMDQ, VAS	Intervention groups showed better results than control; but individualized acupuncture is more effective than standardized acupuncture
Zhang et al. (2017) [229]	DiscogenicSciatica	n = 50, 50 Hz electroacupuncture	n = 50, MFE	NRS, ODI, PGI	The effect of electroacupuncture was superior to that of MFE
Thomas et al. (1994) [230]	CNLBP	n = 7, manual acupuncture; n = 9, 2 Hz low frequency electroacupuncture; n = 11, 80 Hz high frequency electroacupuncture	n = 10, waiting list	ADL related to pain, ROM	All intervention groups showed reduction of pain, more so in low frequency electroacupuncture group in long term
Glazov et al. (2014) [231]	NSCLBP	840 nm laser acupuncture: n = 48, 0.8 Joules high dose; n = 48, 0.2 Joules low dose	n = 48, 0 Joules sham laser acupuncture (without switching on the laser)	NPRS, ODI	Treatment groups showed better result but no difference between sham and laser groups
Shin et al. (2015) [232]	LBP	660 nm laser acupuncture: n = 28	n = 27, sham laser acupuncture (without switching on the laser)	VAS, PPT	Both groups showed improvement in pain but no significant difference outcomes between the two groups

NA = Not Available; ADL = Activities of Daily Life; CPGS = Chronic Pain Grade Scale; HFAQ = Hanover Functional Ability Questionnaire; MFE = Medium-Frequency Electrotherapy; NDI = Neck Disability Index; NRS = Numerical Rating Scale; ODI = Oswestry Disability Index; NPRS = Numerical Pain Rating Scale; PGI = patient global impression; PPT = Pressure Pain Threshold; RDS = Roland Disability Scale; RMDQ = Roland-Morris Disability Questionnaire; ROM = Range of Motion; SBS = Symptom Bothersomeness Scale; SF-36 = Short-Form 36 Health Survey; VAS = Visual Analog Scale; CLBP = chronic low back pain; CNLBP = chronic nociceptive low back pain; CSP = chronic spinal pain; LBP = low back pain; NSCLBP = non-specific chronic low back pain; nm = Nanometer.

Table 2. Selection of acupuncture points of randomized control trials for treatment of lower back pain.

Authors	Local Points	Distant Points	Other Points
Pach et al. (2013) [218]	BL 23, 24, 25	BL 40, 60; GB 34; K 3	-
Molsberger et al. (2002) [219]	BL 23, 25; GB 30	BL 40, 60; GB 34	4 Ashi Points of maximum pain
Weiß et al. (2013) [220]	NA	NA	-
Inoue et al. (2006) [221]	-	-	Single Ashi Point at the most painful point
Giles et al. (2003) [222]	8 to 10 needles were placed in local paraspinal intramuscular maximum pain areas	Approximately 5 needles were placed in distal acupuncture point	-
Haake et al. (2007) [223]	14 to 20 needles were inserted but exact locations were not mentioned		
Brinkhaus et al. (2006) [224]	At least 4 local points: BL 20 to 34; BL 50 to 54; GB 30; GV 3, 4, 5, 6	At least 2 distant points: SI 3; BL 40, 60, 62; K 3, 7; GB 31, 34, 41; LR 3; GV 14, 20	Extraordinary Points: Huatojiaji & Shiqizhuixia
Cho et al. (2013) [225]	Points were chosen according to 3 types of meridian patterns: 1. Gallbladder Meridian: 12, 26, 30, 34, 41 2. Bladder Meridian: 23, 24, 25, 37, 40 3. Mixed Meridian: ST 4, 36; SP 13, 14; GV 3, 4, 5, 24, 26		
Cherkin et al. (2001) [226]	NA	NA	-
Cherkin et al. (2009) [227]	1. Individualized Acupuncture: Averaged of 10.8 needles, chosen from 74 points, half from Bladder meridian 2. Standardized Acupuncture: 8 acupuncture points commonly used for chronic low back pain (GV 3, BL 23 *, BL 40 *, K 3 *, Low Back Ashi Point) 3. Simulated Acupuncture: Using toothpick on acupuncture points		
Yun et al. (2012) [228]	GV 3; BL 23	BL 40; K 3	Low Back Ashi Points, Back-Pain Points ^
Zhang et al. (2017) [229]	BL 25	-	Extraordinary Points: JiaJi * (Ex-B2)
Thomas et al. (1994) [230]	BL 23, 25, 26, 32; GB 30, 34	BL 40, 60; SI 6; ST 36	-
Glazov et al. (2014) [231]	An average of 9 points were used: GV 13%, BL 37%, GB 13%, other meridians 16%, Ashi Points 14%, Extraordinary Points 7%		
Shin et al. (2015) [232]	GV 3, 4, 5; BL 23 *, 24 *, 25 *; GB 30 *	BL 40 *	-

BL = Bladder; GB = Gallbladder; GV = Governor Vessel; K = Kidney; LR = Liver; SP = Spleen; ST = Stomach; NA = Not Available; * = Bilaterally; ^ = Extra Meridian points on the back of hand.

8.1. *In the Wake of Double-Blind Randomised Control Trials (RCTs)*

The double-blind placebo-controlled clinical trial is considered as the gold standard for testing or comparing the efficacy of either new or existing treatments/drugs [233]. The idea was put forward by Austin Bradford Hill back in 1937 [234]. Before the mid-20th century, the practice of informed consent was not mandatory. Patients were often not informed of their involvement in a clinical study and did not realize that they might receive a placebo instead of a real treatment [235].

The main purpose to conduct a clinical RCT is to prevent bias or manipulation of results in medical studies [217,234–236]. Such biases originate from several sources. Patients' awareness of trials might lead to exaggerated expectations and responses [217,235,237–247]. Some clinical researchers might depend heavily on the pharmaceutical industry funding and may not be effectively protected from transmitting their sponsor's bias in favour of a new drug [247,248]. Surveys showed that double-blind methodologies are still not always properly applied to clinical tests [236,249–251].

8.2. *The Placebo Effect*

The question of whether acupuncture merely produces a placebo effect has to be considered in light of numerous studies done in this field. The word "placebo", is a Latin word, usually translated as "I shall please" [237]. According to Shapiro, a placebo is defined as "any therapeutic procedure (or a component of any therapeutic procedure) which is given (1) deliberately to have an effect, or (2) unknowingly and has an effect on a symptom, syndrome, disease, or patient but which is objectively without specific activity for the condition being treated. The placebo is also used as an adequate control in research. The placebo effect is defined as the changes produced by placebos" [252].

As stated by Walter Brown, author of The Placebo Effect in Clinical Practice, the act of seeking and receiving medical care itself is a placebo effect. Some conditions are highly placebo-responsive, which could bring up to as much as 50% relief. The placebo treatment can be used to enhance the benefits of standard treatments. The healing environment, which involves the personal attention and the two-way communication between a patient and a care provider, is a powerful antidote for illness [235]. Miller and Kaptchuk proposed this kind of placebo effect as "contextual healing", in which a specific clinical encounter contributes to therapeutic outcomes [253]. Jay Katz, author of The Silent World of Doctor and Patient, noted that "Physicians and patients may gradually learn that the placebo effect is an integral and inevitable component of the practice of medicine, that it constitutes its art and augments its science" [254]. Kerr et al. expressed "neurophenomenological" as the reason that caused the placebo effect from sham acupuncture due to the palpation and touch by the practitioner and tactile stimulation by sham acupuncture needles [255].

The mechanisms of the placebo analgesic effects include activation of endogenous opioids and dopamine release, and alteration of central processing of pain [238–240]. Expectation of benefit also plays an important role in the efficacy of placebo interventions [238–245]. Henry Beecher in his article "The Powerful Placebo", suggests that placebos can relieve pain arising from physiological causes and have an average significant effectiveness of $35.2 \pm 2.2\%$ [256].

8.3. *Clinical Studies*

The placebo effect produced by sham acupuncture, derives from patients' expectation and bias. Yet, this does not mean that the therapeutic effect of acupuncture is only explained as a placebo intervention. In comparing placebo to no treatment, such as those shown in Table 1, placebo was significantly more effective than no-treatment groups or even standard medical care. This was demonstrated by an impressive series of three-arm studies in German Acupuncture Trials (GERAD) for relief of LBP [223]. Subsequently, the outcome of treatment of chronic LBP by acupuncture was so positive that German insurance companies agreed to cover the cost of such treatments [223,257].

Therefore, it is safe to say that a placebo intervention that produces a real effect is not supposed to be called a "placebo". There must be some physiological or psychological mechanism that explains such effects. Besides tactile stimulation [255], several studies proposed that afferent nerve fibres are involved in response to acupuncture treatment [110,112].

8.4. Acupuncture Points for Lower Back Pain

In Table 2, only six out of 15 RCTs stated precisely which acupuncture points were used for the treatment of LBP. Of these, the most commonly used acupuncture points are GV 3, BL 23, BL 25 and BL 40. GV 3, BL 23 and BL 25 are all local points, while BL 40, located in the popliteal fossa, is a distal point for treating LBP. Other distal points are BL 60 and K 3, they are situated behind the lateral and medial malleolus.

The most commonly used acupuncture points in the treatment of LBP are listed in the literature [232,258]. Lee et al. did an investigation based on 53 clinical studies and came out with a summary of the most frequently used acupuncture points for the treatment of LBP [258]. It clearly shows that both the bladder and gallbladder meridians are the chosen choice for treating LBP with acupuncture, especially BL 23 (51%), follow by BL 25 (43%), BL 24, BL 40, BL 60 and GB 30 (32% each), BL 26 and BL 32 (28% each), and GB 34 (21%). In the opinion of Maciocia, the proper selection of local and distal points is based on the location and the nature of pain, and depends on the condition, if it is either acute or chronic [144].

8.5. Clinical Relevance

According to Robinson [176], acupuncture points BL 23, BL 24 and BL 26 improve circulation to the local tissues and resolve myofascial dysfunction and promote tissue recovery. BL 25 is stimulated to relax the myofascia and free the nerves which are entrapped and irritated. BL 40 may improve circulation and nerve health by reducing myofascial tension caused by neurovascular compression. BL 60 and K 3 are located on each side of the ankle, and represent the distant points for LBP. They contain an extensive sympathetic nerve supply that provides homeostatic effects. GB 30 sits on top of the sciatic nerve and is a good choice to treat sciatica caused by piriformis entrapment syndromes. GB 34, located on the neck of fibular, is a choice point to treat common peroneal (fibular) nerve syndrome. GV 3, which is supplied by the spinal segmental nerve and the somatosomatic as well as somatovisceral reflex connections, has neuromodulatory properties for treating LBP, paraparesis, sciatic pain, genitourinary conditions, and lower gastrointestinal disorders.

9. Mechanism of Acupuncture

What is actually happening the moment an acupuncture needle penetrates the skin [259]? According to Robinson, this interesting phenomenon is due to a higher density of sensory and sympathetic nerve fibres attached to blood vessels in distal than in proximal segments. Such an anatomical arrangement accounts for the relatively stronger autonomous responses associated with distal acupuncture points, especially those at the ends of the channels [176]. Dellon et al. came to the same conclusion concerning the higher concentration of sympathetic innervation in the foot [260].

Manipulation of acupuncture needle results in deformation of connective tissues and thus alters the structure of fibroblasts [197,261–264]. Such micro-injury caused by the puncturing of the acupuncture needle in the skin results in release of ATP [195–201,265,266]. ATP is then further broken down into adenosine and other purines [195–201,265,266]. Both ATP and adenosine act as anti-nociception agents that block pain through purinergic receptors [195–199,265–269].

9.1. Deqi

The pricking sensation caused by stimulation of acupuncture needle is termed Deqi. This refers to the excitation of Qi or vital energy inside meridians. Often patients might experience a combination of various sensations, including numbness, soreness, distention, heaviness, dull pain, or sharp pain during acupuncture needle insertion [270]. Deqi, which was mentioned in the chapter 1 of Huang Di Nei Jing Ling Shu [127], literally means "the arrival of vital energy", which is widely viewed as an important role in the process of achieving therapeutic effectiveness of acupuncture treatment [127,165,271–274]. A functional magnetic resonance imaging (fMRI) study conducted by Napadow et al. shows an increase of blood flow to the penetrated sites that are linked to the sensation of Deqi [275]. Kong et al. found that the different intensity of acupuncture sensations is associated with the effect of analgesia [276]. Spaeth et al. concluded that real acupuncture tends to produce a stronger Deqi sensation and better clinical outcomes as compared to sham acupuncture [277]. However, White et al. indicated that the sensation of Deqi does not impact the efficacy of acupuncture treatment [278].

9.2. *Needle Grasp*

The phenomenon of needle grasp is described as a tug on the needle, like a fish biting on a fishing line, creating a tight mechanical coupling between needle and tissue. Langevin et al. proposed that needle grasp perceived by acupuncturists corresponds to the sensation of Deqi, which is felt by patients. This may play an active role in the therapeutic mechanism of acupuncture [159,279,280]. These authors hypothesize that the manoeuvre of the needle (by rotation or piston movement) causes needle grasp, and hence, Deqi is a result of collagen and elastic fibres winding and tightening around the needle. Such a mechanism is responsible for the increase in pull-out force induced by needle rotation [159,279–281]. The higher density of connective tissues at acupuncture points might explain the occurrence of needle grasp [159].

Needle grasp allows further movements of the needle to pull and deform the connective tissue surrounding the needle, delivering some of its effects through mechanical influence on the connective tissue matrix [159,279–281]. In addition, the manipulation of the acupuncture needle causes remodeling of fibroblasts in the connective tissue [261–264].

9.3. *Afferent Nerve Fibres*

Many RCT studies claimed the lack of significant difference between real and sham acupuncture (Table 1) [224,227,231,232]. This conclusion arose from the fact that both real and sham acupuncture in these RCTs are involved in tactile stimulation [255]. The reason behind such phenomenon is due to the stimulation of the afferent nerve fibres [110,112,282]. Such superficial pressure via sham needling intervention can have significant effects on the brain's limbic system [245,283]. Acupuncture fMRI studies have shown that both tactile stimulation and acupuncture manipulation activate neural activities and thus might have a potential effect on pain modulation [283–286].

The human tactile sensation is thought to be moderated primarily by large myelinated afferents ($A\alpha$ and $A\beta$), while pain and temperature sensations are brought about by small myelinated ($A\delta$ fibre) and unmyelinated (C fibre) afferents [287]. It is therefore plausible that many sham acupunctures, used as control procedures in acupuncture studies, activated this group of afferents and hence produced analgesic effects [110,112]. Zhou et al. concluded that afferent fibres of type II ($A\beta$) and III ($A\delta$) are responsible for transmitting the acupuncture signal, which are important for acupuncture analgesia [168].

9.4. *Acupuncture Analgesic*

The study of acupuncture in pain management and its analgesic effects have been highlighted in the literature [110,112,119,134,136–140,142–144,146,147,151,163,170,176,192,195–201,235,241,288–290]. The gate control theory of pain, which was proposed by Melzack and Wall back in 1965 [93], and later by Melzack, suggested that the stimulation by the acupuncture needle activates the inhibitory brainstem system and therefore blocks pain signals [291]. The release of endogenous opioids [112,119,163,292] and ATP [195–201,265,266] triggered by an acupuncture needle have been well documented by many studies. This suggests a link between acupuncture and signaling mediated by neurotransmitters.

Endorphins are amongst the most studied neurotransmitters in acupuncture research. They are more powerful in pain relief than exogenous morphine [293]. A recent study conducted by Grissa et al. compared the effectiveness of acupuncture versus morphine in the management of acute pain in the emergency department. A reduction of pain by 92% was observed in patients treated with acupuncture, while morphine-treated patients experienced only 78% reduction. In addition, acupuncture-treated patients had a much faster pain recovery time (an average of 16 min compared to 28 min in the morphine control group) [294].

9.5. ATP as Neurotransmitter

Adenosine triphosphate (ATP) was discovered by Karl Lohman in 1929 [295]. In that same year, Drury and Szent-Györgyi described the effects of ATP on heart excitability, lowering of blood pressure and coronary vasodilation [206]. Research by Holton and Holton in 1954 identified ATP as a neurotransmitter in the somatosensory system. They demonstrated that ATP is released from peripheral endings of primary sensory neurons [296]. The signaling function of ATP in peripheral tissues was confirmed by numerous investigations done by Geoffrey Burnstock. This led to the discovery of Purinergic Signaling that consists of neurotransmission by purinergic receptors [297].

In 2009, Burnstock proposed that stimulation of the tissue with acupuncture needle, heat or electrical current triggers the release of a large quantity of ATP from keratinocytes, fibroblasts and other cells in the skin [298]. ATP activates P2X ligand-gated ion channel 3 receptors (P2X3), which are located on sensory nerves. Resulting signals modulate the pathways that lead to the CNS responsible for conscious awareness of pain [265–268,299–302].

9.6. Adenosine-Induced Anti-Nociception

As mentioned before, energy in the form of ATP is one of the essential requirements for our body's function [188]. Adenosine, which is the core molecule of ATP and of nucleic acids, forms a unique link among cell energy, gene regulation, and neuronal excitability [302]. Adenosine is recognised by specific receptors, which regulate neuronal and non-neuronal cellular functions. As a neurotransmitter, adenosine regulates pain transmission in both the spinal cord and in the periphery [303]. Adenosine acts as an endogenous anti-inflammatory agent and as such plays an important role as a signaling molecule in immunity and inflammation [304]. Hence, adenosine is involved in nearly every aspect of cell function.

Recently, in a series of experiments by Goldman et al., adenosine was identified as a mediator of anti-nociceptive properties in acupuncture experiments in mice [195]. In another study conducted by the same group in human subjects, they used tissue microdialysis to demonstrate the increased release of adenosine, adenosine monophosphate (AMP), adenosine diphosphate (ADP), and ATP at stimulated acupuncture points [196]. Both studies show that the concentration of interstitial purines were increased by mechanical stimulation from the acupuncture needle. In contrast, transgenic mice lacking adenosine A1 receptors do not show any sign of pain reduction [195].

Pharmacologically, the anti-nociceptive effect of acupuncture is prolonged by 2 to 2.5 h when the combination of acupuncture and injection of deoxycoformycin (dCF) were introduced [195,199]. Hurt and Zylka suggested that a longer period of pain relief might be achieved by injecting prostatic acid phosphatase (PAP) into the acupuncture points [305]. Both dCF and PAP are agonists of ATP production in response to acupuncture treatment [195,305]. But the opposite is observed when an adenosine receptor antagonist, such as caffeine, is either taken orally or injected at the acupuncture points, which then interfere with the analgesic effect of acupuncture [199,306]. Interestingly, from their observation, Tang et al. concluded that the higher efficacy of acupuncture in China than in western countries could be due to the lower consumption of coffee in China than in Europe and America [268].

10. Discussion

Low back pain is one of the most common musculoskeletal disorders in modern society [1–4]. There are increasing numbers of patients seeking complementary therapies, such as acupuncture, as a mean to supplement the conventional treatments. Many studies have produced conflicting results relating to the efficacy of acupuncture as a method to treat LBP. This is probably due to a small sample sizes, a lack of blinding procedures and improper methodological assessment tools [5,61,65,113,115].

In most RCTs, sham acupuncture was used as a control, either using sham acupuncture needles which do not penetrate the skin, or selecting sham acupuncture points (Table 1). It was interesting to observe the outcomes from the verum and sham acupuncture groups (Table 1). Both groups produced better results than conventional therapies or non-treatment groups and it was obvious that verum acupuncture produced slightly better results than sham acupuncture. The reason behind such a phenomenon could be attributed to tactile stimulation. Both puncturing the skin by acupuncture needle, and stimulation by sham needle on the skin surface, activate the afferent sensory receptors, leading to therapeutic effects.

The high density of nerve endings under acupuncture points could be another reason that contributed to the acupuncture-induced analgesic effects, which yields better results in verum than in the sham acupuncture group. The release of purines, such as ATP and adenosine, which bind to the purinergic receptors, provide a hypothesis to explain the efficacy in acupuncture against pain [110,112,119,134,136–140,142–144,146,147,151,163,170,176,192,195–201,235,241,288–290].

Why is acupuncture effective on some patients, but not on others? Many factors could give rise to such uneven responses. Patients' expectations might play a crucial role in the determination of the outcome of an acupuncture trial. So does the tendency of researchers' strong bias in favour of or against the efficacy of acupuncture, which might affect the overall outcome of a trial.

Combination of acupuncture with other regular therapies produces better results than conventional therapies alone. Therefore, a holistic approach to integrate acupuncture with other types of conventional treatments should be carried out for the benefit of the patients.

Of course our article also has potential limitations. In addition to the mentioned literature, many other high-quality RCTs on acupuncture and LBP have been conducted recently [307–309]. Although, the meta-analysis results of some of the systematic reviews indicated that acupuncture might be an effective treatment for chronic LBP in the short-term, conclusions among the reviews are inconsistent overall.

11. Conclusions

The WHO confirmed in 2002, the effectiveness of acupuncture treatment from controlled clinical trials for 28 diseases, symptoms, and conditions. LBP was one of the conditions that was mentioned in this report [310]. A meta-analysis of 33 RCTs of acupuncture for LBP showed better results than sham acupuncture and no treatment [311]. Meanwhile, the evidence for efficacy of the German Acupuncture Trials (GERAD) of 1162 patients with chronic low back pain compared verum acupuncture, sham acupuncture and a conventional therapy group as the control. The effectiveness of acupuncture, both verum and sham, was almost twice that of conventional therapy 6 months after the trial [223]. Acupuncture is recommended for patients with chronic LBP due to its cost-effectiveness [312] and low adverse effects [313].

The discovery of purines-mediated (both ATP and adenosine) anti-nociceptive effects of acupuncture, has led to a better understanding of molecular events underlying the mechanism of acupuncture in the peripheral nervous system. However, our knowledge of mechanisms associated with acupuncture's analgesic properties remains limited. Integration of acupuncture treatments with conventional therapies, and pharmacological agents should lead to medical strategies without addictive side effects.

Despite shown effectiveness by RCTs and the discovery of potential molecular mechanisms, acupuncture is still not well accepted by the social security services in Austria and many European countries. Such a situation results from health policy and the regulation of the healthcare bodies in different European Union (EU) members. Yet, any treatment producing better outcomes at a lower cost is a desirable step towards more sustainable health systems.

Author Contributions: The manuscript has been written by T.-K.L. as master thesis at the Medical University of Vienna under the supervision of G.L., Head of the TCM Research Center at the Medical University of Graz, Austria. G.L. is also lecturer at the Master Program "Principles and Practice of Traditional Chinese Medicine (TCM)" (Coordinator: Y.M.) at Medical University of Vienna. The scientific work was co-supervised by F.B. from the Gregor Mendel Institute of Vienna.

Acknowledgments: Supported by the Austrian Federal Ministry of Education, Science and Research ("Sino-Austrian TCM Research on Lifestyle-Related Diseases" (2016–2019; project leaders: Yan Ma and Gerhard Litscher)). The manuscript was read and corrected by all authors. The study was partially supported by the Austrian Ministry of Education, Science, and Research and the Eurasia Pacific Uninet as well as the German Academy of Acupuncture (President Bernd Ramme), for which a heartfelt thank you should be expressed.

Abbreviations

5-HT	5-hydroxytryptamine
A1R	Adenosine A1 receptor
ADL	activities of daily life
ADP	adenosine diphosphate
AIDS	acquired immune deficiency syndrome
AMP	adenosine monophosphate
ATP	adenosine triphosphate
BCEC	Biologically Closed Electric Circuits
BMI	body mass index
cAMP	cyclic adenosine monophosphate
CGRP	calcitonin gene-related peptide
CLBP	chronic low back pain
CNLBP	chronic nociceptive low back pain
CNS	central nervous system
CO_2	carbon dioxide
COPD	chronic obstructive pulmonary disease
CSP	chronic spinal pain
CVDs	cardiovascular diseases
DALYs	disability-adjusted life years
dCF	deoxycoformycin
DRG	dorsal root ganglia
EA	electroacupuncture
ECG	electrocardiogram
EEG	electroencephalogram
EU	European Union
fMRI	functional magnetic resonance imaging
GBD	The Global Burden of Disease Study
GERAD	German Acupuncture Trials
GIDs	gastrointestinal disorders
G proteins	guanine nucleotide-binding proteins
GV	Governing Vessel
H^+	protons
H_2O	water
HIV	human immunodeficiency virus
HM	Heart meridian
LBP	lower back pain
MA	manual acupuncture
MFE	Medium-Frequency Electrotherapy
mTrPs	Myofascial Trigger Points
MUS	medically unexplained symptoms

NGF	nerve growth factor
NRS	numerical rating scale
NSAIDs	non-steroidal anti-inflammatory drugs
NSCLBP	non-specific chronic low back pain
P2X3	P2X ligand-gated ion channel 3 receptor
PAP	prostatic acid phosphatase
PGI	patient global impression
PN	primo node
PPT	pressure pain threshold
PV	primo vessel
PVS	primo vascular system
RCTs	randomised control trials
ROM	range of motion
SQID	Superconducting Quantum Interference Device
TCM	Traditional Chinese Medicine
TENS	transcutaneous electric nerve stimulation
TRP	transient receptor potential
TRPA1	transient receptor potential ankyrin 1
TRPV1	transient receptor potential vanilloid 1
VAS	visual analogue scale
WHO	World Health Organisation
YLDs	years lived with disability

References

1. Béatrice Duthey. Background Paper 6.24 Lower Back Pain. 2013. Available online: http://www.who.int/medicines/areas/priority_medicines/BP6_24LBP.pdf (accessed on 5 June 2018).
2. Driscoll, T.; Jacklyn, G.; Orchard, J.; Passmore, E.; Vos, T.; Freedman, G.; Lim, S.; Punnett, L. The global burden of occupationally related low back pain: Estimates from the Global Burden of Disease 2010 study. *Ann. Rheum. Dis.* **2014**, *73*, 975–981. [CrossRef] [PubMed]
3. Hoy, D.; March, L.; Brooks, P.; Blyth, F.; Woolf, A.; Bain, C.; Williams, G.; Smith, E.; Vos, T.; Barendregt, J.; et al. The global burden of low back pain: Estimates from the Global Burden of Disease 2010 study. *Ann. Rheum. Dis.* **2014**, *73*, 968–974. [CrossRef] [PubMed]
4. Van Tulder, M.; Koes, B. Low Back Pain. In *Wall and Melzack's Textbook of Pain*, 6th ed.; McMahon, S., Koltzenburg, M., Tracey, I., Turk, D., Eds.; Churchill Livingstone: Philadelphia, PA, USA, 2013; Chapter 49.
5. Van Tulder, M.; Becker, A.; Bekkering, T.; Breen, A.; Hutchinson, A.; Koes, B.; Laerum, E.; Malmivaara, A. Chapter 3 European guidelines for the management of acute nonspecific lower back pain in primary care. *Eur. Spine J.* **2006**, *15* (Suppl. 2), S169–S191. [CrossRef] [PubMed]
6. Burton, A.K.; Balagué, F.; Cardon, G.; Eriksen, H.R.; Henrotin, Y.; Lahad, A.; Leclerc, A.; Müller, G.; van der Beek, A.J. Chapter 2 European guidelines for prevention in low back pain. *Eur. Spine J.* **2006**, *15* (Suppl. 2), S136–S168. [CrossRef] [PubMed]
7. Yiengprugsawan, V.; Hoy, D.; Buchbinder, R.; Bain, C.; Seubsman, S.; Sleigh, A.C. Low back pain and limitations of daily living in Asia: Longitudinal findings in the Thai cohort study. *BMC Musculoskelet. Disord.* **2017**, *18*, 19. [CrossRef] [PubMed]
8. Norbye, A.D.; Omdal, A.V.; Nygaard, M.E.; Romild, U.; Eldøen, G.; Midgard, R. Do patients with chronic low back pain benefit from early intervention regarding absence from work? *Spine* **2016**, *41*, E1257–E1264. [CrossRef] [PubMed]
9. Kolu, P.; Tokola, K.; Kankaanpää, M.; Suni, J. Evaluation of the effects of physical activity, cardiorespiratory condition, and neuromuscular fitness on direct healthcare costs and sickness-related absence among nursing personnel with recurrent nonspecific low back pain. *Spine* **2017**, *42*, 854–862. [CrossRef] [PubMed]

10. McPhillips-Tangum, C.A.; Cherkin, D.C.; Rhodes, L.A.; Markham, C. Reasons for repeated medical visits among patients with chronic back pain. *J. Gen. Intern Med.* **1998**, *13*, 289–295. [CrossRef] [PubMed]
11. Jöud, A.; Petersson, I.F.; Englund, M. Low back pain: Epidemiology of consultations. *Arthritis Care Res.* **2012**, *64*, 1084–1088. [CrossRef] [PubMed]
12. WHO Methods and Data Sources for Global Burden of Disease Estimates 2000–2011. Available online: http://www.who.int/healthinfo/statistics/GlobalDALYmethods_2000_2011.pdf (accessed on 5 June 2018).
13. Global, regional, and national incidence, prevalence, and years lived with disability for 328 diseases and injuries for 195 countries, 1990–2016: A systematic analysis for the Global Burden of Disease Study 2016. *Lancet* **2017**, *390*, 1211–1259.
14. Global, regional, and national disability-adjusted life-years (DALYs) for 333 diseases and injuries and healthy life expectancy (HALE) for 195 countries and territories, 1990–2016: A systematic analysis for the Global Burden of Disease Study 2016. *Lancet* **2017**, *390*, 1260–1344.
15. WHO Methods and Data Sources for Global Burden of Disease Estimates 2000–2015. WHO: Geneva, Switzerland, January 2017. Available online: http://www.who.int/healthinfo/global_burden_disease/GlobalDALYmethods_2000_2015.pdf (accessed on 5 June 2018).
16. The Institute for Health Metrics and Evaluation (IHME). Available online: http://www.healthdata.org/austria (accessed on 5 June 2018).
17. Hoy, D.; Bain, C.; Williams, G.; March, L.; Brooks, P.; Blyth, F.; Woolf, A.; Vos, T.; Buchbinder, R. A systematic review of the global prevalence of low back pain. *Arthritis Rheum.* **2012**, *64*, 2028–2037. [CrossRef] [PubMed]
18. Frymoyer, J.W.; Cats-Baril, W.L. An overview of the incidences and costs of low back pain. *Orthop. Clin. N. Am.* **1991**, *22*, 263–271.
19. Geusens, P.; De Winter, L.; Quaden, D.; Vanhoof, J.; Vosse, D.; Van den Bergh, J.; Somers, V. The prevalence of vertebral fractures in spondyloarthritis: Relation to disease characteristics, bone mineral density, syndesmophytes and history of back pain and trauma. *Arthritis Res. Ther.* **2015**, *17*, 294. [CrossRef] [PubMed]
20. Kim, K.; Isu, T.; Chiba, Y.; Iwamoto, N.; Yamazaki, K.; Morimoto, D.; Isobe, M.; Inoue, K. Treatment of low back pain in patients with vertebral compression fractures and superior cluneal nerve entrapment neuropathies. *Surg. Neurol. Int.* **2015**, *6* (Suppl. 24), S619–S621. [CrossRef] [PubMed]
21. Michailidou, C.; Marston, L.; De Souza, L.H.; Sutherland, I. A systematic review of the prevalence of musculoskeletal pain, back and low back pain in people with spinal cord injury. *Disabil. Rehabilit.* **2014**, *36*, 705–715. [CrossRef] [PubMed]
22. Määttä, J.H.; Wadge, S.; MacGregor, A.; Karppinen, J.; Williams, F.M. ISSLS prize winner: Vertebral endplate (Modic) change is an independent risk factor for episodes of severe and disabling low back pain. *Spine* **2015**, *40*, 1187–1193. [CrossRef] [PubMed]
23. Jensen, O.K.; Nielsen, C.V.; Sørensen, J.S.; Stengaard-Pedersen, K. Back pain was less explained than leg pain: A cross-sectional study using magnetic resonance imaging in low back pain patients with and without radiculopathy. *BMC Musculoskelet. Disord.* **2015**, *16*, 374. [CrossRef] [PubMed]
24. Daghighi, M.H.; Pouriesa, M.; Maleki, M.; Fouladi, D.F.; Pezeshki, M.Z.; Khameneh, R.M.; Bazzazi, A.M. Migration patterns of herniated disc fragments: A study on 1020 patients with extruded lumbar disc herniation. *Spine J.* **2014**, *14*, 1970–1977. [CrossRef] [PubMed]
25. Kuniya, H.; Aota, Y.; Kawai, T.; Kaneko, K.; Konno, T.; Saito, T. Prospective study of superior cluneal nerve disorder as a potential cause of low back pain and leg symptoms. *J. Orthop. Surg. Res.* **2014**, *9*, 139. [CrossRef] [PubMed]
26. Samini, F.; Gharedaghi, M.; Mahdi Khajavi, M.; Samini, M. The etiologies of low back pain in patients with lumbar disk herniation. *Iran. Red Crescent Med. J.* **2014**, *16*, E15670. [CrossRef] [PubMed]
27. Gorth, D.J.; Shapiro, I.M.; Risbud, M.V. Discovery of the drivers of inflammation induced chronic low back pain: From bacteria to diabetes. *Discov. Med.* **2015**, *20*, 177–184. [PubMed]
28. Fisher, T.J.; Osti, O.L. Do bacteria play an important role in the pathogenesis of low back pain? *ANZ J. Surg.* **2015**, *85*, 808–814. [CrossRef] [PubMed]
29. Hassoon, A.; Bydon, M.; Kerezoudis, P.; Maloney, P.R.; Rinaldo, L.; Yeh, H.C. Chronic low-back pain in adult with diabetes: NHANES 2009–2010. *J. Diabetes Complicat.* **2017**, *31*, 38–42. [CrossRef] [PubMed]
30. Piazzolla, A.; Solarino, G.; Bizzoca, D.; Montemurro, V.; Berjano, P.; Lamartina, C.; Martini, C.; Moretti, B. Spinopelvic parameter changes and low back pain improvement due to femoral neck anteversion in patients

with severe unilateral primary hip osteoarthritis undergoing total hip replacement. *Eur. Spine J.* **2018**, *27*, 125–134. [CrossRef] [PubMed]
31. Yamada, K.; Suzuki, A.; Takahashi, S.; Yasuda, H.; Koike, T.; Nakamura, H. Severe low back pain in patients with rheumatoid arthritis is associated with Disease Activity Score but not with radiological findings on plain X-rays. *Mod. Rheumatol.* **2015**, *25*, 56–61. [CrossRef] [PubMed]
32. El Barzouhi, A.; Vleggeert-Lankamp, C.L.; van der Kallen, B.F.; Lycklama à Nijeholt, G.J.; van den Hout, W.B.; Koes, B.W.; Peul, W.C. Back pain's association with vertebral end-plate signal changes in sciatica. *Spine J.* **2014**, *14*, 225–233. [CrossRef] [PubMed]
33. Wang, C.; Yu, X.; Yan, Y.; Yang, W.; Zhang, S.; Xiang, Y.; Zhang, J.; Wang, W. Tumor necrosis factor-α: A key contributor to intervertebral disc degeneration. *Acta Biochim. Biophys. Sin.* **2017**, *49*, 1–13. [CrossRef] [PubMed]
34. Wang, M.; Yu, J.; Liu, N.; Liu, Z.; Wei, X.; Yan, F.; Yu, S. Low back pain among taxi drivers: A cross-sectional study. *Occup. Med.* **2017**, *67*, 290–295. [CrossRef] [PubMed]
35. Snow, C.R.; Gregory, D.E. Perceived risk of low-back injury among four occupations. *Hum. Factors* **2016**, *58*, 586–594. [CrossRef] [PubMed]
36. Esquirol, Y.; Niezborala, M.; Visentin, M.; Leguevel, A.; Gonzalez, I.; Marquié, J.C. Contribution of occupational factors to the incidence and persistence of chronic low back pain among workers: Results from the longitudinal VISAT study. *Occup. Environ. Med.* **2017**, *74*, 243–251. [CrossRef] [PubMed]
37. Rafeemanesh, E.; Omidi Kashani, F.; Parvaneh, R.; Ahmadi, F. A Survey on Low Back Pain Risk Factors in Steel Industry Workers in 2015. *Asian Spine J.* **2017**, *11*, 44–49. [CrossRef] [PubMed]
38. Sundstrup, E.; Andersen, L.L. Hard physical work intensifies the occupational consequence of physician-diagnosed back disorder: Prospective cohort study with register follow-up among 10,000 workers. *Int. J. Rheumatol.* **2017**, *2017*, 1037051. [CrossRef] [PubMed]
39. Heuch, I.; Heuch, I.; Hagen, K.; Zwart, J.A. Physical activity level at work and risk of chronic low back pain: A follow-up in the Nord-Trøndelag Health Study. *PLoS ONE* **2017**, *12*, e0175086. [CrossRef] [PubMed]
40. Trompeter, K.; Fett, D.; Platen, P. Prevalence of back pain in sports: A systematic review of the literature. *Sports Med.* **2017**, *47*, 1183–1207. [CrossRef] [PubMed]
41. Matesan, M.; Behnia, F.; Bermo, M.; Vesselle, H. SPECT/CT bone scintigraphy to evaluate low back pain in young athletes: Common and uncommon etiologies. *J. Orthop. Surg. Res.* **2016**, *11*, 76. [CrossRef] [PubMed]
42. del Pozo-Cruz, B.; Gusi, N.; Adsuar, J.C.; del Pozo-Cruz, J.; Parraca, J.A.; Hernandez-Mocholí, M. Musculoskeletal fitness and health-related quality of life characteristics among sedentary office workers affected by sub-acute, non-specific low back pain: A cross-sectional study. *Physiotherapy* **2013**, *99*, 194–200. [CrossRef] [PubMed]
43. Billy, G.G.; Lemieux, S.K.; Chow, M.X. Lumbar disc changes associated with prolonged sitting. *PM R* **2014**, *6*, 790–795. [CrossRef] [PubMed]
44. Teichtahl, A.J.; Urquhart, D.M.; Wang, Y.; Wluka, A.E.; O'Sullivan, R.; Jones, G.; Cicuttini, F.M. Physical inactivity is associated with narrower lumbar intervertebral discs, high fat content of paraspinal muscles and low back pain and disability. *Arthritis Res. Ther.* **2015**, *17*, 114. [CrossRef] [PubMed]
45. Krieg, S.M.; Meyer, B. Operative Therapiemöglichkeiten beim Postnukleotomiesyndrom. *Orthopäde* **2016**, *45*, 732–737. [CrossRef] [PubMed]
46. Manchikanti, L.; Manchikanti, K.N.; Gharibo, C.G.; Kaye, A.D. Efficacy of percutaneous adhesiolysis in the treatment of lumbar post surgery syndrome. *Anesthesiol. Pain Med.* **2016**, *6*, E26172. [CrossRef] [PubMed]
47. Kaptan, H.; Kulaksızoğlu, H.; Kasımcan, Ö.; Seçkin, B. The association between urinary incontinence and low back pain and radiculopathy in women. *Open Access Maced. J. Med. Sci.* **2016**, *4*, 665–669. [CrossRef] [PubMed]
48. Ha, I.H.; Lee, J.; Kim, M.R.; Kim, H.; Shin, J.S. The association between the history of cardiovascular diseases and chronic low back pain in South Koreans: A cross-sectional study. *PLoS ONE* **2014**, *9*, e93671. [CrossRef] [PubMed]
49. Heuch, I.; Heuch, I.; Hagen, K.; Zwart, J.A. Does high blood pressure reduce the risk of chronic low back pain? The Nord-Trøndelag Health Study. *Eur. J. Pain* **2014**, *18*, 590–598. [CrossRef] [PubMed]
50. Bohman, T.; Alfredsson, L.; Jensen, I.; Hallqvist, J.; Vingård, E.; Skillgate, E. Does a healthy lifestyle behaviour influence the prognosis of low back pain among men and women in a general population? A population-based cohort study. *BMJ Open* **2014**, *4*, e005713. [CrossRef] [PubMed]

51. Maulik, S.; Iqbal, R.; De, A.; Chandra, A.M. Evaluation of the working posture and prevalence of musculoskeletal symptoms among medical laboratory technicians. *J. Back Musculoskelet. Rehabilit.* **2014**, *27*, 453–461. [CrossRef] [PubMed]
52. Burgel, B.J.; Elshatarat, R.A. Psychosocial work factors and low back pain in taxi drivers. *Am. J. Ind. Med.* **2017**, *60*, 734–746. [CrossRef] [PubMed]
53. Yang, H.; Haldeman, S.; Lu, M.L.; Baker, D. Low back pain prevalence and related workplace psychosocial risk factors: A study using data from the 2010 National Health Interview Survey. *J. Manip. Physiol. Ther.* **2016**, *39*, 459–472. [CrossRef] [PubMed]
54. Rahimi, A.; Vazini, H.; Alhani, F.; Anoosheh, M. Relationship between low back pain with quality of life, depression, anxiety and stress among emergency medical technicians. *Trauma Mon.* **2015**, *20*, E18686. [CrossRef] [PubMed]
55. Smuck, M.; Kao, M.C.; Brar, N.; Martinez-Ith, A.; Choi, J.; Tomkins-Lane, C.C. Does physical activity influence the relationship between low back pain and obesity? *Spine J.* **2014**, *14*, 209–216. [CrossRef] [PubMed]
56. Zhang, T.T.; Liu, Z.; Liu, Y.L.; Zhao, J.J.; Liu, D.W.; Tian, Q.B. Obesity as a risk factor for low back pain: A meta-analysis. *Clin. Spine Surg.* **2018**, *31*, 22–27. [CrossRef] [PubMed]
57. Großschädl, F.; Freidl, W.; Rásky, E.; Burkert, N.; Muckenhuber, J.; Stronegger, W.J. A 35-year trend analysis for back pain in Austria: The role of obesity. *PLoS ONE* **2014**, *9*, e107436. [CrossRef] [PubMed]
58. Farioli, A.; Mattioli, S.; Quaglieri, A.; Curti, S.; Violante, F.S.; Coggon, D. Musculoskeletal pain in Europe: Role of personal, occupational and social risk factors. *Scand. J. Work Environ. Health* **2014**, *40*, 36–46. [CrossRef] [PubMed]
59. Wong, A.Y.; Karppinen, J.; Samartzis, D. Low back pain in older adults: Risk factors, management options and future directions. *Scoliosis Spinal Disord.* **2017**, *12*, 14. [CrossRef] [PubMed]
60. Jesus-Moraleida, F.R.; Ferreira, P.H.; Ferreira, M.L.; Silva, J.P.; Maher, C.G.; Enthoven, W.T.; Bierma-Zeinstra, S.M.A.; Koes, B.W.; Luijsterburg, P.A.J.; Pereira, L.S.M. Back complaints in the elders in Brazil and the Netherlands: A cross-sectional comparison. *Age Ageing* **2017**, *46*, 476–481. [CrossRef] [PubMed]
61. Maher, C.; Underwood, M.; Buchbinder, R. Non-specific low back pain. *Lancet* **2017**, *389*, 736–747. [CrossRef]
62. Arrouas, M.; Fiala, W.; Hanna-Klinger, M.; Hartl, F.; Lampl, P.D.D.C.; Plank, V.; Schlegl, C. Update der evidenz- und konsensusbasierten österreichischen Leitlinien für das Management akuter und chronischer unspezifischer Kreuzschmerzen 2011. *ÖÄZ* **2012**, *2324*, 30–39. Available online: http://www.aekwien.at/aekmedia/UpdateLeitlinienKreuzschmerz_2011_0212.pdf (accessed on 5 June 2018).
63. Krismer, M.; van Tulder, M. Strategies for prevention and management of musculoskeletal conditions. Low back pain (non-specific). *Best Pract. Res. Clin. Rheumatol.* **2007**, *21*, 77–91. [CrossRef] [PubMed]
64. Hoy, D.; Brooks, P.; Blyth, F.; Buchbinder, R. The epidemiology of low back pain. *Best Pract. Res. Clin. Rheumatol.* **2010**, *24*, 769–781. [CrossRef] [PubMed]
65. Salzberg, L.D.; Manusov, E.G. Management options for patients with chronic back pain without an etiology. *Health Serv. Insights* **2013**, *6*, 33–38. [CrossRef] [PubMed]
66. Wáng, Y.X.J.; Wáng, J.Q.; Káplár, Z. Increased low back pain prevalence in females than in males after menopause age: Evidences based on synthetic literature review. *Quant. Imaging Med. Surg.* **2016**, *6*, 199–206. [CrossRef] [PubMed]
67. Schneider, S.; Randoll, D.; Buchner, M. Why do women have back pain more than men? A representative prevalence study in the federal republic of Germany. *Clin. J. Pain* **2006**, *22*, 738–747. [CrossRef] [PubMed]
68. Ochsmann, E.; Rüger, H.; Kraus, T.; Drexler, H.; Letzel, S.; Münster, E. Geschlechtsspezifische Risikofaktoren akuter Rückenschmerzen. *Schmerz* **2009**, *23*, 377–384. [CrossRef] [PubMed]
69. Großschädl, F.; Stolz, E.; Mayerl, H.; Rásky, É.; Freidl, W.; Stronegger, W. Educational inequality as a predictor of rising back pain prevalence in Austria—Sex differences. *Eur. J. Public Health* **2016**, *26*, 248–253. [CrossRef] [PubMed]
70. Kaulagekar, A. Age of menopause and menopausal symptoms among urban women in Pune, Maharashtra. *J. Obstet. Gynaecol. India* **2011**, *61*, 323–326. [CrossRef]
71. Foster, N.E.; Bishop, A.; Bartlam, B.; Ogollah, R.; Barlas, P.; Holden, M.; Ismail, K.; Jowett, S.; Kettle, C.; Kigozi, J.; et al. Evaluating acupuncture and standard care for pregnant women with back pain (EASE Back): A feasibility study and pilot randomised trial. *Health Technol. Assess.* **2016**, *20*, 1–236. [CrossRef] [PubMed]

72. Liddle, S.D.; Pennick, V. Interventions for preventing and treating low-back and pelvic pain during pregnancy. *Cochrane Database Syst. Rev.* **2015**. [CrossRef] [PubMed]
73. Bhardwaj, A.; Nagandla, K. Musculoskeletal symptoms and orthopaedic complications in pregnancy: Pathophysiology, diagnostic approaches and modern management. *Postgrad. Med. J.* **2014**, *90*, 450–460. [CrossRef] [PubMed]
74. Chen, H.M.; Wang, H.H.; Chiu, M.H.; Hu, H.M. Effects of acupressure on menstrual distress and low back pain in dysmenorrheic young adult women: An experimental study. *Pain Manag. Nurs.* **2015**, *16*, 188–197. [CrossRef] [PubMed]
75. Katz, V.L.; Lentz, G.M.; Lobo, R.A.; Gershenson, D.M. *Comprehensive Gynecology*, 5th ed.; Mosby Elsevier: Philadelphia, PA, USA, 2007; Chapter 36.
76. Poomalar, G.K.; Arounassalame, B. The quality of life during and after menopause among rural women. *J. Clin. Diagn Res.* **2013**, *7*, 135–139.
77. Kozinoga, M.; Majchrzycki, M.; Piotrowska, S. Low back pain in women before and after menopause. *Prz. Menopauzalny* **2015**, *14*, 203–207. [CrossRef] [PubMed]
78. Wijnhoven, H.A.; de Vet, H.C.; Smit, H.A.; Picavet, H.S. Hormonal and reproductive factors are associated with chronic low back pain and chronic upper extremity pain in women—The MORGEN study. *Spine* **2006**, *31*, 1496–1502. [CrossRef] [PubMed]
79. Chou, Y.C.; Shih, C.C.; Lin, J.G.; Chen, T.L.; Liao, C.C. Low back pain associated with sociodemographic factors, lifestyle and osteoporosis: A population-based study. *J. Rehabil. Med.* **2013**, *45*, 76–80. [CrossRef] [PubMed]
80. Ahn, S.; Song, R. Bone mineral density and perceived menopausal symptoms: Factors influencing low back pain in postmenopausal women. *J. Adv. Nurs.* **2009**, *65*, 1228–1236. [CrossRef] [PubMed]
81. Yi, Y.; Hwang, B.; Son, H.; Cheong, I. Low bone mineral density, but not epidural steroid injection, is associated with fracture in postmenopausal women with low back pain. *Pain Physician* **2012**, *15*, 441–449. [PubMed]
82. Kitahara, H.; Ye, Z.; Aoyagi, K.; Ross, P.D.; Abe, Y.; Honda, S.; Kanagae, M.; Mizukami, S.; Kusano, Y.; Tomita, M.; et al. Associations of vertebral deformities and osteoarthritis with back pain among Japanese women: The Hizen-Oshima study. *Osteoporos. Int.* **2013**, *24*, 907–915. [CrossRef] [PubMed]
83. Heuch, I.; Heuch, I.; Hagen, K.; Zwart, J.A. Body mass index as a risk factor for developing chronic low back pain: A follow-up in the Nord-Trøndelag Health Study. *Spine* **2013**, *38*, 133–139. [CrossRef] [PubMed]
84. Kulie, T.; Slattengren, A.; Redmer, J.; Counts, H.; Eglash, A.; Schrager, S. Obesity and women's health: An evidence-based review. *J. Am. Board Fam. Med.* **2011**, *24*, 75–85. [CrossRef] [PubMed]
85. WHO. Obesity and Overweight. Available online: http://www.who.int/mediacentre/factsheets/fs311/en/ (accessed on 5 June 2018).
86. Bouchard, C.; Katzmarzyk, P.T. *Physical Activity and Obesity*, 2nd ed.; Human Kinetics: Champaign, IL, USA, 2010; Chapter 78.
87. Shemory, S.T.; Pfefferle, K.J.; Gradisar, I.M. Modifiable risk factors in patients with low back pain. *Orthopedics* **2016**, *39*, e413–e416. [CrossRef] [PubMed]
88. Kwon, M.A.; Shim, W.S.; Kim, M.H.; Gwak, M.S.; Hahm, T.S.; Kim, G.S.; Kim, C.S.; Choi, Y.H.; Park, J.H.; Cho, H.S.; et al. A correlation between low back pain and associated factors: A study involving 772 patients who had undergone general physical examination. *J. Korean Med. Sci.* **2006**, *21*, 1086–1091. [CrossRef] [PubMed]
89. Hayes, M.H.S.; Patterson, D.G. Experimental development of the graphic rating method. *Psychol. Bull.* **1921**, *18*, 98–99.
90. Siegfried, M.; Gerwin, R.D. *Muscle Pain: Understanding the Mechanisms*; Springer: Heiderberg, Germany, 2010; Chapter 1.
91. Merskey, H.; Bogduk, N. *Classification of Chronic Pain*, 2nd ed.; IASP Press: Seattle, WA, USA, 1994.
92. Sherrington, C. *The Integrative Action of the Nervous System*; Yale University Press: New Haven, CT, USA, 1906.
93. Melzack, R.; Wall, P.D. Pain mechanisms: A new theory. *Science* **1965**, *150*, 971–979. [CrossRef] [PubMed]
94. Khadilkar, A.; Odebiyi, D.O.; Brosseau, L.; Wells, G.A. Transcutaneous electrical nerve stimulation (TENS) versus placebo for chronic low-back pain. *Cochrane Database Syst. Rev.* **2008**. [CrossRef] [PubMed]
95. Pert, C.B.; Snyder, S.H. Opiate receptor: Demonstration in nervous tissue. *Science* **1973**, *179*, 1011–1014. [CrossRef] [PubMed]

96. Hughes, J.; Kosterlitz, H.W.; Smith, T.W.; Fothergill, L.A.; Morgan, B.A.; Morris, H.R. Identification of two related pentapeptides from the brain with potent opiate agonist activity. *Nature* **1975**, *258*, 577–580. [CrossRef] [PubMed]
97. Hughes, J.; Kosterlitz, H.W.; Smith, T.W. The distribution of methionine-enkephalin and leucine-enkephalin in the brain and peripheral tissues. *Br. J. Pharmacol.* **1977**, *61*, 639–647. [CrossRef] [PubMed]
98. Nicoll, R.A.; Siggins, G.R.; Ling, N.; Bloom, F.E.; Guillemin, R. Neuronal actions of endorphins and enkephalins among brain regions: A comparative microiontophoretic study. *Proc. Natl. Acad. Sci. USA* **1977**, *74*, 2584–2588. [CrossRef] [PubMed]
99. Simantov, R.; Kuhar, M.J.; Uhl, G.R.; Snyder, S.H. Opioid peptide enkephalin: Immunohistochemical mapping in rat central nervous system. *Proc. Natl. Acad. Sci. USA* **1977**, *74*, 2167–2171. [CrossRef] [PubMed]
100. Tran, V.T.; Chang, R.S.; Snyder, S.H. Histamine H1 receptors identified in mammalian brain membranes with [3H]mepyramine. *Proc. Natl. Acad. Sci. USA* **1978**, *75*, 6290–6294. [CrossRef] [PubMed]
101. Loeser, J.D.; Treede, R.D. The Kyoto protocol of IASP basic pain terminology. *Pain* **2008**, *137*, 473–477. [CrossRef] [PubMed]
102. Purves, D.; Augustine, G.J.; Fitzpatrick, D.; Hall, W.C.; LaMantia, A.S.; McNamara, J.O.; Williams, S.M. *Neuroscience*, 3rd ed.; Sinauer Associates, Inc.: Sunderland, MA, USA, 2004; Chapter 9.
103. Dobkin, B.H. *The Clinical Science of Neurologic Rehabilitation*, 2nd ed.; Oxford University Press: Oxford, UK, 2003; Chapter 8.
104. Usunoff, K.G.; Popratiloff, A.; Schmitt, O.; Wree, A. *Functional Neuroanatomy of Pain*; Springer: Berlin, Germany, 2006; Chapter 1.
105. Lautenbacher, S.; Fillingim, R.B. *Pathophysiology of Pain Perception*; Springer: New York, NY, USA, 2004; Chapter 1.
106. Macintyre, P.E.; Schug, S.A.; Scott, D.A.; Visser, E.J.; Walker, S.M. *Acute Pain Management: Scientific Evidence*, 3rd ed.; Working Group of the Australian and New Zealand College of Anaesthetists and Faculty of Pain Medicine, ANZCA & FPM: Melbourne, Australia, 2010; Chapter 1.
107. Archer, P.; Nelson, L. *Applied Anatomy & Physiology for Manual Therapists*; Lippincott, Williams & Wilkins: Philadelphia, PA, USA, 2013; Chapter 7.
108. Livingston, W.K. *Pain Mechanisms*; Plenum Press: New York, NY, USA, 1976; Chapter 1.
109. Basbaum, A.I.; Bautista, D.M.; Scherrer, G.; Julius, D. Cellular and molecular mechanisms of pain. *Cell* **2009**, *139*, 267–284. [CrossRef] [PubMed]
110. Kagitani, F.; Uchida, S.; Hotta, H. Afferent nerve fibers and acupuncture. *Auton. Neurosci.* **2010**, *157*, 2–8. [CrossRef] [PubMed]
111. Palastanga, N.; Soames, R. *Anatomy and Human Movement*, 6th ed.; Churchill Livingstone: Edinburg, UK, 2012; Chapter 1.
112. Zhao, Z.Q. Neural mechanism underlying acupuncture analgesia. *Prog. Neurobiol.* **2008**, *85*, 355–375. [CrossRef] [PubMed]
113. Qaseem, A.; Wilt, T.J.; McLean, R.M.; Forciea, M.A. Clinical Guidelines Committee of the American College of Physicians. Noninvasive treatments for acute, subacute, and chronic low back pain: A clinical practice guideline from the American College of Physicians. *Ann. Intern Med.* **2017**, *166*, 514–530. [CrossRef] [PubMed]
114. Bernstein, I.A.; Malik, Q.; Carville, S.; Ward, S. Low back pain and sciatica: Summary of NICE guidance. *BMJ* **2017**, *356*, i6748. [CrossRef] [PubMed]
115. Nunn, M.L.; Hayden, J.A.; Magee, K. Current management practices for patients presenting with low back pain to a large emergency department in Canada. *BMC Musculoskelet. Disord.* **2017**, *18*, 92. [CrossRef] [PubMed]
116. Australian Acute Musculoskeletal Pain Guidelines Group. *Evidence-Based Management of Acute Musculoskeletal Pain*; Australian Academic Press: Brisbane, Australia, 2003; Chapter 4. Available online: https://www.nhmrc.gov.au/_files_nhmrc/publications/attachments/cp94_evidence_based_management_acute_musculoskeletal_pain_131223.pdf (accessed on 5 June 2018).
117. Kissin, I. The development of new analgesics over the past 50 years: A lack of real breakthrough drugs. *Anesth. Analg.* **2010**, *110*, 780–789. [CrossRef] [PubMed]
118. Marcus, D.A. *Chronic Pain*; Human Press: Totowa, NJ, USA, 2005; Chapter 2.

119. Maoying, Q.; Mi, W. Acupuncture Analgesia in Clinical Practice. In *Acupuncture Therapy for Neurological Diseases*; Xia, Y., Cao, X.D., Wu, G.C., Cheng, J.S., Eds.; Tsinghua University Press: Beijing, China; Springer: Berlin, Germany, 2010; Chapter 7.
120. World Health Organization. WHO Global Atlas of Traditional, Complementary and Alternative Medicine. WHO Centre for Health Development: Kobe, Japan, 2005. Available online: http://apps.who.int/iris/bitstream/10665/43108/1/9241562862_map.pdf (accessed on 5 June 2018).
121. Cui, J.; Wang, S.B.; Ren, J.H.; Zhang, J.; Jing, J. Use of acupuncture in the USA: Changes over a decade (2002–2012). *Acupunct. Med.* **2017**, *35*, 200–207. [CrossRef] [PubMed]
122. Von Ammon, K.; Frei-Erb, M.; Cardini, F.; Daig, U.; Dragan, S.; Hegyi, G.; Roberti di Sarsina, P.; Sörensen, J.; Lewith, G. Complementary and alternative medicine provision in Europe—First results approaching reality in an unclear field of practices. *Forsch. Komplementmed.* **2012**, *19* (Suppl. 2), 37–43. [CrossRef] [PubMed]
123. Breuer, J.; Reinsperger, I.; Piso, B. *Akupunktur. Einsatzgebiete, Evidenzlage und gesicherte Indikationen. HTA Projektbericht Nr. 78*; Ludwig Boltzmann Institut für Health Technology Assessment: Wien, Austria, 2014.
124. Bundesgesetz über die Gesundheit Österreich GmbH (GÖGG) 132/2006. In Legal Status and Regulation of CAM in Europe. Available online: http://www.cam-europe.eu/dms/files/CAMbrella_Reports/CAMbrella-WP2-part_1final.pdf (accessed on 5 June 2018).
125. World Health Organization. WHO Traditional Medicine Strategy: 2014–2023. World Health Organization, 2013. Available online: http://apps.who.int/iris/bitstream/10665/92455/1/9789241506090_eng.pdf (accessed on 5 June 2018).
126. Unschuld, P.U.; Tessenow, H.; Zheng, J. *Huang Di Nei Jing Su Wen: An Annotated Translation of Huang Di's Inner Classic—Basic Questions*; University of California Press: Berkeley, CA, USA, 2011.
127. *Huang Di Nei Jing Ling Shu*; Unschuld, P.U., Translator; University of California Press: Oakland, CA, USA, 2016.
128. *Nan-Ching (The Classic of Difficult Issues)*; Translated and annotated by Unschuld, P.U.; University of California Press: Berkeley, CA, USA, 1986.
129. *Zhen Jiu Jia Yi Jing (The Systematic Classic of Acupuncture and Moxibustion) by Huangfu Mi*; Yang, S.; Chace, C., Translators; Blue Poppy Press: Boulder, CO, USA, 2004.
130. Unschuld, P.U. *Approaches to Traditional Chinese Medical Literature: Proceedings of an International Symposium on Translation Methodologies and Terminologies*; Kluwer Academic Publishers: Dordrecht, The Netherlands, 1989.
131. Kiple, K.F. *The Cambridge World History of Human Disease*; Cambridge University Press: Cambridge, UK, 1993; Chapter 1.
132. Ma, K.W. Acupuncture: Its place in the history of Chinese medicine. *Acupunct. Med.* **2000**, *18*, 88–99. [CrossRef]
133. White, A.; Ernst, E. A brief history of acupuncture. *Rheumatology* **2004**, *43*, 662–663. [CrossRef] [PubMed]
134. Bivins, R.E. *Acupuncture, Expertise and Cross-Cultural Medicine*; Palgrave Macmillan: Basingstoke, UK, 2000.
135. Reston, J. *Now, About My Operation in Peking*; New York Times: New York, NY, USA, 1971; Volume 1, p. 6. Available online: http://www.nytimes.com/1971/07/26/archives/now-about-my-operation-in-peking-now-let-me-tell-you-about-my.html (accessed on 5 June 2018).
136. Chaves, J.F.; Barber, T.X. Acupuncture Analgesia: A Six-Factor Theory. In *Pain*; Weisenberg, M., Tursky, B., Eds.; Plenum Press: New York, NY, USA, 1976; Chapter 4.
137. Dimond, E.G. Acupuncture anesthesia. Western medicine and Chinese traditional medicine. *JAMA* **1971**, *218*, 1558–1563. [CrossRef] [PubMed]
138. SpoereL, W.E. Acupuncture: Canadian anesthetists report on visit to China. *Can. Med. Assoc. J.* **1974**, *111*, 1123.
139. Bonica, J.J. Acupuncture anesthesia in the People's Republic of China. Implications for American medicine. *JAMA* **1974**, *229*, 1317–1325. [CrossRef] [PubMed]
140. Hamilton, S.G. Anesthesia by acupuncture. *Br. Med. J.* **1972**, *4*, 232–233. [CrossRef] [PubMed]
141. World Health Organization. The Contribution of Traditional Chinese Medicine to Sustainable Development: Keynote Address at the International Conference on the Modernization of Traditional Chinese Medicine. WHO: Singapore, October 2016. Available online: http://www.who.int/dg/speeches/2016/chinese-medicine-sustainable/en/ (accessed on 5 June 2018).
142. Lozano, F. Basic Theories of Traditional Chinese Medicine. In *Acupuncture for Pain Management*; Lin, Y., Hsu, E.S., Eds.; Springer: Heidelberg, Germany, 2014; Chapter 2.

143. Sun, P. *The Treatment of Pain with Chinese Herbs and Acupuncture*, 2nd ed.; Churchill Livingstone: Edinburg, UK, 2011; Chapter 1.
144. Maciocia, G. *The Practice of Chinese Medicine: The Treatment of Diseases with Acupuncture and Chinese Herbs*, 2nd ed.; Churchill Livingstone: Edinburg, UK, 2008; Chapter 39.
145. Du, G.H.; Yuan, T.Y.; Du, L.D.; Zhang, Y.X. The potential of traditional Chinese medicine in the treatment and modulation of pain. *Adv. Pharmacol.* **2016**, *75*, 325–361. [PubMed]
146. Newberg, A.B.; Lee, B.Y.; LaRiccia, P.J. Acupuncture in theory and practice part I: Theoretical basis and physiologic effects. *Hosp. Physician* **2004**, *40*, 11–18.
147. British Medical Association. *Acupuncture: Efficacy, Safety and Practice*; Harwood Academic Publishers: Amsterdam, The Netherlands, 2005; Chapter 2.
148. Beijing College of Traditional Chinese Medicine. *Essentials of Chinese Acupuncture*; Foreign Languages Press: Beijing, China, 1980.
149. World Health Organization. *WHO Standard Acupuncture Point Locations*; World Health Organization: Geneva, Switzerland, 2009.
150. Focks, C. *Atlas of Acupuncture*; Churchill Livingstone: Munich, Germany, 2008.
151. Deadman, P.; Al-Khafaji, M.; Baker, K. A Manual of Acupuncture. *J. Chin. Med. Publ.* **2001**. Available online: https://www.naturmed.de/produkt/a-manual-of-acupuncture-deadman-p-al-khafaji-m-baker-k/ (accessed on 5 June 2018).
152. Kim, B.H. On the Kyungrak System. *J. Acad. Med. Sci. DPR Korea* **1963**, *90*, 1–35.
153. Soh, K.S.; Kang, K.A.; Ryu, Y.H. 50 years of Bong-Han theory and 10 years of primo vascular system. *Evid. Based Complement. Alternat. Med.* **2013**, *2013*, 587827. [CrossRef] [PubMed]
154. Shin, H.S.; Soh, K.S. Electrical method to detect a Bonghan duct inside blood vessels. *New Phys.* **2002**, *45*, 376–378.
155. Stefanov, M.; Potroz, M.; Kim, J.; Lim, J.; Cha, R.; Nam, M.H. The primo vascular system as a new anatomical system. *J. Acupunct. Meridian Stud.* **2013**, *6*, 331–338. [CrossRef] [PubMed]
156. Ciszek, M.; Szopinski, J.; Skrzypulec, V. Investigations of morphological structure of acupuncture points and meridians. *J. Tradit. Chin. Med.* **1985**, *5*, 289–292. [PubMed]
157. Lazorthes, Y.; Esquerré, J.P.; Simon, J.; Guiraud, G.; Guiraud, R. Acupuncture meridians and radiotracers. *Pain* **1990**, *40*, 109–112. [CrossRef]
158. Darras, J.; Albarède, P.; de Vernejoul, P. Nuclear medicine investigation of transmission of acupuncture information. *Acupunct. Med.* **1993**, *11*, 22–28. [CrossRef]
159. Langevin, H.M.; Yandow, J.A. Relationship of acupuncture points and meridians to connective tissue planes. *Anat. Rec.* **2002**, *269*, 257–265. [CrossRef] [PubMed]
160. Heine, H. Anatomical structure of acupoints. *J. Tradit. Chin. Med.* **1988**, *8*, 207–212. [PubMed]
161. Li, A.H.; Zhang, J.M.; Xie, Y.K. Human acupuncture points mapped in rats are associated with excitable muscle/skin-nerve complexes with enriched nerve endings. *Brain Res.* **2004**, *1012*, 154–159. [CrossRef] [PubMed]
162. Ahn, A.C.; Wu, J.; Badger, G.J.; Hammerschlag, R.; Langevin, H.M. Electrical impedance along connective tissue planes associated with acupuncture meridians. *BMC Complement. Altern. Med.* **2005**, *5*, 10. [CrossRef] [PubMed]
163. Ahn, A.C.; Park, M.; Shaw, J.R.; McManus, C.A.; Kaptchuk, T.J.; Langevin, H.M. Electrical impedance of acupuncture meridians: The relevance of subcutaneous collagenous bands. *PLoS ONE* **2010**, *5*, e11907. [CrossRef] [PubMed]
164. Litscher, G.; Wang, L. Biomedical engineering meets acupuncture—Development of a miniaturized 48-channel skin impedance measurement system for needle and laser acupuncture. *Biomed. Eng. Online* **2010**, *9*, 78. [CrossRef] [PubMed]
165. Stux, G.; Pomeranz, B. *Acupuncture: Textbook and Atlas*; Springer: Berlin, Germany, 1987; Chapter 1.
166. Kramer, S.; Winterhalter, K.; Schober, G.; Becker, U.; Wiegele, B.; Kutz, D.F.; Kolb, F.P.; Zaps, D.; Lang, P.M.; Irnich, D. Characteristics of electrical skin resistance at acupuncture points in healthy humans. *J. Altern. Complement. Med.* **2009**, *15*, 495–500. [CrossRef] [PubMed]
167. Litscher, G.; Wang, L.; Gao, X.Y.; Gaischek, I. Electrodermal mapping: A new technology. *World J. Methodol.* **2011**, *1*, 22–26. [CrossRef] [PubMed]

168. Zhou, F.; Huang, D.K.; Xia, Y. Neuroanatomic Basis of Acupuncture Points. In *Acupuncture Therapy for Neurological Diseases*; Tsinghua University Press: Beijing, China; Springer: Berlin, Germany, 2010; Chapter 2.
169. Yao, W.; Yang, H.W.; Yin, N.; Ding, G.H. Mast cell-nerve cell interaction at acupoint: Modeling mechanotransduction pathway induced by acupuncture. *Int. J. Biol. Sci.* **2014**, *10*, 511–519. [CrossRef] [PubMed]
170. Zhang, D.; Ding, G.; Shen, X.; Yao, W.; Zhang, Z.; Zhang, Y.; Lin, J.; Gu, Q. Role of mast cells in acupuncture effect: A pilot study. *Explore* **2008**, *4*, 170–177. [CrossRef] [PubMed]
171. Marcelli, S. Gross anatomy and acupuncture: A comparative approach to reappraise the meridian system. *Med. Acupunct.* **2013**, *25*, 5–22. [CrossRef]
172. Peuker, E.; Cummings, M. Anatomy for the acupuncturist—Facts & fiction 1: The head and neck region. *Acupunct. Med.* **2003**, *21*, 2–8. [PubMed]
173. Peuker, E.; Cummings, M. Anatomy for the acupuncturist—Facts & fiction 2: The chest, abdomen, and back. *Acupunct. Med.* **2003**, *21*, 72–79. [PubMed]
174. Cheng, K.J. Neuroanatomical characteristics of acupuncture points: Relationship between their anatomical locations and traditional clinical indications. *Acupunct. Med.* **2011**, *29*, 289–294. [CrossRef] [PubMed]
175. Shaw, V.; McLennan, A.K. Was acupuncture developed by Han Dynasty Chinese anatomists? *Anat. Rec.* **2016**, *299*, 643–659. [CrossRef] [PubMed]
176. Robinson, N.G. *Interactive Medical Acupuncture Anatomy*; Tenton NewMedia: Jackson, MS, USA, 2016; Section 3, Channel 1.
177. Zhang, W.; Tao, Q.; Guo, Z.; Fu, Y.; Chen, X.; Shar, P.A.; Shahen, M.; Zhu, J.; Xue, J.; Bai, Y.; et al. Systems pharmacology dissection of the integrated treatment for cardiovascular and gastrointestinal disorders by Traditional Chinese Medicine. *Sci. Rep.* **2016**, *6*, 32400. [CrossRef] [PubMed]
178. Myers, T. *Anatomy Trains*, 2nd ed.; Churchill Livingstone: Edinburg, UK, 2009.
179. Finando, S.; Finando, D. Fascia and the mechanism of acupuncture. *J. Bodyw. Mov. Ther.* **2011**, *15*, 168–176. [CrossRef] [PubMed]
180. Kellgren, J.H. A preliminary account of referred pains arising from muscle. *Br. Med. J.* **1938**, *1*, 325–327. [CrossRef] [PubMed]
181. Travell, J.; Rinzler, S.; Herman, M. Pain and disability of the shoulder and arm: Treatment by intramuscular infiltration with procaine hydrochloride. *J. Am. Med. Assoc.* **1942**, *120*, 417–422. [CrossRef]
182. Travell, J.; Simons, D. *Myofascial Pain and Dysfunction: The Trigger Point Manual (Volume 1: Upper Extremities)*, 2nd ed.; Williams & Wilkins: Baltimore, MD, USA, 1998.
183. Travell, J.; Simons, D. *Myofascial Pain and Dysfunction: The Trigger Point Manual (Volume 2: Lower Extremities)*; Lippincott Williams & Wilkins: Philadelphia, PA, USA, 1983.
184. Dorsher, P.T. Myofascial referred-pain data provide physiologic evidence of acupuncture meridians. *J. Pain* **2009**, *10*, 723–731. [CrossRef] [PubMed]
185. Jiang, S.; Zhao, J.S. The historical source of "Trigger Points": Classical ashi points. *World J. Acupunct. Moxibustion* **2016**, *26*, 11–14. [CrossRef]
186. Nugent-Head, A. Ashi points in clinical practice. *J. Chin. Med.* **2013**, *101*, 5–12.
187. Focks, C.; Hosbach, I.; März, U. *Leitfaden Akupunktur, 2. Auflage*; Elsevier: München, Germany, 2014.
188. Tortora, G.J.; Derrickson, B. *Principles of Anatomy & Physiology*, 14th ed.; Wiley: Hoboken, NJ, USA, 2014.
189. Wilson-Pauwels, L.; Stewart, P.; Akesson, E. *Autonomic Nerves*; BC Decker: London, UK, 1997; Chapter 3.
190. Rong, P.; Zhu, B. Mechanism of relation among heart meridian, referred cardiac pain and heart. *Sci. China C Life Sci.* **2002**, *45*, 538–545. [CrossRef] [PubMed]
191. Cheng, J. *Anatomical Atlas of Chinese Acupuncture Points*; Shandong Science and Technology Press: Jinan China, 1982.
192. Maciocia, G. *The Foundations of Chinese Medicine*, 3rd ed.; Elsevier: Edinburg, UK, 2015; Chapter 32.
193. Liu, Z.; Liu, L. *Essential of Chinese Medicine*; Springer: Heidelberg, Germany, 2009; Chapter 5; Volume 2.
194. O'Brien, K.A. Alternative perspectives: How Chinese medicine understands hypercholesterolemia. *Cholesterol* **2010**, *2010*, 723289. [CrossRef] [PubMed]
195. Goldman, N.; Chen, M.; Fujita, T.; Xu, Q.; Peng, W.; Liu, W.; Jebsebm, T.K.; Pei, Y.; Wang, F.; Han, X.; et al. Adenosine A1 receptors mediate local anti-nociceptive effects of acupuncture. *Nat. Neurosci.* **2010**, *13*, 883–888. [CrossRef] [PubMed]

196. Takano, T.; Chen, X.; Luo, F.; Goldman, N.; Zhao, Y.; Markman, J.D.; Nedergaard, M. Traditional acupuncture triggers a local increase in adenosine in human subjects. *J. Pain* **2012**, *13*, 1215–1223. [CrossRef] [PubMed]
197. Goldman, N.; Chandler-Militello, D.; Langevin, H.M.; Nedergaard, M.; Takano, T. Purine receptor mediated actin cytoskeleton remodeling of human fibroblasts. *Cell Calcium* **2013**, *53*, 297–301. [CrossRef] [PubMed]
198. Ren, W.; Tu, W.Z.; Jiang, S.H.; Cheng, R.D.; Du, Y.P. Electroacupuncture improves neuropathic pain: Adenosine, adenosine 5′-triphosphate disodium and their receptors perhaps change simultaneously. *Neural Regen Res.* **2012**, *7*, 2618–2623. [PubMed]
199. Zylka, M.J. Needling adenosine receptors for pain relief. *Nat. Neurosci.* **2010**, *13*, 783–784. [CrossRef] [PubMed]
200. Wang, L.; Sikora, J.; Hu, L.; Shen, X.Y.; Grygorczyk, R.; Schwarz, W. ATP release from mast cells by physical stimulation: A putative early step in activation of acupuncture points. *Evid. Based Complement. Alternat. Med.* **2013**, *2013*, 350949. [CrossRef] [PubMed]
201. Lin, D.; De La Pena, I.; Lin, L.L.; Zhou, S.F.; Borlongan, C.V.; Cao, C.H. The neuroprotective role of acupuncture and activation of the BDNF signalling pathway. *Int. J. Mol. Sci.* **2014**, *15*, 3234–3252. [CrossRef] [PubMed]
202. Szent-Györgyi, A. *Introduction to a Submolecular Biology*; Academic Press: New York, NY, USA, 1960.
203. Szent-Györgyi, A. The Development of Bioenergetics. In *Membrane Structure and Mechanisms of Biological Energy Transduction*; Plenum Press: London, UK, 1973.
204. Szent-Györgyi, A. *Bioenergetics*; Academic Press: New York, NY, USA, 1957.
205. Szent-Györgyi, A. *Bioelectronics*; Academic Press: New York, NY, USA, 1968.
206. Drury, A.N.; Szent-Györgyi, A. The physiological activity of adenine compounds with special reference to their action upon mammalian heart. *J. Physiol.* **1929**, *68*, 213–237. [CrossRef] [PubMed]
207. Oschman, J.L. *Energy Medicine: The Scientific Basis*, 2nd ed.; Elsevier: Edinburg, UK, 2016.
208. Sengupta, B.; Stemmler, M.; Laughlin, S.B.; Niven, J.E. Action potential energy efficiency varies among neuron types in vertebrates and invertebrates. *PLoS Comput. Biol.* **2010**, *6*, E1000840. [CrossRef] [PubMed]
209. Yi, G.S.; Wang, J.; Deng, B.; Hong, S.H.; Wei, X.L.; Chen, Y.Y. Action potential threshold of wide dynamic range neurons in rat spinal dorsal horn evoked by manual acupuncture at ST36. *Neurocomputing* **2015**, *166*, 201–209. [CrossRef]
210. Becker, R.; Selden, G. *The Body Electric*; William Marrow: New York, NY, USA, 1985; Chapter 13.
211. Nordenström, B. *Biologically Closed Electric Circuits*; Nordic Medical Publications: Stockholm, Sweden, 1983; Chapter 18.
212. Cohen, D.; Palti, Y.; Cuffin, B.N.; Schmid, S.J. Magnetic fields produced by steady currents in the body. *Proc. Natl. Acad. Sci. USA* **1980**, *77*, 1447–1451. [CrossRef] [PubMed]
213. McCraty, R. *Science of the Heart*; HeartMath Institute: Boulder Creek, CA, USA, 2015; Volume 2, Chapter 6.
214. Russek, L.; Schwartz, G. Energy cardiology: A dynamical energy systems approach for integrating conventional and alternative medicine. *Advances* **1996**, *12*, 4–24.
215. Adams, J.; Parker, K. *Extracellular and Intracellular Signalling*; Royal Society of Chemistry: Cambridge, UK, 2011; Chapter 1.
216. Adams, J.; Lien, E. *Traditional Chinese Medicine: Scientific Basis for Its Use*; Royal Society of Chemistry: Cambridge, UK, 2013; Chapter 1.
217. Deng, S.; Zhao, X.; Du, R.; He, S.; Wen, Y.; Huang, L.; Tian, G.; Zhang, C.; Meng, Z.; Shi, X. Is acupuncture no more than a placebo? Extensive discussion required about possible bias. *Exp. Ther. Med.* **2015**, *10*, 1247–1252. [CrossRef] [PubMed]
218. Pach, D.; Yang-Strobel, X.; Lüdtke, R.; Roll, S.; Icke, K.; Brinkhaus, B.; Witt, C.M. Standardized versus individualized acupuncture for chronic low back pain: A randomized controlled trial. *Evid. Based Complement. Alternat. Med.* **2013**, *2013*, 125937. [CrossRef] [PubMed]
219. Molsberger, A.F.; Mau, J.; Pawelec, D.B.; Winkler, J. Does acupuncture improve the orthopedic management of chronic low back pain—A randomized, blinded, controlled trial with 3 months follow up. *Pain* **2002**, *99*, 579–587. [CrossRef]
220. Weiss, J.; Quante, S.; Xue, F.; Muche, R.; Reuss-Borst, M. Effectiveness and acceptance of acupuncture in patients with chronic low back pain: Results of a prospective, randomized, controlled trial. *J. Altern. Complement. Med.* **2013**, *19*, 935–941. [CrossRef] [PubMed]

221. Inoue, M.; Kitakoji, H.; Ishizaki, N.; Tawa, M.; Yano, T.; Katsumi, Y.; Kawakita, K. Relief of low back pain immediately after acupuncture treatment—A randomised, placebo controlled trial. *Acupunct. Med.* **2006**, *24*, 103–108. [CrossRef] [PubMed]
222. Giles, L.; Muller, R. Chronic spinal pain: A randomized clinical trial comparing medication, acupuncture, and spinal manipulation. *Spine* **2003**, *28*, 1490–1502. [CrossRef] [PubMed]
223. Haake, M.; Müller, H.H.; Schade-Brittinger, C.; Basler, H.D.; Schäfer, H.; Maier, C.; Endres, H.G.; Trampisch, H.J.; Wolsberger, A. German Acupuncture Trials (GERAC) for chronic low back pain: Randomized, multicenter, blinded, parallel-group trial with 3 groups. *Arch. Intern Med.* **2007**, *167*, 1892–1898. [CrossRef] [PubMed]
224. Brinkhaus, B.; Witt, C.M.; Jena, S.; Linde, K.; Streng, A.; Wagenpfeil, S.; Irnich, D.; Walther, H.-U.; Melchart, D.; Willich, S.N. Acupuncture in patients with chronic low back pain: A randomized controlled trial. *Arch. Intern Med.* **2006**, *166*, 450–457. [CrossRef] [PubMed]
225. Cho, Y.J.; Song, Y.K.; Cha, Y.Y.; Shin, B.C.; Shin, I.H.; Park, H.J.; Lee, H.-S.; Kim, K.-W.; Cho, J.-H.; Chuang, W.S.; et al. Acupuncture for chronic low back pain: A multicenter, randomized, patient-assessor blind, sham-controlled clinical trial. *Spine* **2013**, *38*, 549–557. [CrossRef] [PubMed]
226. Cherkin, D.C.; Eisenberg, D.; Sherman, K.J.; Barlow, W.; Kaptchuk, T.J.; Street, J.; Deyo, R.A. Randomized trial comparing traditional Chinese medical acupuncture, therapeutic massage, and self-care education for chronic low back pain. *Arch. Intern Med.* **2001**, *161*, 1081–1088. [CrossRef] [PubMed]
227. Cherkin, D.C.; Sherman, K.J.; Avins, A.L.; Erro, J.H.; Ichikawa, L.; Barlow, W.E.; Delney, K.; Hawkes, R.; Hamilton, L.; Pressman, A.; et al. A randomized trial comparing acupuncture, simulated acupuncture, and usual care for chronic low back pain. *Arch. Intern Med.* **2009**, *169*, 858–866. [CrossRef] [PubMed]
228. Mingdong, Y.; Na, X.; Mingyang, G.; Jun, Z.; Defang, L.; Yong, L.; Lingling, G.; Jiao, Y. Acupuncture at the back-pain-acupoints for chronic low back pain of peacekeepers in Lebanon: A randomized controlled trial. *J. Muscoskelet. Pain* **2012**, *20*, 107–115. [CrossRef]
229. Zhang, X.; Wang, Y.; Wang, Z.; Wang, C.; Ding, W.; Liu, Z. A randomized clinical trial comparing the effectiveness of electroacupuncture versus medium-frequency electrotherapy for discogenic sciatica. *Evid. Based Complement. Alternat. Med.* **2017**, *2017*, 9502718. [CrossRef] [PubMed]
230. Thomas, M.; Lundberg, T. Importance of modes of acupuncture in the treatment of chronic nociceptive low back pain. *Acta Anaesthesiol. Scand.* **1994**, *38*, 63–69. [CrossRef] [PubMed]
231. Glazov, G.; Yelland, M.; Emery, J. Low-dose laser acupuncture for non-specific chronic low back pain: A double-blind randomised controlled trial. *Acupunct. Med.* **2014**, *32*, 116–123. [CrossRef] [PubMed]
232. Shin, J.Y.; Ku, B.; Kim, J.U.; Lee, Y.J.; Kang, J.H.; Heo, H.; Choi, H.-J.; Lee, J-H. Short-term effect of laser acupuncture on lower back pain: A randomized, placebo-controlled, double-blind trial. *Evid. Based Complement. Alternat Med.* **2015**, *2015*, 808425. [CrossRef] [PubMed]
233. Bothwell, L.E.; Greene, J.A.; Podolsky, S.H.; Jones, D.S. Assessing the gold standard—Lessons from the history of RCTs. *N. Engl. J. Med.* **2016**, *374*, 2175–2181. [CrossRef] [PubMed]
234. Hill, A.B. *Principles of Medical Statistics*, 6th ed.; Oxford University Press: New York, NY, USA, 1955; Chapter 1.
235. Brown, W. *The Placebo Effect in Clinical Practice*; Oxford University Press: Oxford, UK, 2013; Chapters 2–4.
236. Kaptchuk, T.J. The double-blind, randomized, placebo-controlled trial: Gold standard or golden calf? *J. Clin. Epidemiol.* **2001**, *54*, 541–549. [CrossRef]
237. Moerman, D. *Meaning, Medicine, and the "Placebo Effect"*; Cambridge University Press: Cambridge, UK, 2002; Chapter 1.
238. Benedetti, F.; Mayberg, H.S.; Wager, T.D.; Stohler, C.S.; Zubieta, J.K. Neurobiological mechanisms of the placebo effect. *J. Neurosci.* **2005**, *25*, 10390–10402. [CrossRef] [PubMed]
239. Price, D.D.; Finniss, D.G.; Benedetti, F. A comprehensive review of the placebo effect: Recent advances and current thought. *Annu. Rev. Psychol.* **2008**, *59*, 565–590. [CrossRef] [PubMed]
240. Finniss, D.G.; Kaptchuk, T.J.; Miller, F.; Benedetti, F. Biological, clinical, and ethical advances of placebo effects. *Lancet* **2010**, *375*, 686–695. [CrossRef]
241. Bausell, R.B.; Lao, L.; Bergman, S.; Lee, W.L.; Berman, B.M. Is acupuncture analgesia an expectancy effect? Preliminary evidence based on participants' perceived assignments in two placebo-controlled trials. *Eval. Health Prof.* **2005**, *28*, 9–26. [CrossRef] [PubMed]
242. Benedetti, F. What do you expect from this treatment? Changing our mind about clinical trials. *Pain* **2007**, *128*, 193–194. [CrossRef] [PubMed]

243. Linde, K.; Witt, C.M.; Streng, A.; Weidenhammer, W.; Wagenpfeil, S.; Brinkhaus, B.; Willich, S.N.; Melchart, D. The impact of patient expectations on outcomes in four randomized controlled trials of acupuncture in patients with chronic pain. *Pain* **2007**, *128*, 264–271. [CrossRef] [PubMed]
244. Myers, S.S.; Phillips, R.S.; Davis, R.B.; Cherkin, D.C.; Legedza, A.; Kaptchuk, T.J.; Hrbek, A.; Buring, J.E.; Post, D.; Connelly, M.T.; et al. Patient expectations as predictors of outcome in patients with acute low back pain. *J. Gen. Intern Med.* **2008**, *23*, 148–153. [CrossRef] [PubMed]
245. Pariente, J.; White, P.; Frackowiak, R.S.; Lewith, G. Expectancy and belief modulate the neuronal substrates of pain treated by acupuncture. *Neuroimage* **2005**, *25*, 1161–1167. [CrossRef] [PubMed]
246. Colagiuri, B. Participant expectancies in double-blind randomized placebo-controlled trials: Potential limitations to trial validity. *Clin. Trials* **2010**, *7*, 246–255. [CrossRef] [PubMed]
247. Perlis, R.H.; Ostacher, M.; Fava, M.; Nierenberg, A.A.; Sachs, G.S.; Rosenbaum, J.F. Assuring that double-blind is blind. *Am. J. Psychiatry* **2010**, *167*, 250–252. [CrossRef] [PubMed]
248. Hertzman, M.; Adler, L. *Clinical Trials in Psychopharmacology*, 2nd ed.; Wiley-Blackwell: Oxford, UK, 2010; Chapter 18.
249. Hertzman, M.; Feltner, D. *The Handbook of Psychopharmacology Trial*; New York University Press: New York, NY, USA, 1997; Chapter 6.
250. Vickers, A.; Goyal, N.; Harland, R.; Rees, R. Do certain countries produce only positive results? A systematic review of controlled trials. *Control Clin. Trials* **1998**, *19*, 159–166. [CrossRef]
251. Molsberger, A.; Zhou, J.; Boewing, L.; Arndt, D.; Karst, M.; Teske, W.; Drabik, A. An international expert survey on acupuncture in randomized controlled trials for low back pain and a validation of the low back pain acupuncture score. *Eur. J. Med. Res.* **2011**, *16*, 133–138. [CrossRef] [PubMed]
252. Shapiro, A.K. Etiological factors in placebo effect. *JAMA* **1964**, *187*, 712–714. [CrossRef] [PubMed]
253. Miller, F.G.; Kaptchuk, T.J. The power of context: Reconceptualizing the placebo effect. *J. R. Soc. Med.* **2008**, *101*, 222–225. [CrossRef] [PubMed]
254. Katz, J. *The Silent World of Doctor and Patient*; The Free Press: New York, NY, USA, 1984; Chapter 8.
255. Kerr, C.E.; Shaw, J.R.; Conboy, L.A.; Kelley, J.M.; Jacobson, E.; Kaptchuk, T.J. Placebo acupuncture as a form of ritual touch healing: A neurophenomenological model. *Conscious. Cogn.* **2011**, *20*, 784–791. [CrossRef] [PubMed]
256. Beecher, H.K. The powerful placebo. *JAMA* **1955**, *159*, 1602–1606. [CrossRef]
257. Tragende Gründe zum Beschluss des Gemeinsamen Bundesausschusses zur Akupunktur. Press Release by Gemeinsamen Bundesausschusses, Dated 18.04.2006. Available online: https://www.g-ba.de/informationen/beschluesse/295/ (accessed on 5 June 2018).
258. Lee, I.S.; Lee, S.H.; Kim, S.Y.; Lee, H.J.; Park, H.J.; Chae, Y.Y. Visualization of the meridian system based on biomedical information about acupuncture treatment. *Evid. Based Complement. Alternat. Med.* **2013**, *2013*, 872142. [CrossRef] [PubMed]
259. Early Acupuncture, by Mark Parisi. Available online: https://www.offthemark.com/search/?q=early%20acupuncture (accessed on 5 June 2018).
260. Dellon, A.L.; Höke, A.; Williams, E.H.; Williams, C.G.; Zhang, Z.; Rosson, G.D. The sympathetic innervation of the human foot. *Plast. Reconstr. Surg.* **2012**, *129*, 905–909. [CrossRef] [PubMed]
261. Langevin, H.M.; Konofagou, E.E.; Badger, G.J.; Churchill, D.L.; Fox, J.R.; Ophir, J.; Garra, B.S. Tissue displacements during acupuncture using ultrasound elastography techniques. *Ultrasound Med. Biol.* **2004**, *30*, 1173–1183. [CrossRef] [PubMed]
262. Langevin, H.M.; Bouffard, N.A.; Badger, G.J.; Churchill, D.L.; Howe, A.K. Subcutaneous tissue fibroblast cytoskeletal remodeling induced by acupuncture: Evidence for a mechanotransduction-based mechanism. *J. Cell Physiol.* **2006**, *207*, 767–774. [CrossRef] [PubMed]
263. Langevin, H.M.; Bouffard, N.A.; Churchill, D.L.; Badger, G.J. Connective tissue fibroblast response to acupuncture: Dose-dependent effect of bidirectional needle rotation. *J. Altern. Complement. Med.* **2007**, *13*, 355–360. [CrossRef] [PubMed]
264. Fox, J.R.; Gray, W.; Koptiuch, C.; Badger, G.J.; Langevin, H.M. Anisotropic tissue motion induced by acupuncture needling along intermuscular connective tissue planes. *J. Altern. Complement. Med.* **2014**, *20*, 290–294. [CrossRef] [PubMed]
265. Burnstock, G. Physiology and pathophysiology of purinergic neurotransmission. *Physiol. Rev.* **2007**, *87*, 659–797. [CrossRef] [PubMed]

266. Abbracchio, M.P.; Burnstock, G.; Verkhratsky, A.; Zimmermann, H. Purinergic signalling in the nervous system: An overview. *Trends Neurosci.* **2009**, *32*, 19–29. [CrossRef] [PubMed]
267. Yu, J.; Zhao, C.; Luo, X. The effects of electroacupuncture on the extracellular signal-regulated kinase 1/2/P2X3 signal pathway in the spinal cord of rats with chronic constriction injury. *Anesth. Analg.* **2013**, *116*, 239–246. [CrossRef] [PubMed]
268. Tang, Y.; Yin, H.Y.; Rubini, P.; Illes, P. Acupuncture-induced analgesia: A neurobiological basis in purinergic signaling. *Neuroscientist* **2016**, *22*, 563–578. [CrossRef] [PubMed]
269. Zylka, M.J. Pain-relieving prospects for adenosine receptors and ectonucleotidases. *Trends Mol. Med.* **2011**, *17*, 188–196. [CrossRef] [PubMed]
270. Zhou, W.; Benharash, P. Significance of "Deqi" response in acupuncture treatment: Myth or reality. *J. Acupunct. Meridian Stud.* **2014**, *7*, 186–189. [CrossRef] [PubMed]
271. Kong, J.; Gollub, R.; Huang, T.; Polich, G.; Napadow, V.; Hui, K.; Vangel, M.; Rosen, B.; Kaptchuk, T.J. Acupuncture de qi, from qualitative history to quantitative measurement. *J. Altern. Complement. Med.* **2007**, *13*, 1059–1070. [CrossRef] [PubMed]
272. Cheng, X. *Chinese Acupuncture and Moxibustion*, revised ed.; Foreign Languages Press: Beijing, China, 1999; Chapter 14.
273. *Essentials of Chinese Acupuncture*; Beijing College of Traditional Chinese Medicine; Shanghai College of Traditional Chinese Medicine; Nanjing College of Traditional Chinese Medicine; The Acupuncture Institute of the Academy of Traditional Chinese Medicine. (Compiler) Foreign Languages Press: Beijing, China, 1980; Part 3, Chapter 1.
274. Stux, G.; Berman, B.; Pomeranz, B. *Basics of Acupuncture*, 5th ed.; Springer: Berlin, Germany, 2003; Chapter 5.
275. Napadow, V.; Dhond, R.P.; Kim, J.; LaCount, L.; Vangel, M.; Harris, R.E.; Kettner, N.; Park, K. Brain encoding of acupuncture sensation—Coupling on-line rating with fMRI. *Neuroimage* **2009**, *47*, 1055–1065. [CrossRef] [PubMed]
276. Kong, J.; Fufa, D.T.; Gerber, A.J.; Rosman, I.S.; Vangel, M.G.; Gracely, R.H.; Gollub, R.L. Psychophysical outcomes from a randomized pilot study of manual, electro, and sham acupuncture treatment on experimentally induced thermal pain. *J. Pain* **2005**, *6*, 55–64. [CrossRef] [PubMed]
277. Spaeth, R.B.; Camhi, S.; Hashmi, J.A.; Vangel, M.; Wasan, A.D.; Kong, J.; Edwards, R.R.; Gollub, R.L.; Kong, J. A longitudinal study of the reliability of acupuncture deqi sensations in knee osteoarthritis. *Evid. Based Complement. Alternat. Med.* **2013**, *2013*, 204259. [CrossRef] [PubMed]
278. White, P.; Prescott, P.; Lewith, G. Does needling sensation (de qi) affect treatment outcome in pain? Analysis of data from a larger single-blind, randomised controlled trial. *Acupunct. Med.* **2010**, *28*, 120–125. [CrossRef] [PubMed]
279. Langevin, H.M.; Churchill, D.L.; Cipolla, M.J. Mechanical signaling through connective tissue: A mechanism for the therapeutic effect of acupuncture. *FASEB J.* **2001**, *15*, 2275–2282. [CrossRef] [PubMed]
280. Langevin, H.M.; Churchill, D.L.; Fox, J.R.; Badger, G.J.; Garra, B.S.; Krag, M.H. Biomechanical response to acupuncture needling in humans. *J. Appl. Physiol.* **2001**, *91*, 2471–2478. [CrossRef] [PubMed]
281. Langevin, H.M.; Churchill, D.L.; Wu, J.; Badger, G.J.; Yandow, J.A.; Fox, J.R.; Krag, M.H. Evidence of connective tissue involvement in acupuncture. *FASEB J.* **2002**, *16*, 872–874. [CrossRef] [PubMed]
282. Zhu, J.; Kennedy, D.N.; Cao, X. Neural Transmission of Acupuncture Signal. In *Acupuncture Therapy for Neurological Diseases*; Xia, Y., Cao, X.D., Wu, G.C., Cheng, J.S., Eds.; Tsinghua University Press: Beijing, China; Springer: Berlin, Germany, 2010; Chapter 3.
283. Hui, K.K.; Liu, J.; Marina, O.; Napadow, V.; Haselgrove, C.; Kwong, K.K.; Kennedy, D.N.; Markris, N. The integrated response of the human cerebro-cerebellar and limbic systems to acupuncture stimulation at ST 36 as evidenced by fMRI. *Neuroimage* **2005**, *27*, 479–496. [CrossRef] [PubMed]
284. Tang, W.J.; Li, J.; Zhang, J.H.; Yi, T.; Wang, S.W.; Dong, J.C. Acupuncture treatment of chronic low back pain reverses an abnormal brain default mode network in correlation with clinical pain relief. *Acupunct. Med.* **2013**, 1–7. [CrossRef]
285. Chen, X.; Spaeth, R.B.; Retzepi, K.; Ott, D.; Kong, J. Acupuncture modulates cortical thickness and functional connectivity in knee osteoarthritis patients. *Sci. Rep.* **2014**, *4*, 6482. [CrossRef] [PubMed]
286. Shi, Y.; Liu, Z.; Zhang, S.; Li, Q.; Guo, S.; Yang, J.; Wu, W. Brain network response to acupuncture stimuli in experimental acute low back pain: An fMRI study. *Evid. Based Complement. Alternat. Med.* **2015**, *2015*, 210120. [CrossRef] [PubMed]

287. Kandel, E.; Schwartz, J.; Jessel, T.; Siegelbaum, S.; Hudspeth, A.J. *Principles of Neural Science*, 5th ed.; McGraw-Hill: New York, NY, USA, 2013; Chapter 22.
288. Pomeranz, B.; Chiu, D. Naloxone blockade of acupuncture analgesia: Endorphin implicated. *Life Sci.* **1976**, *19*, 1757–1762. [CrossRef]
289. Lee, A.D.; Hsu, E.S. Mechanisms of Acupuncture Analgesia. In *Acupuncture for Pain Management*; Lin, Y., Hsu, E.S., Eds.; Springer: Heidelberg, Germany, 2014; Chapter 4.
290. Li, P.; Chiang, C.Y. The Analgesic Effects of Acupuncture. In *The Mechanism of Acupuncture Therapy and Clinical Case Studies*; Cheung, L., Li, P., Wong, C., Eds.; Taylor & Francis: London, UK, 2001; Chapter 4.
291. Melzack, R. Akupunktur und Schmerzbeeinflussung. *Anaesthesist* **1976**, *25*, 204–207. [PubMed]
292. Pomeranz, B.; Berman, B. Scientific Basis of Acupuncture. In *Basics of Acupuncture*, 5th ed.; Stux, G., Berman, B., Pomeranz, B., Eds.; Springer: Berlin, Germany, 2003; Chapter 2.
293. Dung, H. *Acupuncture: An Anatomical Approach*, 2nd ed.; CRC Press: London, UK, 2014; Chapter 9.
294. Grissa, M.H.; Baccouche, H.; Boubaker, H.; Beltaief, K.; Bzeouich, N.; Fredj, N.; Msolli, M.A.; Boukef, R.; Bouida, W.; et al. Acupuncture vs intravenous morphine in the management of acute pain in the, ED. *Am. J. Emerg. Med.* **2016**, *34*, 2112–2116. [CrossRef] [PubMed]
295. Lohmann, K. Über die Pyrophosphatfraktion im Muskel. *Naturwissenschaften* **1929**, *17*, 624–625.
296. Holton, F.A.; Holton, P. The capillary dilator substances in dry powders of spinal roots; a possible role of adenosine triphosphate in chemical transmission from nerve endings. *J. Physiol.* **1954**, *126*, 124–140. [CrossRef] [PubMed]
297. Burnstock, G. Purinergic nerves. *Pharmacol. Rev.* **1972**, *24*, 509–581. [PubMed]
298. Burnstock, G. Acupuncture: A novel hypothesis for the involvement of purinergic signalling. *Med. Hypotheses* **2009**, *73*, 470–472. [CrossRef] [PubMed]
299. Burnstock, G. P2X receptors in sensory neurones. *Br. J. Anaesth.* **2000**, *84*, 476–488. [CrossRef] [PubMed]
300. Burnstock, G. Pathophysiology and therapeutic potential of purinergic signaling. *Pharmacol. Rev.* **2006**, *58*, 58–86. [CrossRef] [PubMed]
301. Burnstock, G.; Verkhratsky, A. *Purinergic Signalling and the Nervous System*; Springer: Berlin, Germany, 2012; Chapter 8.
302. Masino, S.; Boison, D. *Adenosine: A Key Link between Metabolism and Brain Activity*; Springer: Heidelberg, Germany, 2013.
303. Sawynok, J.; Liu, X.J. Adenosine in the spinal cord and periphery: Release and regulation of pain. *Prog. Neurobiol.* **2003**, *69*, 313–340. [CrossRef]
304. Bours, M.J.; Swennen, E.L.; Di Virgilio, F.; Cronstein, B.N.; Dagnelie, P.C. Adenosine 5′-triphosphate and adenosine as endogenous signaling molecules in immunity and inflammation. *Pharmacol. Ther.* **2006**, *112*, 358–404. [CrossRef] [PubMed]
305. Hurt, J.K.; Zylka, M.J. PAPupuncture has localized and long-lasting antinociceptive effects in mouse models of acute and chronic pain. *Mol. Pain* **2012**, *8*, 28. [CrossRef] [PubMed]
306. Fujita, T.; Feng, C.; Takano, T. Presence of caffeine reversibly interferes with efficacy of acupuncture-induced analgesia. *Sci. Rep.* **2017**, *7*, 3397. [CrossRef] [PubMed]
307. Montes, L.A.; Valenzuela, M.J. Effectiveness of low back pain treatment with acupuncture. *Biomedica* **2017**, *38*, 54–60. [CrossRef] [PubMed]
308. Leem, J.; Kim, H.; Jo, H.G.; Jeon, S.R.; Hong, Y.; Park, Y.; Seo, B.; Cho, Y.; Kang, J.W.; Kim, E.J.; et al. Efficacy and safety of thread embedding acupuncture combined with conventional acupuncture for chronic low back pain: A study protocol for a randomized, controlled, assessor-blinded, multicenter clinical trial. *Medicine* **2018**, *97*, e10790. [CrossRef] [PubMed]
309. Vitoula, K.; Venneri, A.; Varrassi, G.; Paladini, A.; Sykioti, P.; Adewusi, J.; Zis, P. Behavioral therapy approaches for the management of low back pain: An up-to-date systematic review. *Pain Ther.* **2018**, *16*. [CrossRef] [PubMed]
310. Zhang, X. *Acupuncture: Review and Analysis of Controlled Clinical Trials*; World Health Organization: Geneva, Switzerland, 2002. Available online: http:www.iama.edu/OtherArticles/acupunctureWHOfullreport.pdf (accessed on 5 June 2018).
311. Manheimer, E.; White, A.; Berman, B.; Forys, K.; Ernst, E. Meta-analysis: Acupuncture for low back pain. *Ann. Intern Med.* **2005**, *142*, 651–663. [CrossRef] [PubMed]

312. Taylor, P.; Pezzullo, L.; Grant, S.J.; Bensoussan, A. Cost-effectiveness of acupuncture for chronic nonspecific low back pain. *Pain Pract.* **2014**, *14*, 599–606. [CrossRef] [PubMed]
313. Wu, J.; Hu, Y.; Zhu, Y.; Yin, P.; Litscher, G.; Xu, S. Systematic review of adverse effects: A further step towards modernization of acupuncture in China. *Evid. Based Complement. Alternat. Med.* **2015**, 432467. [CrossRef] [PubMed]

16

The Effect of Acupuncture on Visual Function in Patients with Congenital and Acquired Nystagmus

Tilo Blechschmidt, Maike Krumsiek and Margarita G. Todorova *

Department of Ophthalmology, University of Basel, Mittlere Strasse 91, CH-4031 Basel, Switzerland; tilo.blechschmidt@usb.ch (T.B.); maike.krumsiek@usb.ch (M.K.)

* Correspondence: margarita.todorova@usb.ch

Academic Editors: Gerhard Litscher and William Chi-shing Cho

Abstract: Background: The aim of this study is to examine the short-term effect of visual function following acupuncture treatment in patients with congenital idiopathic nystagmus and acquired nystagmus (CIN and AN). **Methods:** An observational pilot study on six patients with confirmed diagnosis of nystagmus (three CIN and three AN patients (2♀, 4♂; mean age 42.67; SD ± 20.57 y)), was performed. Acupuncture treatment was done following a standardized protocol applying needle-acupuncture on the body and the ears. The treatment was scheduled with 10 sessions of 30 min duration over five weeks. To assess the effect of the treatment, we performed before, between, and after acupuncture objective measurement of the BCVA (EDTRS charts), contrast vision (CSV-1000, Vector Vision), nystagmography (Compact Integrated Pupillograph), complemented by evaluation questionnaires. A placebo non-acupuncture control group (Nr: 11, 22 eyes; 8♀, 3♂; mean age: 33.34 y (SD ± 7.33 y)) was taken for comparison. **Results:** The results showed that, following acupuncture treatment, CIN and AN patients showed improvement (SD± mean) in their binocular BCVA (baseline: 0.45 ± 0.36; between: 0.53 ± 0.34 and post-treatment: 0.51 ± 0.28), and in their monocular contrast sensitivity (baseline: 11.29 ± 12.35; between: 11.43 ± 11.45 and post-treatment: 14.0 ± 12.22). The post-/baseline-difference showed a significant improvement in contrast vision and in BCVA for CIN and AN patients, but not for controls (p = 0.029 and p = 0.007, respectively). The effect of the eye showed also, within CIN and AN, significant values for the examined parameters in the post-/baseline difference (p = 0.004 and $p \leq 0.001$). Evaluated only binocularly, the respective between-/baseline and post-/baseline difference in the CIN and AN group showed significant values ($p < 0.045$). Two AN patients reported reduction of oscillations. Among general subjective symptoms, our patients reported reduction of tiredness and headache attacks, improvement of vision, and shorter sleep onset time. **Conclusion:** The applied acupuncture protocol showed improvement in the visual function of nystagmus patients and thus, in their quality of life. Further studies are mandatory to differentiate which group of nystagmus patients would benefit more from acupuncture.

Keywords: acupuncture; nystagmus; contrast vison; visual function; nystagmography

1. Introduction

Nystagmus refers to a heterogeneous group of diseases, characterized by an involuntary rhythmic oscillation of the eyes. The resulting excessive movement of images on the fovea leads to a reduction of central vision. The onset time and the waveform characteristics of the nystagmus, categorize it into: congenital idiopathic nystagmus (CIN), which usually appears at birth or in early infancy; and acquired nystagmus (AN), presenting later in life. Contrary to the variety of distinctive waveforms described in recordings of the eye movements of CIN patients, the nystagmus waveforms are simpler in patients with AN. CIN can be idiopathic or associated with visual sensory abnormalities, as for instance, with congenital cataracts, retinal or optic nerve dystrophy/ hypoplasia, or it can be part of neurological disease or syndrome [1,2]. In order to exclude any underlying ocular or systemic pathology, in children with nystagmus, further electrophysiological laboratory tests—together with neurological work-up and neuro-radiological imaging—may be necessary. Neurological disease should be ruled out when the nystagmus is asymmetric in direction, unilateral by nature, or when its characteristics have changed over time.

Generally, treatment options for nystagmus include a refractive error correction and pharmacological and surgical interventions. Spectacles and contact lenses for correction of the underlying refractive error are the first choice to reduce optical aberrations and enlarge the retinal image and visual field, thus improving the quality of the retinal image [3–5]. Pharmacological agents used for nystagmus mitigation—such as GABA and glycine agonists—have proven to be effective in patients with CIN [6]. However, in cases of obviously abnormal head posture, eye muscle surgery remains an important option in order to shift the null-zone of the nystagmus into primary gaze, and thus to alleviate the neck/ocular torticollis [7–9].

Acupuncture treatment is still considered a non-mainstream therapeutic approach. Yet, its positive effect has been shown in a variety of degenerative and psychosomatic diseases, following cerebral and peripheral ischemia, and it was also effectively used to improve blood flow. For instance, in a mice model of Parkinson's disease, the application of electro-acupuncture has proven to be effective in slowing the degeneration of dopaminergic neurons in the ventral midbrain [10]. Acupuncture has been also applied in various diseases involving psychosomatic status: such as anxiety, depression, and sleep disturbances [11]. There are also previous reports on the application of acupuncture in patients with nystagmus: vibratory and electrical stimulation of the face and neck were found to improve foveal fixation and thus, visual acuity in patients with CIN [12]. Blekher et al. reported a reduction of frequency and a decrease of slow phase velocities, as well as an improvement of foveolar fixation, following acupuncture in patients with CIN [13].

Particularly significant is the fact that patients with nystagmus often present unstable cerebral and vertebral blood flow [14]. As traditional acupuncture stimulation has shown its positive effect on systemic blood flow [15,16], it seems to be a promising supporting treatment in patients with nystagmus, as well.

The quality of life of patients with nystagmus is greatly dependent on the fluctuations of their nystagmus speed and velocity, and thus on the central fixation. Any attempt to stabilize their fixation, therefore, seems to be of benefit for them.

With this background in mind, we aimed at examining the effect of needle acupuncture on the body and the ears of nystagmus patients, following standardized acupuncture protocol. In addition, we evaluated which specific nystagmus patients the acupuncture drew greater benefit from the treatment.

2. Materials and Methods

This was an observational pilot study, in which all subjects received acupuncture, in order to determine a preliminary short-term efficacy or proof of principle of a standardized acupuncture protocol. The patients were recruited through the Department of Ophthalmology at the University of Basel (T.M.G.; B.T.).

The acupuncture protocol was developed for a group of nystagmus diseases, based on the extensive clinical experience of an ophthalmologist and a licensed, qualified, and well-trained acupuncturist (B.T.). A placebo non-acupuncture control group (Nr: 11, 22 eyes; 8♀, 3♂; mean age: 33.34 y (SD $\pm$ 7.33 y)) was taken for comparison, as the treatment is still controversial.

All procedures took place in the acupuncture unit at the Department of Ophthalmology at the University of Basel between July 2014 and May 2015. The study and data accumulation were in conformity with institutional requirements, and in accordance with the statements and principles of the declaration of Helsinki, as well as all governmental regulations.

2.1. Subjects

Patients suffering from congenital idiopathic nystagmus and acquired nystagmus (CIN and AN), followed at the Department of Ophthalmology (University of Basel, Basel, Switzerland), were enrolled in the study.

According to the clinical, diagnostic, and orthoptic findings, the patients were divided into the following groups:

- Patients with clinical characteristics of congenital idiopathic nystagmus (CIN), $N = 3$ (6 eyes),
- Patients with phenotypic characteristics of acquired nystagmus (AN), $N = 3$ (6 eyes).

Inclusion criteria for all patients were: congenital idiopathic nystagmus and acquired nystagmus; Caucasian origin.

Exclusion criteria were: above inclusion criteria not fulfilled; presence of ocular and/or systemic pathology other than nystagmus; currently using antidepressants, alcohol, or drugs; unwillingness to participate in the study, hyper-reactivity to acupuncture treatment.

Alarming signs and symptoms excluding any participation in the study and indicating instead further neurological, neurosensory, and imaging work-up were: history of onset after the age of four months, dissociated (asymmetric) form of nystagmus, preserved optokinetic nystagmus, presence of afferent pupillary defect, papilledema, and neurological symptoms like vertigo and nausea.

All nystagmus patients fulfilling our inclusion criteria underwent detailed ophthalmic examination including: refraction, best-corrected visual acuity at 2.5 m distance (BCVA), contrast vision at 2.5 m distance, nystagmography (Compact Integrated Pupillograph), intraocular pressure (Goldmann applanation tonometer), slit-lamp examination, biomicroscopy, and fundoscopy.

For each patient, BCVA was measured at distance with a standard decimal visual acuity Snellen charts. Contrast vision was evaluated at distance using a CSV-1000 colour vision test (CSV-1000, Vector Vision). The nystagmography was performed using compact integrated pupillograph (CIP, AMTech) and performed by the same experienced orthoptist (K.M.). Since the visual function in nystagmus patients could change from day to day or even during the day—and is thus linked to the nystagmus frequency, amplitude, and foveation periods during nystagmus—all examinations were performed in the morning. Also, in order to have reproducible measurements completed, the nystagmus was measured monocularly, in primary gaze, keeping fixation for distance. In this way, any additional effect of convergence on nystagmus characteristics could be excluded, as well. The patient was asked to keep both eyes during the examination open. Nystagmus latency was defined as delay between the onset of target movement and the initiation of target movement and nystagmus velocity was defined as the time taken to complete the saccade, once it was initiated.

Subjectively, the effect of acupuncture was evaluated using evaluation questionnaires in regard to changes in visual acuity, contrast sensitivity, as well as the presence of oscillopsias and their change following acupuncture.

For a fair comparison, our non-acupuncture control group also underwent measurements of: refraction, BCVA at 2.5 m distance, contrast vision at 2.5 m distance, intraocular pressure (Goldmann applanation tonometer), slit-lamp examination, biomicroscopy, and fundoscopy.

The acupuncture method followed a modified standardized protocol [17]: The acupuncture protocol consists of 10 sessions of 30 min duration, administered twice a week over a period of five weeks.

The scheduling of each patient and the complete orthoptic examinations were performed by the same experienced orthoptist (K.M.). Before the initial treatment appointment, the acupuncturist gave the patient a brief introduction outlining the duration and the course of treatment, as well as the possible complications. Each scheduled treatment session was initiated only after a short conversation with the patient and his answers to questions concerning his condition after the previous treatment and his present general condition.

2.2. Needle Acupuncture of the Body and the Ears

Sterile and disposable single-use needles of different sizes were used, namely Seirin B type needle No.3 (0.20) × 15 mm, No.5 (0.25) × 40 mm, No.8 (0.30) × 30 mm, Seirin Pyonex Press Needles P type 0.22 × 1,6 (Seirin Corporation, Shizuoka, Japan); Dong Bang needle DB106 (0.20) × 15, DB105G (0.20) × 25, Dong Bang Press Needles 0.20 × 2 × 1.0 (Dong Bang Acupuncture, Inc., Chungnam, Korea). The established protocol indicates the specific pre-selected points for all participants, needling depths, and manipulation techniques. The needles were applied by the same certified and experienced acupuncturist (BT). The standard points for all subjects were located around the eyes, on the head, ears, back, abdomen, arms, hands, lower legs, and toes and include: GV-20 (Bai Hui), ExHN-3 (Yin Tang), CV-6 (Qi Hai), UB-18 (Gan Shu), UB-20 (Pi Shu), UB-23 (Shen Shu), GB-20 (Feng Chi), LI-4 (He Gu), HT-7 (Shen Men), SI-3 (Hou Xi), LV-3 (Tai Chong), GB-34 (Yang Ling Quan), GB-37 (Guang Ming), SP-6 (San Yin Jiao), ST-36 (Zu San Li); local points: UB-1 (Jing Ming), ST-1 (Cheng Qi), ExHN-7 (Qiu Hou); ear points: Eye Point (24a), Liver Zone (97), Zero Point, Brainstem, and Point de Jerome (29b). Additionally, semi-permanent-needles were localized at following ear points: Liver Zone (29), Zero Point, and Brainstem. The needles were applied according to a standardized protocol (Figure 1, Table 1). Individual choice of acupuncture points was not allowed in contrary to the common Chinese Medicine (CM). Likewise, due to standardization, the number of applied needles exceeded the common practices of CM. The needle application sites were determined with respect to the CM standards. The aim was to produce an irradiating needle sensation ('de qi'), if possible. The needles at LI-4 (He Gu), CV-6 (Qi Hai), LV-3 (Tai Chong), and all ear needles were manually stimulated once in each session after 15 min (+/−5 min). Additional CM therapeutic techniques—like electro-stimulation, heat lamps, music during treatment, etc.—were not applied.

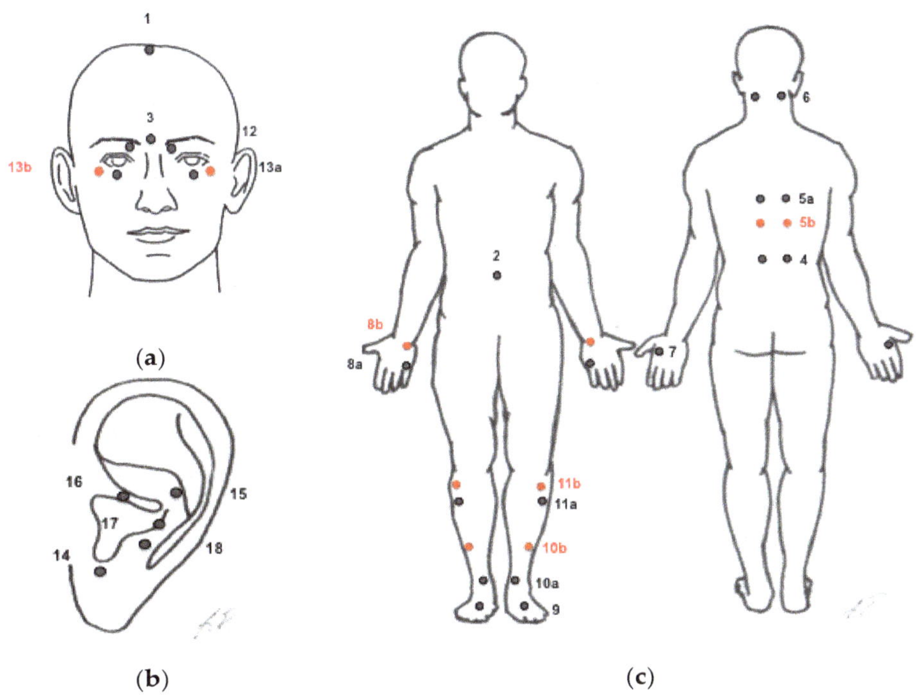

Figure 1. Needle acupuncture of the body and the ears was performed following standardized protocol (Table 1). The approximate location of the needles on the face and the ears are presented on (**a**,**b**); and on the body - on (**c**). The needles at LI-4 (He Gu), CV-6 (Qi Hai), LV-3 (Tai Chong), and all ear needles were manually stimulated once in each session after 15 min (+/−5 min). Treatment 1 (labelled in black) alternated with treatment 2 (labelled in red, see also in Table 1).

Table 1. All acupuncture points, the alternation in treatment (labeled in red, see also in Figure 1) and the stimulation duration. Standardized needles acupuncture protocol was applied as shown in Figure 1.

Acupuncture Study Protocol			
Treatment Modality	**Treatment 1 (a)**	**Treatment 2 (b)**	**Laterality**
Needle Nr:	**Alternating with Treatment 2**	**Alternating with Treatment 1**	
1	GV20 (Bai Hui)		Median
2	CV6 (Qi Hai)		Median
3	Ex-HN 3 (Yin Tang)		Median
4	UB23 (Shen Shu)		BL
5 (a/b)	UB18 (Gan Shu)	UB20 (Pi Shu)	BL
6	GB20 (Feng Chi)		BL
7	LI4 (He Gu)		BL
8 (a/b)	SI3 (Hou Xi)	HT7 (Shen Men)	BL
9	LV3 (Tai Chong)		BL
10 (a/b)	SP6 (San Yin Jiao)	GB 37 (Guang Ming)	BL
11 (a/b)	GB 34 (Yang Ling Quan)	ST36 (Zu San Li)	BL
12	UB1 (Jing Ming)		BL
13 (a/b)	ST1 (Cheng Qi)	EX-HN7 (Qiu Hou)	BL
Additional Ear Acupuncture Points (Alternately, Starting with the Right Ear)			
14	Eye Point (24a)		UL
15	Liver Zone (97)		UL
16	Zero Point		UL
17	Brainstem		UL
18	Point de Jerome (29 b)		UL
+ One Semi-Permanent Needle (Press Tack Needle) (Alternately, Starting with the Left Ear, Points in the Order Specified Bellow):			
15	Liver Zone (97)		UL
16	Zero Point		UL
17	Brainstem		UL
Needle Stimulation (after 15 min) at the Following Points:			
1	GV20 (Bai Hui)		s. above
2	CV6 (Qi Hai)		s. above
7	LI4 (He Gu)		s. above
9	LV3 (Tai Chong)		s. above
14–18	Ear Points		s. above
Duration of Needle Stimulation:			
30 min			

2.3. Statistical Analysis

A statistical package IBM SPSS Statistics 22 was applied. To evaluate the effect of acupuncture on visual functions, a univariate ANOVA test was performed. In our statistical model, the group was taken as a fixed factor. Each pair of the tested objective methods (best-corrected visual acuity (BCVA, Snellen charts)), contrast vision (CSV-1000, Vector Vision), amplitude, and frequency of nystagmus (Nystagmography, Compact Integrated Pupillograph CIP, AMTech), was treated as a dependent variable.

The acupuncture effect on patients was analyzed at baseline (1: baseline), after five acupuncture sessions (2: between treatment), and at the end of the acupuncture protocol (3: post-treatment). Our results are presented as the mean difference for each of the tested parameters, with the respective standard deviation.

In addition, for each nystagmus patients and for each control subject, the difference between-/pre-treatment was calculated by extracting the between treatment value from the pre-treatment one (2-1). Correspondingly, the post-/baseline-treatment difference was calculated extracting the post-treatment value from the baseline-treatment one (3-1). The effect of acupuncture was assessed comparing the between-/baseline-treatment difference against the post-/baseline-treatment difference within nystagmus patients. P-values of less than 0.05 are considered statistically significant.

3. Results

An observational pilot study on six patients with clinical picture and confirmed diagnosis of nystagmus (three CIN and three AN patients (2♀, 4♂; mean age 42.67; SD ± 20.57 y)), was performed. A placebo non-acupuncture control group (Nr: 11, 22 eyes; 8♀, 3♂; mean age: 33.34 y (SD ± 7.33 y)) was taken, for comparison. The clinical characteristics of the patients are given in Table 2.

Table 2. Clinical characteristics of patients included in the study.

Patient		Nystagmus Characteristics, Ophthalmic/Systemic Diagnosis	Subjective Findings: Before versus after Acupuncture Treatment		
Nr:	Age (y), Gender		BCVA	Contrast Vision	Oscillations
Case 1	51, m	Consecutive exotropia and decompensated latent nystagmus after Botox injection (2014) and strabismus surgery, left eye (2015) for congenital esotropia, latent nystagmus, and dissociated vertical deviation.	Monocular and binocular improvement	Stable	Reduction
Case 2	23, m	Congenital idiopathic nystagmus. Hyperopia. Macular hypoplasia.	Binocular improvement	RE > LE improvement	No
Case 3	20, m	Horizontal pendular nystagmus, latent compound. Accommodative convergence excess esotropia and amblyopia, left eye. Optic disc hypoplasia. Status after surgery for neuroepithelial cyst, right lateral ventricle. Occipital para-ventricular: atrophy and gliosis	Worsening	Improvement	No
Case 4	70, f	Acquired torsional down-beat nystagmus after brain stem ischemia.	Stable	Stable	Reduction
Case 5	39, m	Congenital idiopathic nystagmus. Oculocutaneous Albinism.	Slight improvement	Stable	No
Case 6	26, f	Pendular nystagmus. Multiple sclerosis.	Slight improvement	Slight improvement	Reduction

A subjective improvement of visual function, following the acupuncture treatment, was stated by all nystagmus patients. Evaluated in subgroups, two AN patients and one CIN patient reported reduction of oscillations (Table 2). Among the subjective general symptoms, our patients reported on reduction of tiredness and headache attacks, improvement in vision, and shorter sleep onset time.

Objectively, CIN and AN patients showed improvement (SD± mean) in their binocular BCVA (baseline: 0.45; ±0.36; between: 0.53; ±0.34 and post-treatment: 0.51; ±0.28), in monocular contrast sensitivity (baseline: 11.29 ± 12.35; between: 11.43 ± 11.45 and post- treatment: 14.0 ± 12.22; Figure 2a). Evaluating the between-/baseline-treatment difference against the post-/baseline-treatment difference, we found within CIN and AN patients a statistically significant increase in visual acuity ($p = 0.002$) and a statistically significant trend in improvement in contrast vision ($p = 0.099$; Figure 2b).

Compared to controls, CIN and AN patients showed a significant improvement in their contrast sensitivity and in their BCVA for the post-/baseline-treatment difference ($p = 0.029$ and $p = 0.007$, respectively). The effect of the eye also showed significant values between both groups for the examined parameters in the post-/baseline-treatment difference ($p = 0.004$ and $p \leq 0.001$). These data pointed towards a different relation, when both the eye and the group effects were taken into account. Thus, we proceeded with evaluation of the examined parameters between groups in relation to the examined eye. Within CIN and AN patients, now we could document improvement in their binocular BCVA and contrast sensitivity for both, the between-/baseline-treatment difference, as well as for the post-/baseline-treatment difference with respective values, as follows: 0.044, 0.029; 0.061; 0.006. Here, the corresponding monocular values did not reach statistically significant values ($p > 0.005$).

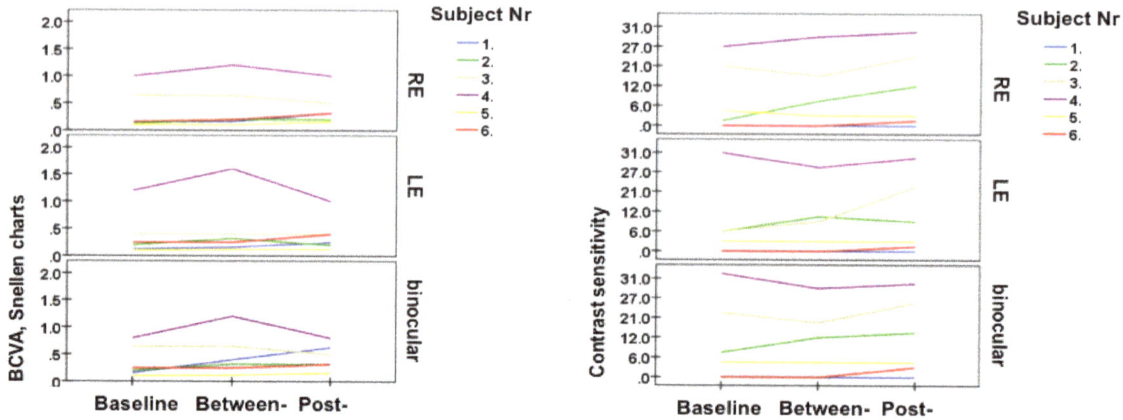

(a) (b)

Figure 2. Line diagrams representing the individual patient's examination data (presented separately for the RE: right eye; for the LE: left eye and for both eyes: binocular); (**a**) BCVA, Snellen charts; (**b**) Contrast sensitivity. The acupuncture effect was analyzed at the beginning (1: baseline-), after five acupuncture sessions (2: between) and at the end of the acupuncture treatment (3: post-).

All six CIN and AN patients demonstrated reduction of the mean amplitude and frequency of the nystagmus, following acupuncture (Table 3). No change of the direction of the nystagmus was recorded in any patient.

Table 3. Summarized nystagmography results of all patients before- and after acupuncture treatment. In order to reduce the influence of the head position and the effect of convergence, each patient was asked to keep both eyes during the examination open while the measurement was performed monocularly, in primary gaze, keeping fixation for distance.

Patient Nr/Age/Gender	Eye	Saccades within 4 Sec. (before-/after Acupuncture)	Amplitude, ° (before-/after Acupuncture)	Velocity, Sec. (before-/after Acupuncture)	Subjective Evaluation after a "Washout" Time Following Acupuncture
1/51/m	RE LE	16/11 9/10	9/8 4/4.5	4/4 4/4	Stable since acupuncture
2/23/m	RE LE	36/18 24/25	6.5/3.5 6/7	4/4 4/4	No control examination has been done
3/20/m	RE LE	20/7 17/27	9/7 18/11	4/4 4/4	Still stable three months after acupuncture
4/70/f	RE LE	Not possible objectively to be analyzed, however reduced oscillations following acupuncture			Stable since acupuncture
5/39/m	RE	Not possible to analyze/11	Not possible to analyze/6.5	4/4	No control examination has been done
	LE	Not possible to analyze/15	Not possible to analyze/17	4/4	
6/26/f	RE LE	17/17 17/17	4.5/4 5.5/5	4/4 4/4	Stable since acupuncture

As an example, in the case with CIN, hyperopia and macula hypoplasia (patient 2, Table 2) the waveform characteristics changed from horizontal conjugate nystagmus with pendular velocity to jerk disconjugate nystagmus, with descending velocity slow phase more pronounced on the right eye (Figure 3a). Here, even if no oscillations were reported, the reduction of the nystagmus amplitude and frequency explained the subjective and objective improvement of monocular and binocular visual acuity of the patient, as well as in the contrast vision. As it is shown in Figure 3a, the frequency and the amplitude of nystagmus (No. saccades/amplitude/velocity) improved much following acupuncture treatment: from 19/6.5°/3.5 s, right and 15/9°/3.5 s, left to 6/6°/3.5 s, right and 2/7°/3.5 s, left. On the contrary, in the case with pendular nystagmus and multiple sclerosis (patient 6, Figure 3b), no improvement in the velocity of nystagmus was measured, but in the amplitude, on the left. Here, by 15 objectively stable saccades at baseline and at post-treatment, a slight reduction in the amplitudes from 4.5° to 4° on the right eye and from 5.5° to 5° on the left eye was recorded (Figure 3b). In addition, the patient reported subjectively on reduction of the oscillations, as well as on improvement in her binocular and monocular vision and contrast sensitivity (Table 2).

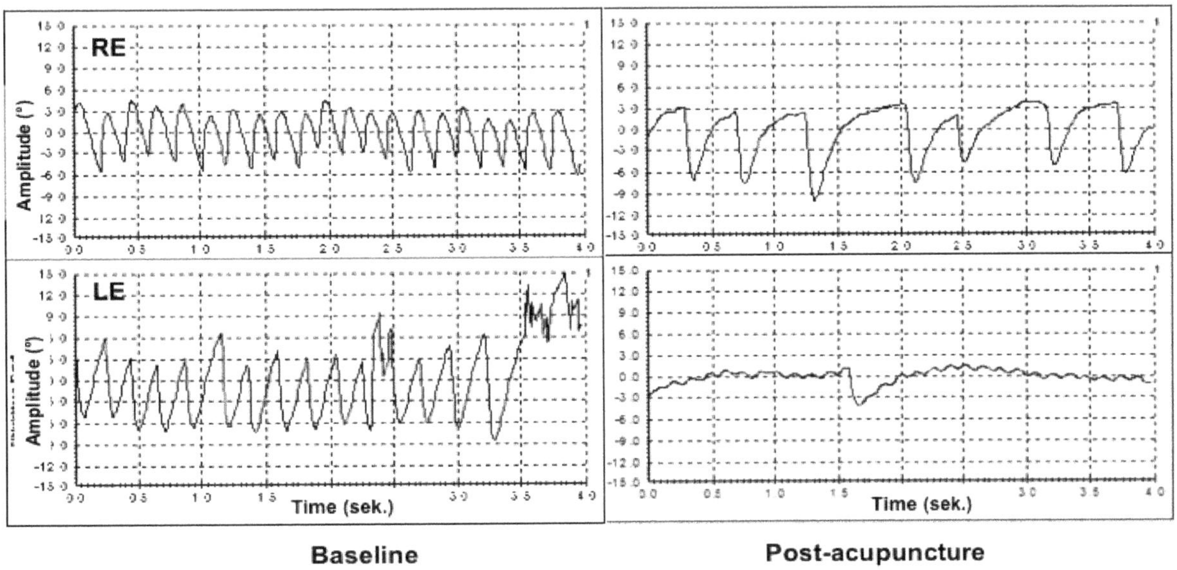

(a)

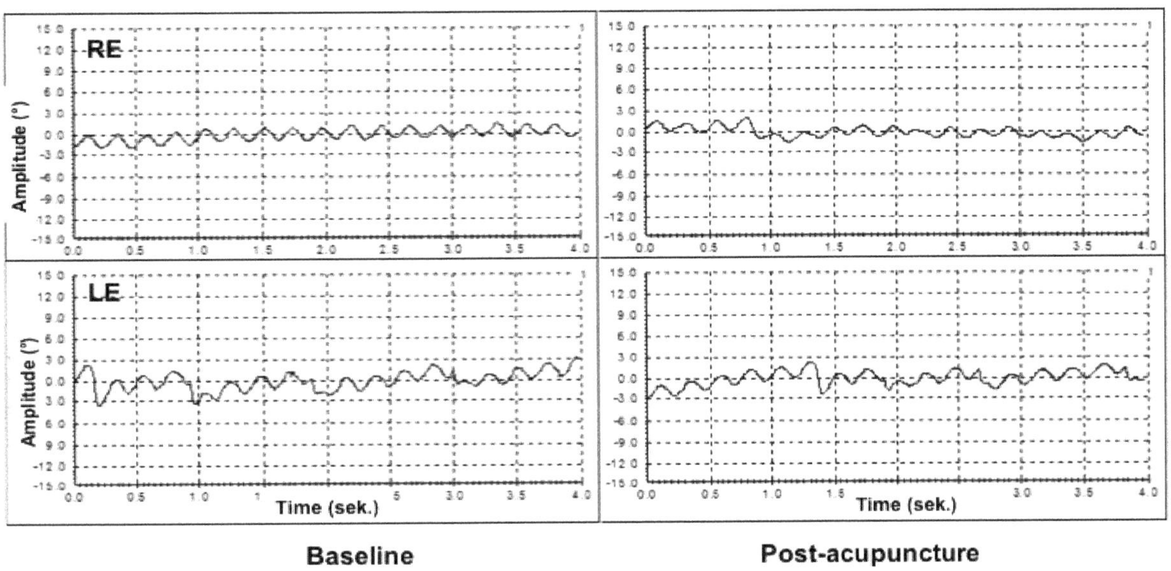

(b)

Figure 3. Nystagmography pictures in two patients (**a**); (**b**) baseline and following acupuncture treatment, as described bellow.

Figure 3a shows an example of nystagmography pictures of a 23-year-old male patient with congenital idiopathic nystagmus, hyperopia, and macula hypoplasia. The patient reported no oscillations. The nystagmography showed, however, a significant reduction of the nystagmus amplitude and the velocity of nystagmus (No. saccades/amplitude/velocity) improved significantly following acupuncture treatment: from 19/6.5°/3.5 s, right and 15/9°/3.5 s, left to 6/6°/3.5 s, right and 2/7°/3.5 s, left. The findings confirm his subjective and objective improvement of monocular and binocular visual acuity, and contrast sensitivity.

Figure 3b shows an example of nystagmography pictures of a 26-year-old female patient with idiopathic pendular nystagmus as part of multiple sclerosis. Even if no improvement in the velocity of nystagmus (15 saccades at baseline and at post-treatment) was measured, an amplitude reduction from 4.5° to 4 on the right eye and from 5.5° to 5° on the left eye could be found. This finding explains the subjectively reported oscillations' reduction, as well as vision- and contrast sensitivity improvement (Table 2).

Neither ocular, nor systemic adverse effects, were reported by any nystagmus patient. All patients included in the study indicated a willingness to repeat the acupuncture treatment.

4. Discussion

Results of our pilot study on patients suffering from nystagmus, confirmed subjective and objective improvement in their visual function, following standardized acupuncture protocol. Our data also demonstrated a dose-response relation: post-acupuncture, the effect of on visual acuity and contrast vision is more pronounced than the effect between-acupuncture, always using the baseline data for comparison.

This is not an unexpected finding, since previous reports on nystagmus patients treated with acupuncture also measured improvement of their foveal visual acuity and contrast sensitivity [12,13]. However, the studies reported until now have been performed on patients with CIN [12,13]. Here, the study of Blekher et al., examined the effects of acupuncture of the neck and face, reporting a reduction of frequency and a decrease of slow phase velocities, as well as an improvement of foveolar fixation, following acupuncture in patients with CIN. The improvement of these foveation periods has been thought to enhance visual acuity. Thus, the pathophysiologic mechanism of the improvement of the underlying CIN was supposed to be produced through the afferent stimulation of the reticular formation and vestibular nucleus via acupuncture of the neck and the face [12].

A novel finding in the present study was the fact that AN patients seemed to benefit from the acupuncture more. A possible explanation for this finding might be the labile nature of the CIN: the nystagmus may be exacerbated with visual effort or when fixating an imaginary target, and on the contrary may reduce with inattention or fatigue. It is noteworthy that the placement of the eyes in convergence gaze angle frequently dampens the nystagmus, which in fact is used as a treatment modality applying prism correction or divergence surgery. The latter explains why the binocular effect on visual function over time was more pronounced in our study and stays in agreement with previous studies. Nevertheless, to exclude the influence of the gaze direction and near fixation on nystagmography, and following the manufacturer's protocol (CSV-1000, Vector Vision; CIP, AMTech), we examined all six patients with the gaze directed for distance, keeping both eyes opened, while performing nystagmography monocularly.

We also found that even if the direction of the nystagmus showed no difference in either of nystagmus subgroups, patients with AN showed reduction in the nystagmus amplitude and frequency, and thus in oscillations, following acupuncture treatment. As a consequence, their central vision and contrast sensitivity seems to have improved more. On the contrary, patients with CIN showed almost stable amplitude and frequency of their nystagmus pattern.

Since patients with nystagmus often present unstable blood flow [14,16], the effect of acupuncture on systemic and ocular blood flow seems to explain in part the present finding. In agreement, studies on electro-acupuncture in rabbits with vertebrobasilar insufficiency showed improvement in their vestibulo-ocular reflex, through improvement of the basilar artery hemodynamic, inner ear blood flow, and blood viscosity [15]. Moreover, the traditional acupuncture stimulation has shown its positive effect on systemic blood flow, an effect, which supposedly is in part mediated by the central nervous system [16].

Even though in different ways, both nystagmus subgroups benefited from the acupuncture treatment. Acupuncture induced more foveation in CIN while mainly mitigating ocular-blood flow disturbances in AN patients. In this regard, our conclusions remain to be elucidated and elaborated upon in further studies.

5. Conclusions

Briefly, the applied acupuncture protocol showed improvement of the visual function and systemic condition of our nystagmus patients and was well tolerated. However, the long-term effect of this complementary therapy needs to be evaluated in further studies.

Acknowledgments: We are grateful to Rossiana Bojinova for editing the manuscript, to Hansjörg Rudin for drawing the pictures to Figure 1, and to Andy Schötzau for his support in statistical analysis.

Author Contributions: All authors have full access to all data from the study and are responsible for the data integrity and the analysis accuracy. T.B. and M.G.T. conceived and designed the experiments; T.B. and M.K. performed the experiments; M.G.T. and M.K. analyzed the data; T.B. contributed materials; M.G.T and T.B. wrote the paper.

References

1. Gelbart, S.S.; Hoyt, C.S. Congenital nystagmus: A clinical perspective in infancy. *Graefes Arch. Clin. Exp. Ophthalmol.* **1988**, *226*, 178–180. [CrossRef] [PubMed]
2. Weiss, A.H.; Biersdorf, W.R. Visual sensory disorders in congenital nystagmus. *Ophthalmology* **1989**, *96*, 517–523. [CrossRef]
3. Abadi, R.V. Visual performance with contact lenses and congenital idiopathic nystagmus. *Br. J. Physiol. Opt.* **1979**, *33*, 32–37. [PubMed]
4. Biousse, V.; Tusa, R.J.; Russell, B.; Azran, M.S.; Das, V.; Schubert, M.S.; Ward, M.; Newman, N.J. The use of contact lenses to treat visually symptomatic congenital nystagmus. *J. Neurol. Neurosurg. Psychiatry* **2004**, *75*, 314–316. [CrossRef] [PubMed]
5. Beuschel, R.; Todorova, M.G. Okulokutaner Albinismus. *Focus* **2016**, *7/8*, 52–54.
6. McLean, R.; Proudlock, F.; Thomas, S.; Degg, C.; Gottlob, I. Congenital nystagmus: Randomized, controlled, double-masked trial of memantine/gabapentin. *Ann. Neurol.* **2007**, *61*, 130–138. [CrossRef] [PubMed]
7. Abadi, R.V.; Whittle, J. Surgery and compensatory head postures in congenital nystagmus. A longitudinal study. *Arch. Ophthalmol.* **1992**, *110*, 632–635. [CrossRef] [PubMed]
8. Bagheri, A.; Farahi, A.; Yazdani, S. The effect of bilateral horizontal rectus recession on visual acuity, ocular deviation or head posture in patients with nystagmus. *J. AAPOS* **2005**, *9*, 433–437. [CrossRef] [PubMed]
9. Dell'Osso, L.F.; Tomsak, R.L.; Thurtell, M.J. Two hypothetical nystagmus procedures: Augmented tenotomy and reattachment and augmented tendon suture (Sans tenotomy). *J. Pediatr. Ophthalmol. Strabismus* **2009**, *46*, 337–344. [CrossRef] [PubMed]
10. Liang, X.B.; Liu, X.Y.; Li, F.Q.; Luo, Y.; Lu, J.; Zhang, W.M.; Wang, X.M.; Han, J.S. Long-term high-frequency electro-acupuncture stimulation prevents neuronal degeneration and up-regulates BDNF mRNA in the substantia nigra and ventral tegmental area following medial forebrain bundle axotomy. *Brain Res. Mol. Brain Res.* **2002**, *108*, 51–59. [CrossRef]
11. Chung, K.F.; Yeung, W.F.; Yu, Y.M.; Yung, K.P.; Zhang, S.P.; Zhang, Z.J.; Wong, M.T.; Lee, W.K.; Chan, L.W. Acupuncture for residual insomnia associated with major depressive disorder: A placebo- and sham-controlled, subject- and assessor-blind, randomized trial. *J. Clin. Psychiatry* **2015**, *76*, e752–e760. [CrossRef] [PubMed]
12. Sheth, N.V.; Dell'Osso, L.F.; Leigh, R.J.; Van Doren, C.L.; Peckham, H.P. The effects of afferent stimulation on congenital nystagmus foveation periods. *Vis. Res.* **1995**, *35*, 2371–2382. [CrossRef]

13. Blekher, T.; Yamada, T.; Yee, R.D.; Abel, L.A. Effects of acupuncture on foveation characteristics in congenital nystagmus. *Br. J. Ophthalmol.* **1998**, *82*, 115–120. [CrossRef] [PubMed]
14. Yamamoto, K.; Kubo, T.; Matsunaga, T. Effects of asymmetric vertebral blood flow upon the vestibulo-ocular reflex of the rabbit. *Eur. Arch. Otorhinolaryngol.* **1985**, *241*, 195–202. [CrossRef]
15. Zheng, Z.; Song, K.Y.; Hu, X.M.; Yu, F.; Deng, X.Z.; Zhang, Q.; Wen, G.W.; Cao, X.M. Experimental study of electroacupuncture improving the obstruction of vestibular microcirculation in vertebrobasilar insufficiency and the effect on vestibulo-ocular reflex. *Zhongguo Ying Yong Sheng Li Xue Za Zhi* **2006**, *22*, 99–104. [PubMed]
16. Takamoto, K.; Hori, E.; Urakawa, S.; Sakai, S.; Ishikawa, A.; Kohno, S.; Ono, T.; Nishijo, H. Cerebral hemodynamic responses induced by specific acupuncture sensations during needling at trigger points: A near-infrared spectroscopic study. *Brain Topogr.* **2010**, *23*, 279–291. [CrossRef] [PubMed]
17. Blechschmidt, T.; Krumsiek, M.; Todorova, M.G. Improvement in Visual Function in Patients with Inherited Diseases of the Retina Following Acupuncture Treatment. *Klin. Monatsbl. Augenheilkd.* **2016**, *233*, 416–423. [CrossRef] [PubMed]

Permissions

All chapters in this book were first published by MDPI; hereby published with permission under the Creative Commons Attribution License or equivalent. Every chapter published in this book has been scrutinized by our experts. Their significance has been extensively debated. The topics covered herein carry significant findings which will fuel the growth of the discipline. They may even be implemented as practical applications or may be referred to as a beginning point for another development.

The contributors of this book come from diverse backgrounds, making this book a truly international effort. This book will bring forth new frontiers with its revolutionizing research information and detailed analysis of the nascent developments around the world.

We would like to thank all the contributing authors for lending their expertise to make the book truly unique. They have played a crucial role in the development of this book. Without their invaluable contributions this book wouldn't have been possible. They have made vital efforts to compile up to date information on the varied aspects of this subject to make this book a valuable addition to the collection of many professionals and students.

This book was conceptualized with the vision of imparting up-to-date information and advanced data in this field. To ensure the same, a matchless editorial board was set up. Every individual on the board went through rigorous rounds of assessment to prove their worth. After which they invested a large part of their time researching and compiling the most relevant data for our readers.

The editorial board has been involved in producing this book since its inception. They have spent rigorous hours researching and exploring the diverse topics which have resulted in the successful publishing of this book. They have passed on their knowledge of decades through this book. To expedite this challenging task, the publisher supported the team at every step. A small team of assistant editors was also appointed to further simplify the editing procedure and attain best results for the readers.

Apart from the editorial board, the designing team has also invested a significant amount of their time in understanding the subject and creating the most relevant covers. They scrutinized every image to scout for the most suitable representation of the subject and create an appropriate cover for the book.

The publishing team has been an ardent support to the editorial, designing and production team. Their endless efforts to recruit the best for this project, has resulted in the accomplishment of this book. They are a veteran in the field of academics and their pool of knowledge is as vast as their experience in printing. Their expertise and guidance has proved useful at every step. Their uncompromising quality standards have made this book an exceptional effort. Their encouragement from time to time has been an inspiration for everyone.

The publisher and the editorial board hope that this book will prove to be a valuable piece of knowledge for researchers, students, practitioners and scholars across the globe.

List of Contributors

Ji Hwan Lee
Department of Physiology, College of Korean Medicine, Kyung Hee University, Seoul 02453, Korea
Department of Science in Korean Medicine, Graduate School, Kyung Hee University, Seoul 02453, Korea

Woojin Kim
Department of Physiology, College of Korean Medicine, Kyung Hee University, Seoul 02453, Korea
Department of Science in Korean Medicine, Graduate School, Kyung Hee University, Seoul 02453, Korea
Department of East-West Medicine, Graduate School, Kyung Hee University, Seoul 02453, Korea

Juan Gang
Department of East-West Medicine, Graduate School, Kyung Hee University, Seoul 02453, Korea

Young-Ho Jin and Eunhee Yang
Department of Physiology, College of Medicine, Kyung Hee University, Seoul 02453, Korea

Ye-Chae Hwang, In-Seon Lee and Younbyoung Chae
Acupuncture & Meridian Science Research Center, College of Korean Medicine, Kyung Hee University, Seoul 02447, Korea

Yeonhee Ryu
KM Fundamental Research Division, Korea Institute of Oriental Medicine, Daejeon 34054, Korea

Ye-Seul Lee
Department of Anatomy and Acupoint, College of Korean Medicine, Gachon University, Seongnam 13306, Korea

Tzu-Hsuan Wei
Department of Chinese Medicine, China Medical University Hospital, Taichung 40447, Taiwan

Ching-Liang Hsieh
Department of Chinese Medicine, China Medical University Hospital, Taichung 40447, Taiwan
Chinese Medicine Research Center, China Medical University, Taichung 40402, Taiwan
Graduate Institute of Acupuncture Science, College of Chinese Medicine, China Medical University, Taichung 40402, Taiwan

Ji-Won Lee and Song-Yi Kim
College of Korean Medicine, Gachon University, Seongnam 13120, Korea

Jun-Hwan Lee
Clinical Medicine Division, Korea Institute of Oriental Medicine, Daejeon 34054, Korea
Korean Medicine Life Science, University of Science & Technology (UST), Campus of Korea Institute of Oriental Medicine, Daejeon 34054, Korea

Mengyun Sui, Long Xue and Xiaohua Ying
NHC Key Laboratory of Health Technology Assessment, School of Public Health, Fudan University, Dongan Road 130, Shanghai 200032, China

David F. Mayor
Department of Allied Health Professions and Midwifery, School of Health and Social Work, University of Hertfordshire, Hatfield AL10 9AB, UK

Lara S. McClure and J. Helgi Clayton McClure
Northern College of Acupuncture, York YO1 6LJ, UK

Joana Teixeira and Maria João Santos
ICBAS- Institute of Biomedical Sciences Abel Salazar, University of Porto, 4050-313 Porto, Portugal

Luís Carlos Matos
Faculdade de Engenharia da Universidade do Porto, Rua Dr. Roberto Frias, s/n 4200-465 Porto, Portugal

Jorge Pereira Machado
ICBAS- Institute of Biomedical Sciences Abel Salazar, University of Porto, 4050-313 Porto, Portugal
LABIOMEP—Porto Biomechanics Laboratory, University of Porto, 4200-450 Porto, Portugal

James David Adams, Jr.
University of Southern California, School of Pharmacy, 1985 Zonal Avenue, Los Angeles, CA, 90089-9121, USA

Narda G. Robinson
Department of Clinical Sciences, Colorado State University, Fort Collins, CO 80526, USA

Xiaojuan Shang and Luquan Chen
Department of Traditional Chinese Medicine, Beijing Tongren Hospital, Capital Medical University, Beijing 100730, China

Daniela Litscher
TCM Research Center Graz, Research Unit of Biomedical Engineering in Anesthesia and Intensive Care Medicine, and Research Unit for Complementary and Integrative Laser Medicine, Medical University of Graz, 8036 Graz, Austria

Gerhard Litscher
Department of Traditional Chinese Medicine, Beijing Tongren Hospital, Capital Medical University, Beijing 100730, China
TCM Research Center Graz, Research Unit of Biomedical Engineering in Anesthesia and Intensive Care Medicine, and Research Unit for Complementary and Integrative Laser Medicine, Medical University of Graz, 8036 Graz, Austria
Department of Anesthesiology, Beijing Tongren Hospital, Capital Medical University, Beijing 100730, China
Department of Acupuncture and Moxibustion, Dongfang Hospital Affiliated to Beijing University of Chinese Medicine, Beijing 100078, China

Lu Wang
Department of Traditional Chinese Medicine, Beijing Tongren Hospital, Capital Medical University, Beijing 100730, China
TCM Research Center Graz, Research Unit of Biomedical Engineering in Anesthesia and Intensive Care Medicine, and Research Unit for Complementary and Integrative Laser Medicine, Medical University of Graz, 8036 Graz, Austria
Department of Anesthesiology, Beijing Tongren Hospital, Capital Medical University, Beijing 100730, China

Yanxia Sun and Chuxiong Pan
Department of Anesthesiology, Beijing Tongren Hospital, Capital Medical University, Beijing 100730, China

Cun-Zhi Liu
Department of Acupuncture and Moxibustion, Dongfang Hospital Affiliated to Beijing University of Chinese Medicine, Beijing 100078, China

Henry Xiao and Christopher Zaslawski
School of Life Sciences, University of Technology Sydney, Ultimo, NSW 2007, Australia

Janette Vardy
Sydney Medical School, University of Sydney, Camperdown, NSW 2006, Australia
Concord Cancer Centre, Concord Repatriation General Hospital, Concord, NSW 2137, Australia

Byeongsang Oh
School of Life Sciences, University of Technology Sydney, Ultimo, NSW 2007, Australia
Sydney Medical School, University of Sydney, Camperdown, NSW 2006, Australia
Northern Sydney Cancer Centre, Royal North Shore Hospital, St Leonards, NSW 2065, Australia

Shuo-Ping Tseng
Department of Chinese Medicine, Tainan Municipal Hospital, Tainan 700, Taiwan

Yu-Ching Hsu
Department of Chinese Medicine, Tainan Hospital, Ministry of Health and Welfare, Tainan 701, Taiwan

Ching-Ju Chiu
Institute of Gerontology, College of Medicine, National Cheng Kung University, Tainan 701, Taiwan

Shang-Te Wu
Department of Internal Medicine and Neurology, Kuo General Hospital, Tainan 700, Taiwan

Masashi Watanabe, Natsumi Saito and Tadashi Ishii
Department of Education and Support for Regional Medicine, Department of Kampo Medicine, Tohoku University Hospital, 1-1 Seiryou-machi, Aoba-ku, Sendai, Miyagi 980-8574, Japan

Soichiro Kaneko, Shin Takayama and Takehiro Numata
Department of Education and Support for Regional Medicine, Department of Kampo Medicine, Tohoku University Hospital, 1-1 Seiryou-machi, Aoba-ku, Sendai, Miyagi 980-8574, Japan
Comprehensive Education Center for Community Medicine, Graduate School of Medicine, Tohoku University, 2-1 Seiryou-machi, Aoba-ku, Sendai, Miyagi 980-8575, Japan

Satoshi Konno, Tomoyuki Yambe and Yasuyuki Shiraishi
Institute of Development, Aging and Cancer, Tohoku University, 4-1 Seiryo-machi, Aoba-ku, Sendai, Miyagi 980-8575, Japan

Takashi Seki
Division of Cyclotron Nuclear Medicine, Cyclotron and Radioisotope Center, Tohoku University, 6-3 Aoba, Aramaki, Aoba-ku, Sendai, Miyagi 980-8578, Japan

Norihiro Sugita
Department of Management Science and Technology, Graduate School of Engineering, Tohoku University, 6-6-05 Aramaki Aza Aoba, Aoba-ku, Sendai, Miyagi 980-8579, Japan

Makoto Yoshizawa
Research Division on Advanced Information Technology, Cyberscience Center, Tohoku University, 6-3 Aramaki Aza Aoba, Aoba-ku, Sendai, Miyagi 980-8578, Japan

Nobuo Yaegashi
Department of Obstetrics and Gynecology, Graduate School of Medicine, Tohoku University, 1-1 Seiryou-machi, Aoba-ku, Sendai, Miyagi 980-8574, Japan

David F. Mayor
Department of Allied Health Professions and Midwifery, School of Health and Social Work, University of Hertfordshire, Hatfield AL10 9AB, UK

Tiaw-Kee Lim
University Postgraduate Education of Principles and Practice of Traditional Chinese Medicine, Medical University of Vienna, 1090 Vienna, Austria

Yan Ma
University Postgraduate Education of Principles and Practice of Traditional Chinese Medicine, Medical University of Vienna, 1090 Vienna, Austria
Institute of Pathophysiology and Allergy Research, Center for Pathophysiology, Infectiology and Immunology, Medical University of Vienna, 1090 Vienna, Austria

Frederic Berger
Gregor Mendel Institute of Molecular Plant Biology GmbH, Austrian Academy of Sciences, 1030 Vienna, Austria

Gerhard Litscher
University Postgraduate Education of Principles and Practice of Traditional Chinese Medicine, Medical University of Vienna, 1090 Vienna, Austria
Research Unit of Biomedical Engineering in Anesthesia and Intensive Care Medicine, Research Unit for Complementary and Integrative Laser Medicine, and TCM Research Center Graz, Medical University of Graz, 8036 Graz, Austria

Tilo Blechschmidt, Maike Krumsiek and Margarita G. Todorova
Department of Ophthalmology, University of Basel, Mittlere Strasse 91, CH-4031 Basel, Switzerland

Index

O

P

R

S

T

U

V

Printed in the USA
CPSIA information can be obtained
at www.ICGtesting.com
LVHW080036211023
761596LV00010BA/1792

9 781646 466344